Maths, Physics and Clinical Measurement for Anaesthesia and Intensive Care

Maths, Physics and Clinical Measurement for Anaesthesia and Intensive Care

Edited by

Hozefa Ebrahim
Consultant in Anaesthesia and Intensive Care Medicine, University Hospitals Birmingham Foundation NHS Trust, UK

David Ashton-Cleary
Consultant in Anaesthesia and Intensive Care Medicine, Royal Cornwall Hospitals NHS Trust

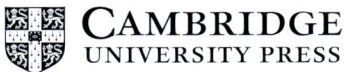

CAMBRIDGE
UNIVERSITY PRESS

University Printing House, Cambridge CB2 8BS, United Kingdom

One Liberty Plaza, 20th Floor, New York, NY 10006, USA

477 Williamstown Road, Port Melbourne, VIC 3207, Australia

314–321, 3rd Floor, Plot 3, Splendor Forum, Jasola District Centre, New Delhi – 110025, India

79 Anson Road, #06-04/06, Singapore 079906

Cambridge University Press is part of the University of Cambridge.

It furthers the University's mission by disseminating knowledge in the pursuit of education, learning, and research at the highest international levels of excellence.

www.cambridge.org
Information on this title: www.cambridge.org/9781108731454
DOI: 10.1017/9781108758505

© Cambridge University Press 2019

This publication is in copyright. Subject to statutory exception and to the provisions of relevant collective licensing agreements, no reproduction of any part may take place without the written permission of Cambridge University Press.

First published 2019

Printed in Singapore by Markono Print Media Pte Ltd

A catalogue record for this publication is available from the British Library.

ISBN 978-1-108-73145-4 Paperback

Cambridge University Press has no responsibility for the persistence or accuracy of URLs for external or third-party internet websites referred to in this publication and does not guarantee that any content on such websites is, or will remain, accurate or appropriate.

....

Every effort has been made in preparing this book to provide accurate and up-to-date information that is in accord with accepted standards and practice at the time of publication. Although case histories are drawn from actual cases, every effort has been made to disguise the identities of the individuals involved. Nevertheless, the authors, editors, and publishers can make no warranties that the information contained herein is totally free from error, not least because clinical standards are constantly changing through research and regulation. The authors, editors, and publishers therefore disclaim all liability for direct or consequential damages resulting from the use of material contained in this book. Readers are strongly advised to pay careful attention to information provided by the manufacturer of any drugs or equipment that they plan to use.

First and foremost, my utmost gratitude to Dr Syedna Mohammed Burhanuddin and Dr Syedna Mufaddal Saifuddin for all their wisdom and guidance throughout my life. Words are not enough to show my appreciation, but I hope that my actions in my clinical and personal life will make you proud. Thank you.

And of course, to my loving family, Tasneem, Mustafa and Farida. Together, all our journeys are easier.

HE

To my parents and sister for a lifetime of love and support. To my loving wife, Gemma, and Elowyn, our little scientist.

DAC

Contents

List of Contributors viii
Preface ix
Acknowledgements x
List of Abbreviations xi

1 **Data Analysis and Medical Statistics** 1
Andrew Biffen and David Ashton-Cleary

2 **Basic Physics and Electronics** 25
Emma Foster and Hozefa Ebrahim

3 **Heat, Temperature and Humidity** 38
Hozefa Ebrahim and Sean Chadwick

4 **Behaviour of Fluids** 53
Hozefa Ebrahim, Sunita Balla and James Rudge

5 **Gas Measurement and Supply** 70
Jonathan Paige

6 **Gas Concentration Measurement** 87
Catriona Frankling

7 **Blood Gas Analysis** 97
David Connor

8 **Vapours and Vaporizers** 113
Ed Copley

9 **Ventilators and Breathing Systems** 130
Dan Shuttleworth and Nick Dodds

10 **Safety in the Clinical Environment** 146
Lauren Weekes and David Ashton-Cleary

11 **Blood Pressure Measurement** 159
Laura Beard and David Ashton-Cleary

12 **Cardiac Output Monitoring** 174
Hozefa Ebrahim and Alistair Burns

13 **Cardiac Support Equipment** 187
Katie Ramm and Laura May

14 **Ultrasound and Doppler** 207
David Ashton-Cleary

15 **Atomic Structure, Radiation, Imaging and Lasers** 226
David Ashton-Cleary and Jumana Hussain

16 **Electro-biophysiology** 246
Vijay Venkatesh and David Ashton-Cleary

Index 257

List of contributors

Hozefa Ebrahim (Editor)
Consultant in Anaesthesia and Intensive Care Medicine, University Hospitals Birmingham, UK

David Ashton-Cleary (Editor)
Consultant in Anaesthesia and Intensive Care Medicine, Royal Cornwall Hospitals NHS Trust, UK

Sunita Balla
Specialist Registrar in Anaesthesia, West Midlands Deanery, UK

Laura Beard
Specialist Registrar in Anaesthesia, West Midlands Deanery, UK

Andrew Biffen
Consultant in Anaesthesia, Plymouth Hospitals NHS Trust, UK

Alistair Burns
Consultant in Anaesthesia, University Hospitals Birmingham, UK

Sean Chadwick
Consultant in Anaesthesia and Intensive Care Medicine, Herefordshire County Hospital, UK

David Connor
Consultant in Anaesthesia and Intensive Care Medicine, Royal Cornwall Hospitals NHS Trust, UK

Ed Copley
Consultant in Anaesthesia, Northamptonshire, UK

Nick Dodds
Specialist Registrar in Anaesthesia and Intensive Care Medicine, Severn Deanery, UK

Emma Foster
Advanced Trainee in Anaesthesia and Intensive Care Medicine, Christchurch Hospital, South Island, New Zealand

Catriona Frankling
Specialist Registrar in Anaesthesia, West Midlands Deanery, UK

Jumana Hussain
Consultant in Radiology: Paediatrics and Nuclear Medicine, Buckinghamshire Healthcare Trust, UK

Laura May
Consultant in Anaesthesia, University Hospitals Coventry and Warwick, UK

Jonathan Paige
Specialist Registrar in Anaesthesia and Intensive Care Medicine, West Midlands Deanery, UK

Katie Ramm
Specialist Registrar in Anaesthesia, West Midlands Deanery, UK

James Rudge
Specialist Registrar in Anaesthesia, West Midlands Deanery, UK

Dan Shuttleworth
Specialist Registrar in Anaesthesia and Intensive Care Medicine, West Midlands Deanery, UK

Vijay Venkatesh
Specialist Registrar in Anaesthesia, West Midlands Deanery, UK

Lauren Weekes
Specialist Registrar in Anaesthesia, Royal Devon and Exeter NHS Foundation Trust, UK

Preface

There is little doubt that many, if not most, of the topics included in this book are amongst those which people shy away from: physics and mathematics do not hold universal appeal for those working in anaesthesia and intensive care medicine. Our motivation for putting this book together is born out of a personal fascination with this subject matter. We're pragmatists though; whilst we certainly hope you find the book interesting, we don't expect you to come away from it quite as passionate about the topics as we are! Over the years though, we have both taken a great deal of satisfaction in seeing colleagues enjoy that "Eureka moment" as we enthuse about a tricky corner of the syllabus during a bit of informal teaching in theatre. That's what we've tried to capture on these pages. You might get the sense that anaesthesia and intensive care medicine would be much easier to manage if you'd loved A-level mathematics and physics. This book aims to provide that level of knowledge in a much more palatable form and with only the relevant areas for clinical practice included: not a quadratic equation or slide-rule in sight!

H.E. & D.A-C.
December 2018

Acknowledgements

Writing a book like this involves hard work from a huge number of people. Sadly, only a small number of these people are named on the front of the book. First and foremost, we must thank our chapter authors; without their knowledge, energy and enthusiasm, we couldn't have produced such a broad range of topics. We therefore thank Andrew Biffen, Emma Foster, Sean Chadwick, Sunita Balla, James Rudge, Jonathan Paige, Catriona Frankling, David Connor, Ed Copley, Dan Shuttleworth, Nick Dodds, Lauren Weekes, Laura Beard, Alistair Burns, Laura May, Katie Ramm, Jumana Hussain and Vijay Venkatesh. Without them, there would have been no book! Thank you, authors, for your knowledge but, particularly, for presenting the information in a way that makes learning enjoyable. Special thanks also go to Ellie Whittingham, our illustrator. She has tirelessly and skilfully produced over 200 illustrations to help us communicate the more complex concepts to you. In a similar vein, we particularly thank Yakuta Hassanali for her graphic design work in creating an aesthetically pleasing and easy-to-understand layout for our text. We, of course, thank Catherine, Jessica, Maeve, Charlotte, Zoë and many others at Cambridge University Press. Without their hard work and patience, the book in your hands would have remained a collection of thoughts, ideas and word processor files.

We have both been blessed to have had some amazing teachers throughout our careers. Some stood in front of the lecture theatre, some taught us at the bedside and in theatre, and some taught us without knowing it. We have learnt from our seniors as well as our juniors. We are who we are because of our teachers. For Hozefa, thanks must go to Professor John Holman, who inspired the physicist in him. Despite being a chemistry teacher, his style of teaching physics lit a flame inside that burns to this day. For Dave, the enthusiasm of the Reverend Mr Nigel Rawlinson and Dr Ray Sinclair continues to inspire him to teach, explain and demystify the tricky stuff every day. To name all our teachers would be impossible – but we will never forget you.

To our readers – thanks for giving us motive. We hope you enjoy learning from this book as much as we enjoyed producing it. However, that may involve a little pain too – stick at it!

For allowing us to use their data and photographs, we would like to thank:

- BOC Healthcare, Guildford, UK
- Public Health England, Personal Dosimetry Service, Didcot, UK
- Precision UK Ltd, Stockport, UK
- Dr Barney Scrace, Specialist Registrar, Anaesthesia & Critical Care, Royal Cornwall Hospitals NHS Trust

And last but not least, our cheerleaders – thanks to Gemma and Elowyn Ashton-Cleary, and Tasneem, Mustafa and Farida Ebrahim. Thanks for always standing by our side, for constantly encouraging us and for putting up with the late nights. You are our inspiration. Thank you!

Abbreviations

AAGBI	Association of Anaesthetists of Great Britain and Ireland	EMG	electromyogram
AC	alternating current	FAST	focused abdominal sonography in trauma
ADC	apparent diffusion coefficient	FDA	Federal Drug Administration (USA)
ALARP	as low as reasonably possible	FEMG	frontal electromyography
ANOVA	analysis of variance	FEV_1	forced expiratory volume in 1 second
AP	anaesthetic proof	FGF	fresh gas flow
APG	anaesthetic proof – category G	FiO_2	fractional inspired concentration of oxygen
APL	adjustable pressure limiting (valve)	FLAIR	fluid attenuated inversion recovery
APRV	airway pressure relief ventilation	FO_2Hb	fractional oxyhaemoglobin content
AR	absolute risk	FRCA	Fellowship of the Royal College of Anaesthetists
ARDS	acute respiratory distress syndrome		
ARR	absolute risk reduction	FVC	forced vital capacity
ASA	American Society of Anesthesiologists	GCP	Good Clinical Practice
ATP	adenosine triphosphate	GCS	Glasgow coma scale
AVSU	area valve service unit	GWP	global warming potential
BiVAD	bi-ventricular assist device	Hb	haemoglobin
BMI	body mass index	β-HCG	human chorionic gonadotropin
BPEG	British Pacing and Electrophysiology Group	HFNO	high-flow nasal oxygen
CD	compact disc	HFOV	high-frequency oscillatory ventilation
CI	confidence interval	HIFU	high-intensity focused ultrasound
CIM	critical illness myopathy	HME	heat and moisture exchanger
CINM	critical illness neuromyopathy	HR	hazard ratio
CIP	critical illness polyneuropathy	HR	heart rate
CM5	clavicle–manubrium–V5	HV	high voltage
CMAP	compound muscle action potential	I:E	inspiration:expiration ratio
CO	cardiac output	IABP	intra-aortic balloon pump
CONSORT	Consolidated Standards of Reporting Trials	ICD	implanted cardioverter defibrillator
		ICU	intensive care unit
		IEC	International Electrotechnical Commission
COSHH	Control of Substances Hazardous to Health	IQ	intelligence quotient
CPAP	continuous positive airway pressure	IQR	interquartile range
CPB	cardiopulmonary bypass	IRMER	Ionizing Radiation (Medical Exposure) Regulations
CPR	cardiopulmonary resuscitation		
CWD	continuous wave Doppler	LASER*	light amplification by stimulated emission of radiation
DBP	diastolic blood pressure		
DC	direct current	LED	light-emitting diode
DC	damping coefficient	LVAD	left-ventricular assist device
DHCA	deep hypothermic circulatory arrest	LVOT	left-ventricular outflow tract
DINAMAP	device for indirect non-invasive automatic MAP	MAC	minimum alveolar concentration
DNA	deoxyribonucleic acid		
DVD	digital versatile disc		
DWI	diffusion-weighted imaging		
$ECCO_2R$	extra-corporeal carbon dioxide removal		
ECG	electrocardiogram		
ECLS	extra-corporeal life support		
ECMO	extra-corporeal membranous oxygenation		
EEG	electroencephalogram		

* The acronyms LASER and SCUBA are fully incorporated into everyday speech as regular words and therefore we will be using sentence case capitalization in the text as opposed to full capitalization which is customary for acronyms

Abbreviations

MAP	mean arterial pressure	RNA	ribonucleic acid
MRgFUS	magnetic-resonance-guided focused ultrasound	RR	relative risk
		RVAD	right-ventricular assist device
MRI	magnetic resonance imaging	SaO_2	arterial oxygen saturation
MUP	motor unit potential	SBP	systolic blood pressure
NASPE	North American Society of Pacing and Electrophysiology	SCUBA*	self-contained underwater breathing apparatus
Nd:YAG	Neodymium-doped yttrium–aluminium–garnet	SD	standard deviation
		SELV	safety extra low voltage
NDT	non-destructive testing	SEM	standard error of the mean
NICE	National Institute for Health and Care Excellence	SHC	specific heat capacity
		SI	Système Internationale
NNH	number needed to harm	SIL	sound intensity level
NNT	number needed to treat	SNAP	sensory nerve action potential
NPV	negative predictive value	SPECT	single-photon emission computed tomography
OCD	obsessive compulsive disorder		
ODM	oesophageal Doppler monitor	SPL	sound pressure level
OR	odds ratio	SpO_2	pulse-oximetry oxygen saturation
PAC	pulmonary artery catheter	SSEP	somato-sensory evoked potential
PaO_2	arterial partial pressure of oxygen	STIR	short-T1 inversion recovery
P_AO_2	alveolar partial pressure of oxygen	STP	standard temperature and pressure
PCO_2	partial pressure of carbon dioxide	SVP	saturated vapour pressure
PCV	pressure-control ventilation	SVR	systemic vascular resistance
PEA	pulseless electrical activity	SVV	stroke volume variation
PEEP	positive end-expiratory pressure	TGC	timed gain compensation
PET	positron emission tomography	TIVA	total intravenous anaesthesia
PO_2	partial pressure of oxygen	TOE	trans-oesophageal echocardiography
PONV	post-operative nausea and vomiting	TURP	trans-urethral resection of the prostate
PPV	positive predictive value	VCV	volume-control ventilation
PRF	pulse repetition frequency	VF	ventricular fibrillation
PWD	pulsed-wave Doppler	VIE	vacuum-insulated evaporator
PZT	lead zirconate titanate	VT	ventricular tachycardia
RCD	residual current device	VTI	velocity–time integral

Chapter 1

Data Analysis and Medical Statistics

Andrew Biffen and David Ashton-Cleary

Learning Objectives

- To acquire an understanding of how statistical considerations shape design and implementation of clinical studies
- To be able to define a specific research question with due consideration to potential bias, ethical considerations and appropriate randomization
- To recognize different types of data and select appropriate measures of central tendency and spread which describe the data
- To understand probability theory and select and use appropriate tests of statistical significance
- To gain an overall understanding of the clinical application of statistics, its strengths and its limitations, and to critique statistical analyses of academic papers

Chapter Content

- Study design and data collection
- Descriptive statistics
- Summary statistics
- Deductive statistics
- Application to clinical practice

Scenario

You are anaesthetizing for a list of total knee replacements and wonder whether there is evidence as to whether femoral nerve block makes any difference to post-operative pain. You conduct a literature review and turn up some studies.

How would you approach evaluation of the evidence? What makes a good trial? How would you design a trial yourself if you found the evidence to be insufficient to answer your question?

Introduction

The first medical statistics book published in Britain appeared in 1931. Since that time, scores of anaesthetists have relegated their knowledge of statistics to a brief window immediately prior to an examination. Engagement with statistics is important in our ongoing appraisal of available evidence; particularly in a time when medical reversal (new research which contradicts established practice) and research fraud means we should be well equipped to interpret published studies.

Study Design and Data Collection

A bad study design begets bad results. Bad results derive from bad data or the wrong data. Therefore, before embarking on a study, it is important to pay heed to some key questions:

- What is the research question?
- What variables need to be measured?
- What is the main outcome variable?
- Are we aiming to deliver an intervention (experimental) or purely perform observation?
- Is a comparison group needed?
- What will be the duration of the study?
- How much will it cost?

Defining the clinical research question is the first step in devising a study (or reviewing the literature). One method to consider is PICO. This model raises key aspects to consider in formulating the question:

- P – patient/population
- I – intervention
- C – comparison
- O – outcome

For example, 'in major trauma patients over the age of 18 years (P) does the administration of tranexamic acid (I) rather than placebo (C) reduce mortality (O)?'

Studies can be classified as either observational or experimental.

Observational Studies

As suggested by the name, observational studies involve observing what happens (without interfering). There are three key types of observational study.

1. Cross-sectional Study

This is a snapshot, e.g. a survey. As such, it cannot determine the direction of causation but such studies are cheap and easy to perform. They may be:

- Descriptive – looking at the prevalence or incidence of a condition
- Analytic – studying variables among groups

2. Cohort Study

This may be prospective or retrospective. The aim is to identify the factors which influence the chance of a particular outcome occurring. To do so prospectively, we would take a group of people and follow them up over a period of time; we are looking to see whether exposure to a particular factor affects an outcome of interest.

Pros

- Can study several outcomes from the same risk factor
- Clear time-order of events
- Less potential for bias than case–control studies
- Suitable for studying rare risk factors

Cons

- Lengthy follow-up required
- Study participants may drop out or change relevant habits

3. Case–Control Study

This starts with a case group that have a condition of interest, for example hypercholesterolaemia. A group of matched individuals without the condition is then recruited to act as the controls. The control individuals are matched to the case individuals on a range of factors, for example gender and age. Prior exposure to risk factors is determined, to look for associations with a chosen outcome. The potential risk factors should be chosen in advance of the study and be clearly defined. By definition, these studies are retrospective.

Pros

- Relatively cheap, easy and quick to perform
- Suitable for studying rare conditions

Cons

- Recall bias – case-patients may remember certain aspects better than control-individuals
- Not suitable for studying rare risk factors

Experimental Studies

Unlike observational studies, experimental studies depend on an intervention being carried out. They are a prospective comparison of two or more treatments, one of which forms the control (this may be the current, standard treatment or a placebo). Having chosen the treatments to compare, we must decide on the outcome measures. Primary and secondary endpoints should be determined in advance.

Outcome Measures and Their Uncertainty

Outcome measures, sometimes referred to as endpoints, are the specific factors quantified to demonstrate effect within a study. The primary outcome relates to the main objective of the study. Secondary endpoints may also be studied. They should be clearly defined in advance (sometimes referred to as, *a priori*; from the Latin, 'from the earlier'; in other words, determined before the experiment).

The CONSORT (Consolidated Standards of Reporting Trials) statement provides recommendations for best-practice reporting of randomized trials. Item number six from their checklist of information to include when reporting a trial relates to outcomes [1]. Namely, that outcome measures (both primary and secondary) should be 'completely defined pre-specified . . . , including how and when they were assessed'. This is important to avoid data being indiscriminately analyzed after the study and yielding chance findings. As an example, the article 'Gone fishing in a fluid trial' by Hjortrup *et al.* intentionally demonstrates the flaw associated with post-hoc analysis of data [2]. They proved a mortality benefit with being born under the Zodiac sign, Pisces, when taking part in a trial of intravenous fluids!

Uncertainty around outcome measures could arise from combined endpoints, e.g. a composite of mortality, cardiovascular events and stroke.

Sampling

In order to determine what size of study sample is required, a power calculation will be performed by the statistician at the study design phase. This topic is dealt with in more detail in the section on hypothesis testing later in the chapter. In essence, it accounts for the predicted magnitude of the effect of the intervention or treatment (e.g. does a new treatment reduce mortality by 2% or 20%) along with a few other factors to determine the sample size required for the study.

Generally speaking, it is not possible to collect data from the entire target population. Therefore, a sample is used, and statistical inference applied. The aim is to have a sample that is representative of the population of interest. This can be achieved by various sampling methods (Table 1.1).

Table 1.1 Various methods of sampling the population

Simple random sampling	Random selection from the population
Systematic random sample	Random first recruit, e.g. 19th admission to ICU this year, then interval sampling thereafter. The interval is determined as population size divided by sample size, e.g. sample of 200 from 1,000 ICU admissions means sampling every fifth patient.
Stratified random sample	Pooled sample from a number of random samples from several strata within the population, e.g. random sample of women, of men, of smokers, etc. Size of samples from each stratum determined by relative size within population: if smoking prevalence is 10%, the final pool will contain smokers and non-smokers in a 1:9 ratio as well.
Cluster sample	Simple random sample from groups within the population which are otherwise expected to be homogeneous, e.g. random sample of post-cardiac arrest patients, admitted to different ICUs.
Consecutive sample	Every eligible individual is recruited from the start of the study period until the required sample size is achieved.

Having obtained our sample, for a prospective study it is then necessary to allocate patients to the intervention and control groups. Allocation is a separate process to sampling but is also undertaken in a random manner. Randomization is used to ensure that any differences between the groups within the study are due to chance, i.e. to reduce the chance of statistical error. This can be done using a random-number table. Due to the nature of randomization, it may be necessary to undertake block randomization in order to maintain equal numbers of subjects in each group.

Blinding refers to obscuring to which group each patient has been assigned. It is not always possible, for example in the case of a study comparing having surgery or not. However, it is a powerful method to avoid bias (see below). Blinding can refer to study participants (patients) or investigators. Where neither party is aware which arm the participant is in, the study is double-blinded. A study which is not blinded is 'open' or 'open-label'.

Bias

Bias refers to a situation that results in a difference between study results and reality. There are numerous ways by which bias may be introduced. Bias may lead to overestimation or underestimation of an effect.

Selection Bias

The study population is not representative of the actual population. This should be reduced through appropriate randomization. Sub-types include:

- Ascertainment: when the sample is not randomly selected
- Attrition: differences in those lost to follow-up to those not
- Response: differences between volunteers to a study and non-volunteers
- Survivorship: study participants have to survive long enough to receive the intervention of note, but survival is measured from an earlier time

Information Bias

The incorrect recording of measurements, to include:

- Central tendency: responses on a Likert scale (1–5 Strongly disagree/Strongly agree) tend to merge to the centre (neither agree nor disagree)

- Lead-time: the advent of new diagnostic tests results in patients entered into a study later being diagnosed earlier in the disease process, leading to an apparent increase in survival – not due to the intervention
- Measurement: from an inaccurate or badly calibrated measuring device
- Misclassification: wrongly classifying an outcome variable
- Observer: also known as assessment bias – when an observer over- or under-reports a variable
- Reporting: study participants may give answers they think the investigator wants to hear or withhold information they (wrongly) believe to be irrelevant

Publication Bias

A tendency of journals only to publish papers with positive results. There is more detail on this in respect of meta-analysis and systematic review towards the end of the chapter.

Confounding

A confounding variable affects both the independent and the dependent variables but is not part of the exposure-outcome causal pathway. Female patients have a higher incidence of PONV and only female patients undergo gynaecological procedures but such procedures do not directly predispose to PONV: gender is a confounding variable here (Figure 1.1).

Confounding effects are controlled for at the design stage of a study by restriction, matching or randomization and at the data analysis stage by stratification or adjustment.

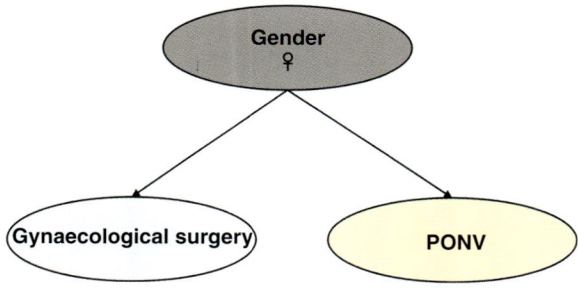

Figure 1.1 Confounding variables; causality indicated by arrows

Other Considerations

Crossover occurs when each group acts as both the control and treatment group within the same study. This can lead to a range of inaccuracies in the final data. Care must be taken to ensure any drug effects are not carried over to the control period. This is ensured by including a suitable wash-out period between the two arms of the study.

Intention-to-treat analysis involves analyzing all data as if any subjects that were lost are still in the study. Subjects may be lost for a number of reasons, e.g. refusal, moving house, dying. The analysis of all subjects aims to achieve a more true-to-life estimate of any treatment effect. In addition, maintenance of the sample size ensures that the power of the study is not diminished by the loss of subjects.

All clinical trials must undergo consideration by an ethics committee. Trials must abide by the Declaration of Helsinki. In addition, training in Good Clinical Practice (GCP) standards is important for individuals involved in research, to ensure that they have a full understanding of their responsibilities as part of the research team.

Descriptive Statistics

Having undertaken the observation phase of a study, you will hopefully have a large number of values: your data. The next step is to characterize and describe the data. This is important in two distinct ways. Firstly, it is helpful to gain a very crude understanding of any patterns in the values. If you have measured the heights of a class of school children, is there a typical range of heights for that age group or is this group unusually tall for their age? Secondly, what type of data have you collected? This directly informs what types of statistical analyses are appropriate to use in gaining a greater understanding of the meaning behind your data. In reality, you ought to understand this aspect at the planning stage of your study but determining data types and matching them to statistical tests is a crucial skill in critical appraisal of medical evidence: the literature is scattered with studies which misidentify the data type or use the incorrect statistical test or often both.

Data Types

Variables are classified as follows:

Qualitative or Categorical

- Dichotomous: data which can only have two categories, e.g. gender, malignant vs. benign, weight >40 kg vs. weight <40 kg
- Nominal: the data have more than two categories but these have no intrinsic order, e.g. different types of lung cancers observed in a study of mine workers
- Ordinal (or ranked): the data fall into several categories which have an intrinsic order but, importantly, cannot have a value assigned to them, e.g. ASA score, GCS.

Categorical data can cause some confusion. The categories should be thought of as having a 'label', not a value, but this can be easily forgotten, particularly with ordinal variables which, by definition, use numbers as the labels; you cannot perform quantitative analysis on observations of GCS – a mean GCS of 8.7 is meaningless.

Quantitative or Metric

- Discrete: the data reflect whole-number counts, e.g. number of patients responding to a treatment, platelet count
- Continuous: the possible number of measured variables is only limited by the resolution of the measuring equipment, e.g. height, temperature, BMI

Quantitative data are easy to spot; they have units of measurement. Sometimes these are not always reported or used in everyday practice, which can lead to misidentifying the variable type. BMI is a good example of this – the units are $kg\,m^{-2}$ but these are colloquially omitted.

Continuous variables can be subclassified to interval and ratio variables. By definition, a ratio variable is one where zero denotes none of that quantity. Consider temperature as an example. Kelvin is the ratio variable for temperature; 20 K is twice as hot as 10 K. By contrast, an interval variable has a relative zero point, e.g. temperature measured in degrees Celsius. Whilst the interval between 10 °C and 20 °C equates to that between 30 °C and 40 °C, 20 °C is not twice as hot as 10 °C; 10 °C and 20 °C actually equate to 283.15 K and 293.15 K so clearly one is not twice as hot as the other.

Data Representation

In simple terms, data can be depicted in rows and columns – a table or, more formally, a contingency table. This form of presentation is the basis for undertaking chi-squared analysis (see later). Graphical depictions of the data can be a more intuitive representation of the interdependence between two variables. The simplest types are those which demonstrate the frequency distribution for the values. There are two distinct types. For qualitative data, a bar chart is used (Figure 1.2). The height of the bars corresponds to the number in each category. The order of the bars along the x-axis is arbitrary (except in the case of ordinal/ranked data). By convention, the bars do not 'touch', which emphasizes the fact that the groups represented by the bars are not numerically contiguous.

By contrast, quantitative data are represented as a histogram (Figure 1.3). For continuous values, the data are first split into groups, sometimes called 'bins'. For example, age data from a population may be grouped

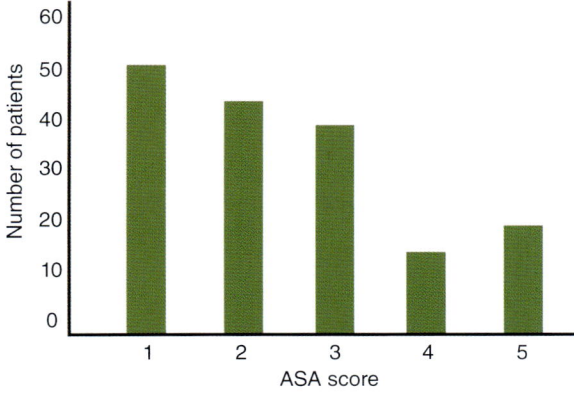

Figure 1.2 A bar chart of patients by ASA score

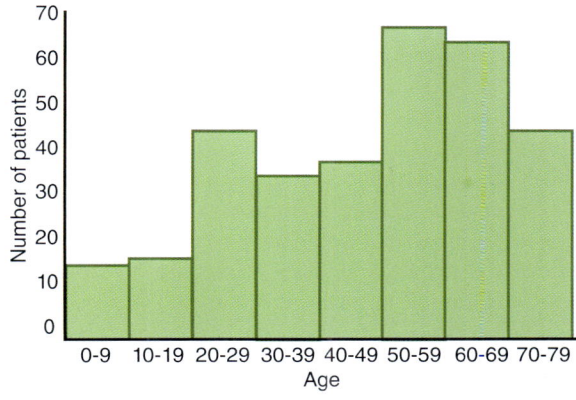

Figure 1.3 A histogram of patients' ages

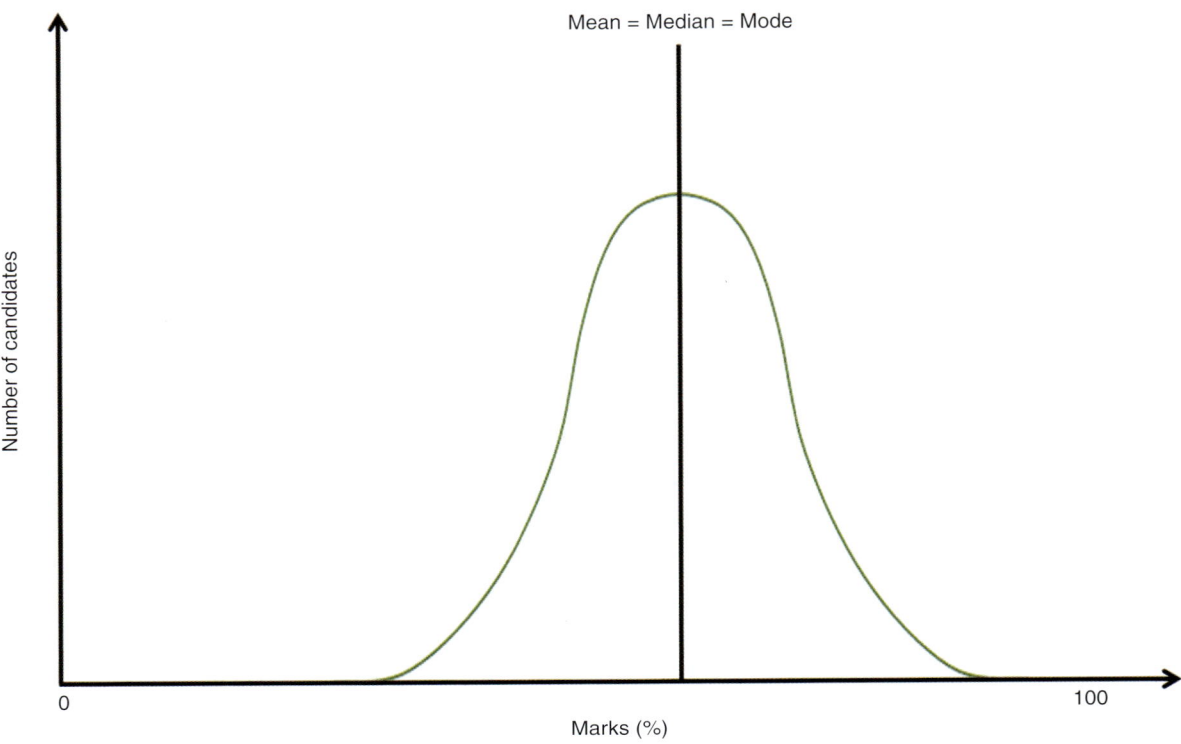

Figure 1.4 The normal distribution of a set of FRCA scores for a group of candidates

into bins of 40–49.9 years, 50–59.9 years and so on. The bins represent contiguous sections of the x-axis and so the bars touch on a histogram and clearly have an order of sequence. Because each patient in each bin in our example could have an age anywhere within the range of the bin, it is the bar area rather than just the height which is proportional to the frequency of patients falling within the bin.

The most familiar distribution for natural phenomena, e.g. height, weight or IQ, is the *normal distribution*, sometimes referred to as a 'bell curve' on account of the characteristic shape (Figure 1.4). It is a symmetrical distribution around the most common value which, in the case of a truly normal distribution, is simultaneously the median, mode and mean (see later).

Other data sets are asymmetrical. This can be the case for variables that would be expected to demonstrate a normal distribution and this is often due to the effects of a small sample size where outliers in the population can distort the distribution. This is referred to as *skew*. Skew can be negative or positive and this simply refers to where the outliers lie on the x-axis. In a positive skew, the outliers lie towards the right of the x-axis (and the bulk of the population more towards the left) and vice versa for a negative skew. Some find it counterintuitive that the description of skew seems to refer to where the outliers are, rather than the bulk of the sample. A useful aide memoire is that the 'skew' produces a 'skewer-like' projection off the side of the bell curve. Thus, in a positive skew, the 'skewer' points to the right of the x-axis and vice versa. Figure 1.5 demonstrates the distribution of marks from two further sittings of the FRCA – the solid line shows positive skew, the dashed line shows negative skew. For a positive skew, mode < median < mean whereas for a negative skew, mode > median > mean (as a rule of thumb).

If skew results from sample-size issues, a larger sample will tend to reduce the skew. This is simply due to the fact that a larger sample is more likely to also include a few outliers at the opposite end of the x-axis. For example, if we recorded the blood pressure of all patients attending a cardiology outpatient clinic, we might find a high proportion of patients with a high blood pressure and only a few with normal or low values; a negative skew. If we take a larger population, for example everyone walking into the hospital (outpatients, staff and visitors), we would expect to mostly encounter normotensive individuals and a

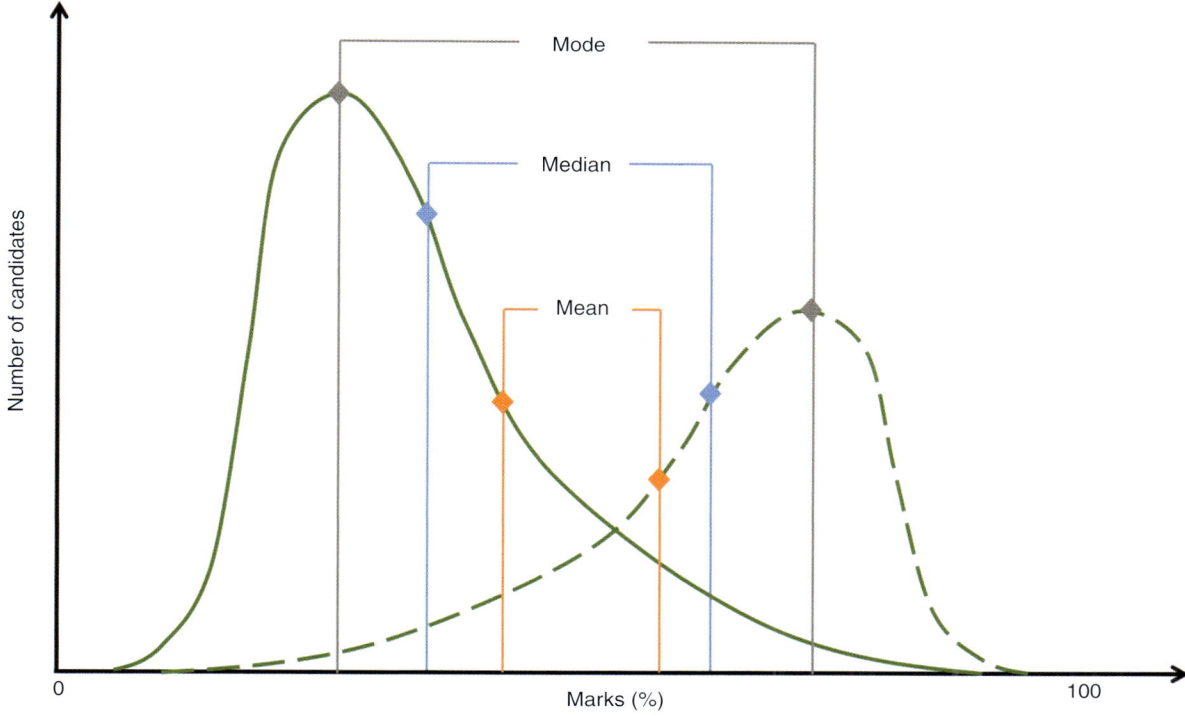

Figure 1.5 Skewed distributions – solid line is positively skewed, dotted line is negatively skewed

group of healthy, cycling enthusiasts/anaesthetists with lower blood pressures. The cyclists would balance the clinic patients and a normal distribution would be expected.

The characteristics of a normal distribution are mathematically a little more complex. Firstly, the median must equal the mean. The 'tails' of a normal distribution are summarized by the standard deviation (see later) and kurtosis. Determining the kurtosis is a complex calculation, yielding a unitless pure number. A value of 3 suggests a normal distribution (mesokurtic); higher values (leptokurtic) suggest extreme outliers, long fat tails and a narrow, thin central peak; whereas lower values (platykurtic) suggest no outliers, i.e. short thin tails and a broad, flat central peak. A calculated skew of zero is a characteristic of a normal distribution but it does not guarantee it; it could result from a balance of a short, fat tail on one end of the distribution and a long, thin tail on the other. Specific tests such as the Kolmogorov–Smirnov test can test the normality of a distribution directly.

The Exponential Distribution

One particular form of skewed distribution is the exponential distribution (Figure 1.6). In this distribution, all outliers are in one direction (an extreme positive skew in the case of a negative exponential). The exponential distribution is also known as the negative exponential distribution because of the mathematical relationship which describes it; it includes a negative exponent. To explain what that means, it's worth looking at a common example from the FRCA syllabus. After a bolus dose of an intravenous medication, such as propofol, the reduction from the peak blood concentration follows a negative exponential relationship. The concentration of propofol at any specified time after the bolus, (C_t), can be found as a function of the initial concentration (C_0) and the time between C_0 and C_t. Here is the maths: the initial concentration is multiplied by the mathematical constant, 'e', raised by an 'exponent' (hence the name of the relationship) of $-kt$, which is the rate constant (k) times the time elapsed (t):

$$C_t = C_0 \times e^{-kt}$$

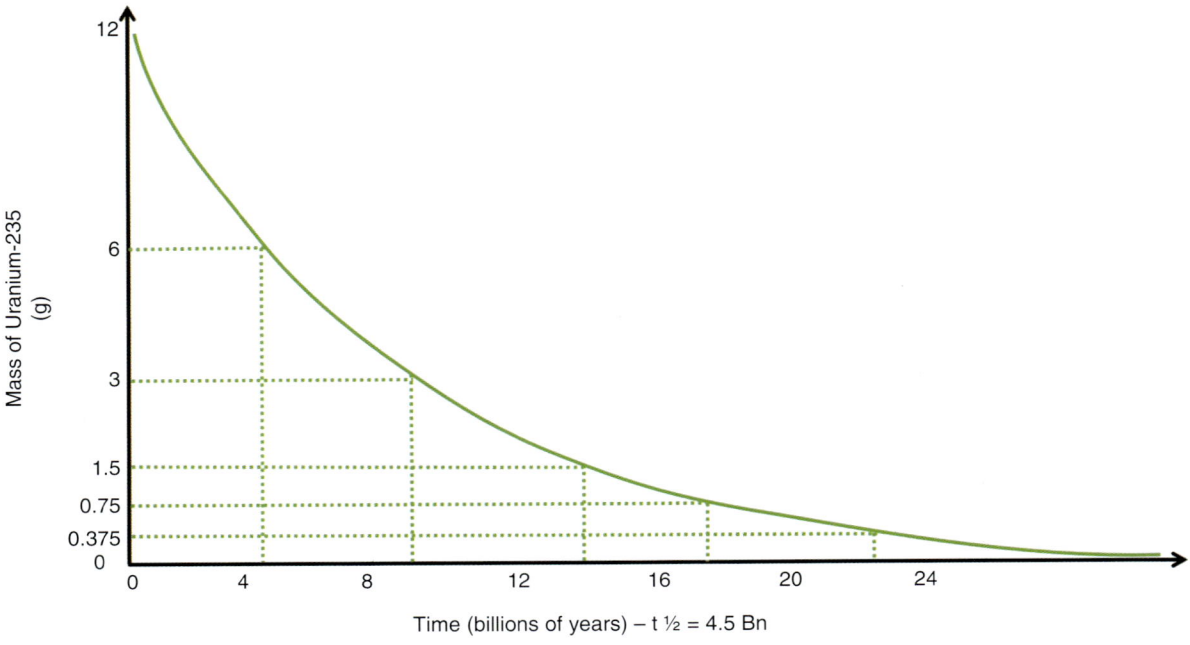

Figure 1.6 The exponential distribution; decay of a 12-g sample of uranium-235

Of course, as any good FRCA candidate knows, the pharmacological reality is a little more complex and the actual mathematical relationship describes the interplay of exponential decay between other pharmacokinetic compartments, resulting in a biexponential relationship.

Euler's number, e, is a mathematic constant named in honour of Swiss mathematician Leonhard Euler. It is the number whose natural logarithm = 1. Like 0, 1, i and π, it is one of the five irrational numbers in mathematics (ones which are not ratios of integers). It was actually discovered by fellow Swiss mathematician, Joseph Bernoulli, when he was studying the financial concept of compound interest. It is also known as Napier's number (who first described natural logarithms). Euler's number is different from Euler's constant (also known as the Euler–Mascheroni constant).

All statistical distributions can be described by a mathematical relationship but the exponential relationship is worthy of the particular focus we have just paid it, due to its clinical and medical physics applications, such as pharmacokinetic phenomena and radioactive decay (see Chapter 15). An everyday example is the computer-controlled pumps used for total intravenous anaesthesia. These perform these exponential calculations in real time.

Summary Statistics

To mathematically describe the data, we need to use *summary statistics*. Probably the first area of interest is the part of the data set which contains the most-frequently-occurring value, for example, the commonest weight within a group of surgical patients. Measures of central tendency, such as averages (see below), allow us to do this, and measures of spread, such as standard deviation, then allow a mathematical description of how the rest of the sample relates to these central values. These statistics are useful for ordinal (qualitative) and all quantitative data (Table 1.2).

The measures of central tendency most commonly used are the averages. The term 'average' is used a little loosely. Technically, it includes mean, median and mode although it is often simply used as a synonym for the mean.

The mode is very straightforward to work out; it is simply the most frequently occurring value in the data set. Consequently, it is not affected by outliers but,

Table 1.2 Appropriate measures of central tendency for different data types

	Mode	Median	Mean
Categorical nominal	Yes	No	No
Categorical ordinal	Yes	Yes	No
Quantitative discrete	Yes	Yes	Yes
Quantitative continuous	No	Yes	Yes

equally, it barely describes any of the data. The only common application of the mode is in describing multi-modal distributions. Age of onset of type-1 diabetes is an example of a bimodal distribution; there is a peak between 5 and 9 years and between 10 and 14 years of age. Continuous data are difficult to describe with the mode. Imagine a truly continuous sample of patient weights, accurate to grams. It is almost inconceivable that even two patients would weigh the same to this level of accuracy so the sample would have no mode.

The median is the middle value in the range when the data are sorted into ascending order. It is not particularly affected by skewed data sets, which is why it is the average of choice for non-normally distributed data. However, as with the mode, it does ignore most of the data apart from those at the centre.

To obtain the mean, all values are added together and divided by the number of values. This has the advantage that all data are incorporated in the measure. This is also its disadvantage as skewed data are poorly described by the mean; you should only use it with normally distributed data. It cannot be used with ordinal data.

A note on discrete data and calculating the mean. This might seem counterintuitive as you may well end up with a non-integer result, e.g. 0.7 of a patient. It is, however, perfectly correct to say that, for example, an average of 28.7 patients are admitted to an ICU per month. That's not quite the same as saying that, in an average month, 28.7 patients are admitted. We don't know what 'an average month' is and that phrase would imply the month is the average 'thing' and we therefore would have to account for what we mean by 0.7 of a patient.

Measure of Spread

Measures of spread help to describe how the remainder of the data relate to the central portion and, in turn, reflect the validity of the measure of central tendency. A widely spread data set suggests the presence of outliers, the potential for skew and hence an unreliable measure of central tendency.

The range simply describes the difference in value between the smallest and largest value in the sample. It is not affected by where the rest of the data lie between those limits. As such, it tells us nothing about skew (asymmetry of the bell curve) or kurtosis (the narrowness of the bell); both of these are measures of central spread. That said, outlier data do dramatically affect the validity of the range as a description of the rest of the data.

Quartiles, as the name suggests, divide the data set into four portions, in exactly the same way that the median divides the data in halves. Quartile 1 includes the first 25% of the data from the smallest value. Quartile 2 includes the next 25% up to the median, and so on. The interquartile range (IQR) is the difference between the lower limit of quartile 2 and the upper limit of quartile 3 – the middle 50% of the data. This therefore excludes any outliers but can still be affected by a skew. By definition, of course, the IQR fails to reflect 50% of the data – the upper 25% and lower 25%. The IQR and median are the basis for a box-and-whisker plot (Figure 1.7). The box contains the IQR and is bisected by a line representing the median. The whiskers extend out to the maximum and minimum values. The figure also demonstrates the effect of skew on the appearance of the plot (Group B in Figure 1.7 has a negative skew).

To describe the distribution of data within these wider bands of ranges and quartiles, we can describe their position mathematically in relation to the mean. Simple measures are the absolute variation and variance but these are somewhat simplistic and do not provide a particularly useful number (so much so, you may not even have heard of them before). The standard deviation (SD) overcomes these technical issues. In turn, it can also be used to quantitatively describe the shape of a distribution (see earlier). Mathematically it is calculated as:

$$SD = \sqrt{\frac{\sum(x - \bar{x})^2}{n - 1}}$$

Where x = each value, $\bar{x}$ = mean, n = number of values. Standard deviation is only suited to continuous data and should only be used for normally distributed data. The mean ± 2 SD defines a range which will contain 95.4% of all data points if the data is normally distributed.

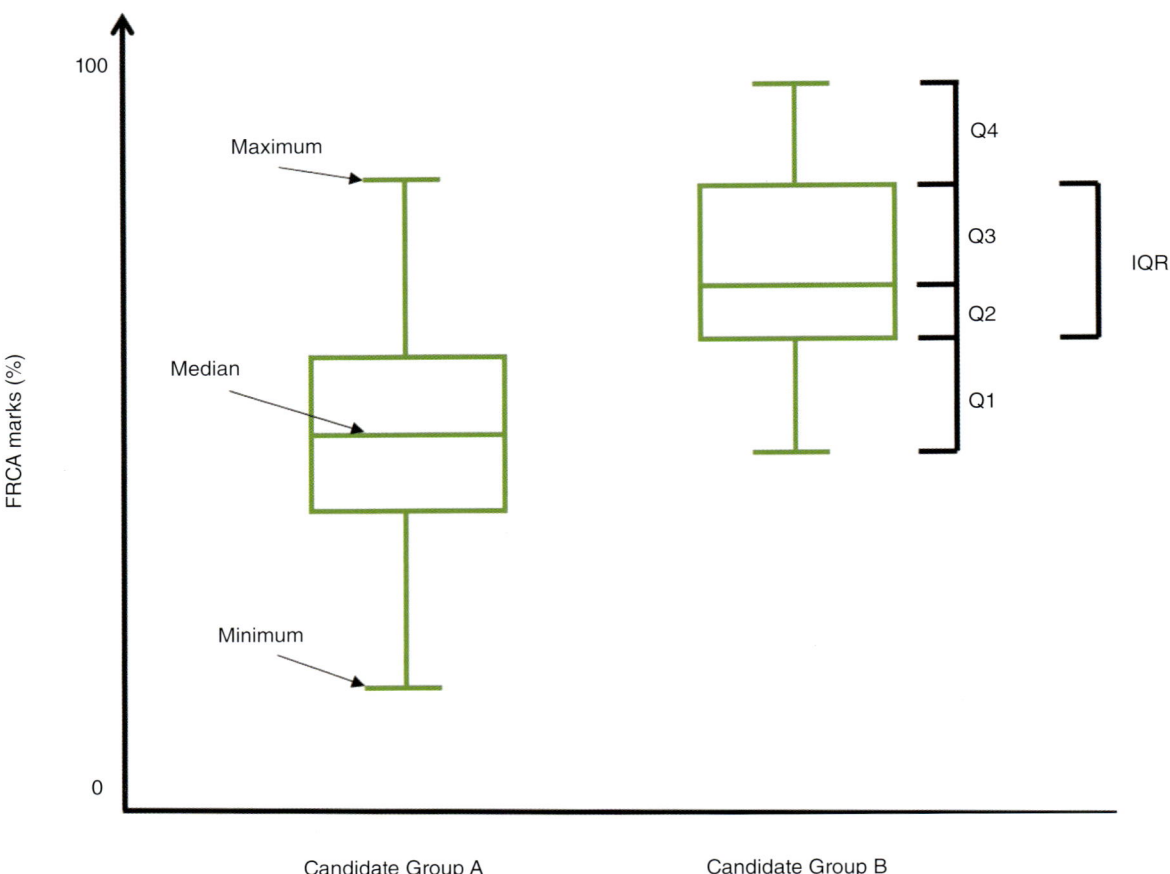

Figure 1.7 Box-and-whisker plot of FRCA scores for two different groups. The components of the box-and-whisker plot are demonstrated for Group B's plot

Statistics vs. Parameters

It is worth mentioning that we have talked principally about statistical terms so far. Statistics are descriptors of a sample. They are often then extrapolated to a population. For example, if we measure all the heights of a class of medical students we could generate a mean height. That mean is a 'parameter' of the class – it is the population mean for that group because we have measured every individual in the population (the population being the class). If we want to use that result as a surrogate for all UK 18-year-old adults, we refer to it as a statistic because it is calculated from a sample, not the whole population of UK 18-year-olds. Just remember: **s**tatistics for **s**amples, **p**arameters for whole **p**opulations. We can calculate the difference between any given statistic and the corresponding parameter by calculating the standard error. The most common example is the standard error of the mean (SEM). The larger the sample, the smaller the SEM – the closer you come to sampling the entire population, the closer the sample mean approximates to the population mean and the SEM tends towards zero:

$$SEM = \frac{\sigma}{\sqrt{n}}$$

The standard deviation of the population (σ) is obviously not often known and so the sample SD is usually substituted but this renders the SEM an approximation:

$$SEM \approx \frac{SD}{\sqrt{n}}$$

Table 1.3 summarizes the measures of spread and for which types of variables they can be applied.

Table 1.3 Applicability of measures of spread

	Range	IQR	SD
Categorical nominal	No	No	No
Categorical ordinal	Yes	Yes	No
Quantitative	Yes	Yes	Yes

Association and Correlation

The interrelation of two variables can be demonstrated using a scatter plot. This can demonstrate a positive or a negative association, otherwise referred to as proportional or inversely proportional, respectively. The term 'directly proportional' is specific to those associations where zero in one variable coincides with zero in the other. Weight and BMI are directly proportional (0 kg will result in 0 kg m^{-2}) but weight and age are just proportional (a baby does not have zero weight). A scatter plot will only give a qualitative idea of the strength of any association. To quantify it, a correlation coefficient is calculated. This is a measure of the average distance of all points from an imaginary straight line drawn through the plot (Figure 1.8). Normally distributed data (referred to as parametric data) can be tested with Pearson's correlation coefficient. Non-parametric data are tested with Spearman's rank correlation coefficient.

The coefficient is reported as the Pearson's r value or Spearman's ρ (rho). A value of <0.2 represents no correlation; 0.2–0.4 is a weak correlation, perhaps worth further research. A strong correlation is 0.6–0.8 and, in fact, some would say 0.8–1.0 is too good to be true and should be scrutinised. A positive value demonstrates that as one variable increases, so does the other; for example, the lifetime incidence of lung cancer increases as the lifetime smoking exposure increases. A negative value implies the opposite; glomerular filtration rate decreases as age increases.

Remember that correlation is not indicative of causation. Furthermore, it is important not to be misled by significance testing, i.e. a *p-value* reported with a correlation coefficient. A large sample, in particular, can easily produce a very statistically significant *p*-value for a weak correlation. More on significance testing and *p*-values later.

Agreement

Agreement refers to how similar two sets of matched observations are. For nominal data, Cohen's or

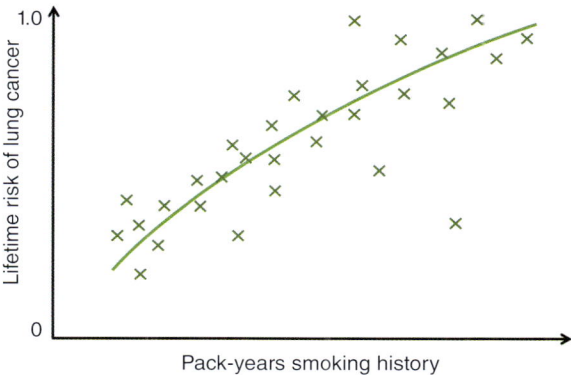

Figure 1.8 Scatter plot and line of best fit, demonstrating the relationship between smoking exposure and lung cancer risk

Fleiss's kappa statistic is calculated. For example, in comparing diagnosis of chest X-ray changes as either consolidation, heart failure, abscess or atelectasis, we could quantify how well two independent radiologists agreed on the diagnosis for each patient using Cohen's kappa. If there were more than two radiologists, Fleiss's kappa must be used. If the data are continuous, the intra-class correlation coefficient is used. For example, we can compare the agreement of two blood gas analyzers to quantify $PaCO_2$, a continuous variable, with this test. The range of possible values for agreement tests are similar to those used for coefficients of correlation (see above) so, for example, a kappa of 1.0 means perfect agreement.

For continuous variables, it is possible to display agreement graphically on a Bland–Altman plot (Figure 1.9). For each pair of values (e.g. PaO_2 of sample 1 measured in machine A and machine B), the difference between the two machines is plotted on the *y*-axis. The mean of the two values gives the *x*-coordinate. The mean value for all *y*-axis coordinates is plotted as a horizontal line called the *bias*. The further the bias is from zero, the more one machine is tending to overestimate the value compared to the other machine. The bias ± 1.96 SD gives two other lines, the limits of agreement. These express how likely it is that agreement is simply due to chance – the closer the limits, the less likely that agreement is a chance phenomenon. This plot has another useful feature; because the *x*-axis relates to the size of the value, the plot can describe differing levels of agreement at different values for the variable. In our example, the plot demonstrates that the two machines have good agreement at higher PaO_2 values but disagree at low values.

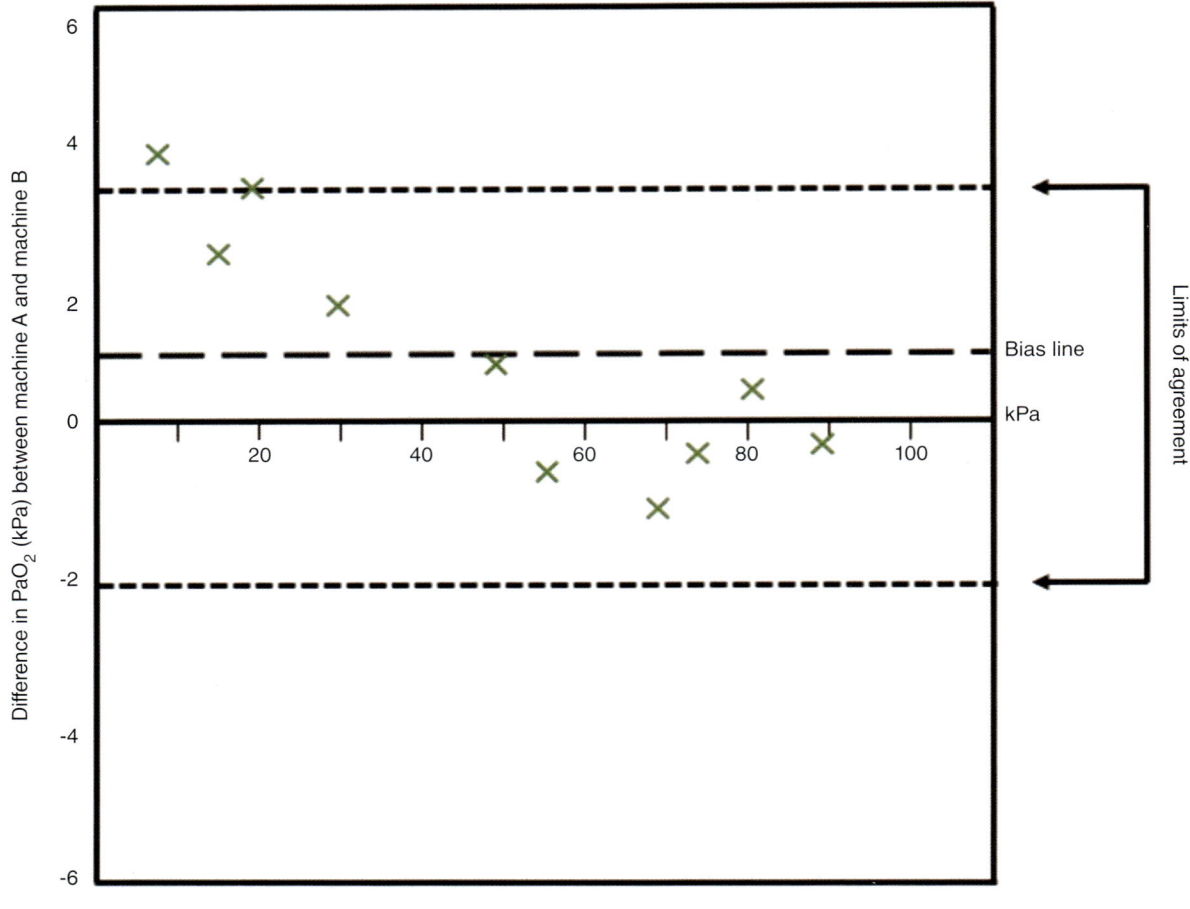

Figure 1.9 Bland–Altman plot of two blood gas analyzers

Sensitivity, Specificity, Negative Predictive Value and Positive Predictive Value

Whilst discussing methods to evaluate diagnostic tests, a related topic is that of sensitivity and specificity as well as negative and positive predictive value. The sensitivity of a test expresses its ability to correctly *detect* the presence of a condition, usually expressed as a percentage. The specificity, meanwhile, denotes the test's ability to correctly confirm the *absence* of a condition. For example, a sensitivity of 100% tells us a new test for influenza virus detects every single case of the disease. If the specificity is 80%, it tells us that 80% of healthy individuals are correctly identified as such but it also suggests 20% erroneously test positive for the virus. Mathematically, these are calculated as:

$$\text{Sensitivity} = \frac{\text{True positives}}{(\text{True positives} + \text{False negatives})}$$

$$\text{Specificity} = \frac{\text{True negatives}}{(\text{True negatives} + \text{False positives})}$$

In medical statistical terms, tests with sensitivity or specificity of 90% or more are considered as robust. Much is made of 'rules of thumb' for specificity being a good 'rule in' (SpIn) of a disease, whereas a sensitive test is good as a 'rule out' (SnOut). The original study used to determine either a very high sensitivity or specificity of a test needs to be methodologically perfect for the SpIn/SnOut rule to be applicable. Often, they are small studies and are based in populations at risk for the condition so are prone to bias. In reality, a test can only really be evaluated with a joint consideration of both aspects.

The positive and negative predictive values (PPV, NPV) are subtly different because they evaluate the ability of a test to accurately predict the outcome. Thus, when we talk about 'true positive' and 'false positive' events in this context, it refers to the test predicting a positive result, which is later confirmed by the gold-standard test; and the test predicting a positive result, which is not confirmed by the gold-standard test. A similar logic applies to defining true negatives and false negatives. Superficially, the mathematical definitions seem similar to those of sensitivity and specificity, particularly if these differing definitions for true/false positives/negatives are not considered:

$$PPV = \frac{\text{True positives}}{(\text{True positives} + \text{False positives})}$$

$$NPV = \frac{\text{True negatives}}{(\text{True negatives} + \text{False negatives})}$$

From a philosophical perspective, the key difference is actually that NPV and PPV reflect the prevalence (Prev) of a condition in the population (not just the sample) and a more helpful mathematical definition is in terms of this and the sensitivity (Sens) and specificity (Spec):

$$PPV = \frac{\text{Sensitivity} \times \text{Prevalence}}{(\text{Sens} \times \text{Prev}) + ((1 - \text{Spec}) \times (1 - \text{Prev}))}$$

$$NPV = \frac{\text{Specificity} \times (1 - \text{Prevalence})}{((1 - \text{Sens}) \times \text{Prev}) + (\text{Spec} \times (1 - \text{Prev}))}$$

Regression

With correlation earlier, we determined how strong the association was between change in one variable with respect to change in another. Regression is the process which allows us to quantify and mathematically describe that relationship. Firstly, it is important to determine whether causality is likely, otherwise it can be easy to overinterpret the clinical significance of a correlation. The established criteria to judge this were defined by Bradford Hill in the 1960s and include [3]:

- Consistency and reproducibility
- Temporality: the effect must follow exposure to the trigger
- Biological gradient: greater exposure to the trigger should lead to a greater effect
- Plausibility: within reasonable limits of knowledge, there ought to be a fair explanation as to how the trigger might cause the effect

Linear regression involves establishing whether or not the relationship between the variables can be described by a straight line on a scatter plot of the data. The mathematical equation of this line is then described and the statistical significance of the relationship is also determined.

The familiar equation for a straight line forms the basis for linear regression equations:

$$y = mx + c$$

In this equation, y is known as the dependent variable; this is the variable determined through experimentation and must be quantitative-continuous. The variable controlled in the experiment, denoted x in the equation, is known as the independent variable (this can be of any data type). For example, if we wanted to know the average height of school children we could group them by age (the independent variable, plotted on the x-axis) and then measure their heights and plot the average height for each year of age on the y-axis to show how height *depends* on age. In the equation, c denotes where the line crosses the y-axis (the y-intercept). There will then be some constant (denoted by m) which describes the maths required to get from a value of x to the corresponding value of y.

In many real-world situations, there are actually multiple independent variables which influence the value of the dependent variable and multiple linear regression analysis is required here. Where multiple variables depend on multiple independent variables, multivariate analysis is required. For example, a study of cardiovascular health may examine those factors contributing to incidence of high cholesterol and high blood pressure. Multiple regression could be performed to look at the effect of age, gender and smoking history on hypertension. We could then repeat the analysis for the same risks and their contribution to hypercholesterolaemia. Multivariate analysis would simultaneously analyze the impact of all three risks on both outcomes which would give a more complete understanding of the interaction of the high cholesterol and hypertension.

How the linear regression line is mathematically fitted amongst the data points is where statisticians really earn their money and there are numerous techniques to achieve this accurately. The coefficient of determination, R^2, quantifies how well the model has succeeded – the 'goodness-of-fit'. A higher number for this value indicates a better fit of the line and equation to the data points; 0.0 is no fit, 1.0 denotes an exact fit.

Logistic regression is a particular method suited to scenarios where the dependent variable is binary, rather than continuous. In simple terms, the dependent variable of interest is converted to a value representing the probability of it occurring. This is then plotted on the y-axis, against the independent variable on the x-axis. For example, logistic regression could be used to describe the link between pack-years of smoking and death due to cancer. Here, the dependent variable (death due to cancer) either occurs or doesn't; a binary outcome. The process of logistic regression allows the probability of a cancer-related death to be predicted from an individual's smoking history. Goodness-of-fit measures for logistic regression are based on chi-squared analysis. Examples include Cox and Snell, Homer-Lemeshow, and Pearson. There is little consensus as to which is best and there are many, many more tests available.

The Poisson distribution is a model for discrete data, i.e. counts. It forecasts the probability of a particular number of events in a specified time frame, provided the average rate of occurrences is known and that each occurrence is independent of others. For example, the probability that 10 new patients arrive at the emergency department in the next hour can be predicted if the average attendance rate is known. Poisson regression (sometimes known as log-linear regression) can be used to determine the relationship between a dependent variable which follows a Poisson distribution and linear-distributed independent variables.

Deductive Statistics

Probability

Probability is the basis of inferential statistics. It informs the way in which we test data and whether or not we accept the outcomes of a study as plausible. In basic terms, probability is a way of quantifying the chance of an event occurring. There are two principal ways of approaching the philosophy of probability: subjectivism and objectivism.

Subjectivism is so called because it relies on subjective assessment of the probability of an event occurring, based on prior events, experiments or distributions. The commonest implementation of this idea is Bayes' theorem or Bayesian statistics. For example, you might be wondering if you trust your junior colleague to perform laryngoscopy. You ask them their first-pass success rate and they tell you this is 90% having performed 100 anaesthetics. You feel encouraged but then you learn the next patient had a previous grade 3 laryngoscopy. Now you ask your colleague for more evidence of their experience with difficult intubations. They tell you that they have only intubated 10 patients with this level of airway difficulty and their first-pass success rate was only 30%. This 30% success rate is referred to as the *prior probability*. There are other factors to consider. For example, there is a probability that the patient will not be as difficult as at the previous attempt. Combining all these factors, we calculate the *conditional probability*. In our example, the conditional probability is the probability of successful intubation in the event that the patient is indeed a grade 3 laryngoscopy. Whether our colleague succeeds or not allows us to calculate the *posterior probability*, which looks back and accounts for the effects of the most recent attempt on their probability of success with the next intubation. The posterior probability becomes the prior probability for their next attempt.

Objectivism, meanwhile, provides the basis for what we might regard as the 'everyday' medical statistical approach. Objectivism or frequentist statistical methods take probability to be a property of a defined system or experiment. It takes no account of prior events to forecast the probability, relying solely on the evidence deduced from an experiment to test the hypothesis. Equally, however, prior to the experiment, the hypothesis can only be assigned two possible probabilities – the hypothesis is true (probability = 1) or false (probability = 0). A Bayesian approach, meanwhile, is based around the idea that it is possible to predict the true probability that the hypothesis is correct at the start of the experiment, based on prior knowledge. By definition, however, this means Bayesian statistical methods are not repeatable as one experiment informs the probability predictions for the next iteration. Furthermore, calculating the prior probability of the next experiment relies on subjective interpretation of the available data. An objectivist approach is founded on the idea that the same result can be obtained by repeating the experiment as often as you wish. The principal focus of our discussions here will be the traditional frequentist or objectivist approach.

Quantifying Probability

As we've already alluded to, probability can be quantified between two extremes from 0.0 (impossible) to 1.0 (certain). Having quantified a probability in this way, it becomes possible to mathematically describe probabilities and the interaction of multiple events. Where the probability of an event = p, the probability of the event not occurring = $1 - p$. For a combination of independent events, each with their own defined probabilities, these are multiplied:

Probability of A and B occurring = $pA \times pB$

For mutually exclusive events, their probabilities are added:

Probability of A or B occurring = $pA + pB$

For non-mutually exclusive events, their individual probabilities are added, as for mutually exclusive events, but the probability of both occurring is subtracted:

Probability of A or B = $pA + pB - (pA \times pB)$

Let's put that into practice. We could do a review of the quality outcomes after our anaesthetics. We might find that, out of the last 100 patients anaesthetized, five suffered nausea and vomiting. On the basis of this review, we could tell our next patient that the probability of them experiencing post-operative nausea and vomiting (PONV) is:

$$p = 0.05$$

This can also be expressed as a percentage, which some patients may find more intuitive to understand. A certainty (probability of 1.0) equates to 100%. A probability of 0.05 is equal to 5 in 100, or 5%.

The probability of not experiencing PONV is therefore:

$$p = 1 - 0.05 = 0.95 \text{ (or 95\%)}$$

The same review might also demonstrate the probability of experiencing significant post-operative pain, when we anaesthetize specifically for laparoscopic surgery, is 0.02. Now we can tell our laparoscopic cholecystectomy patient how likely they are to have both pain and PONV:

$$p = 0.05 \times 0.02 = 0.001 \text{ (or 0.1\%)}$$

That's for the pessimistic patient though; someone who only wants to know the chance of everything going wrong! The realist is probably more interested in the probability of either being sick or sore. These are non-mutually exclusive as being sick doesn't stop you having pain:

$$p = 0.05 + 0.02 - (0.05 \times 0.02) = 0.069 \text{ (or 6.9\%)}$$

To predict the probability of pain after gall-bladder surgery, irrespective of surgical technique, we need the probability of pain after laparotomy – assume our data gives this as 0.03. A patient can either be exposed to the pain probability associated with laparoscopy or the probability of pain associated with laparotomy (if the procedure has to be converted) but not both: these are mutually exclusive events so their probability is added.

$$p = 0.02 + 0.03 = 0.05 \text{ (or 5\%)}$$

Risk, Hazard, Odds and Their Ratios

From probability, the natural progression is to unpick the definition of the terms risk, hazard and odds, which are very often muddled. These are important concepts as they help us to make useful descriptions of the probability of events as applied to real-life phenomena.

Risk is the simplest of these, now that we have an understanding of probability. **Absolute risk** (AR) is synonymous with probability, i.e. the number of times a particular outcome occurs divided by the total number of all outcome occurrences. This is the same as the probability but it is helpful to restate that here again before we discuss relative risk or risk ratio. The **risk ratio** (RR) or **relative risk** (equivalent terms and so also denoted RR) is the ratio of two risks! This is best explained with an example. We have two groups of patients. To one we give a new statin drug, the other a placebo. Our 'event' would be a cholesterol

Table 1.4 Numbers of patients in each treatment group with and without high cholesterol

	Cholesterol >5.0 mmol l^{-1}	Cholesterol <5.0 mmol l^{-1}
Treatment	15	85
Placebo	40	60

of >5.0 mmol l^{-1}. Table 1.4 (above) illustrates the outcome of our study.

The risk expresses the probability of the event (hypercholesterolaemia) and is calculated for each group (treatment and placebo) as the number of events divided by all outcomes (events and non-events):

$$\text{Risk for treatment group} = \frac{15}{(15 + 85)} = 0.15$$

$$\text{Risk for placebo group} = \frac{40}{(40 + 60)} = 0.40$$

The RR compares the risk of hypercholesterolaemia in the two treatment arms and, in doing so, evaluates the success of the treatment in altering the outcome of the cholesterol test. It is calculated as follows:

$$\text{RR} = \frac{0.15}{0.40} = 0.38$$

This means that the risk of developing hypercholesterolaemia with the new drug is 38% of the risk encountered if you take the placebo. An RR (or risk ratio) of less than 1.0 tells us the event (hypercholesterolaemia, in this example) is less likely in the treatment group. An RR of 1.0 implies no effect of the treatment, and an RR of >1.0 would actually suggest the treatment causes hypercholesterolaemia.

Number needed to treat (NNT) is the reciprocal of the absolute risk reduction (ARR) and quantifies the effectiveness of a treatment. The ARR in the example above is 0.25 (risk in the placebo group (0.40) minus the risk in the treatment group (0.15)); thus, the NNT is 1/0.25 = 4. Four people need to be treated with the drug for one of them to benefit from it. Had our calculation resulted in a negative number, then we would be looking at the number needed to harm (NNH); this is useful for considering side-effect data.

Odds and odds ratios (ORs) are subtly different from risk. Odds expresses the rate of events versus non-events in each group; risk expresses the events versus all outcomes. Those are not the same thing.

For a prospective study, the exposure of both groups to various risk factors for an outcome is known and this means risk and RRs can be used (odds and ORs can also be used but an OR tends to exaggerate the strength of an effect when compared to an RR). Because the risk profile of both groups is not usually known for retrospective work, we cannot use RR. If we were going to do a case–control study (retrospective) to evaluate the effectiveness of our statin drug, we couldn't calculate an RR. Why is that? We'd conduct our study by identifying people with a high cholesterol and matching them with people with a normal cholesterol. Then we'd determine if the patients in each group happened to be on our new statin to see if use of the drug was associated with the outcome. But we wouldn't know how many people outside the study were taking the statin but had normal cholesterol (except for the few we might have selected as part of our control group by pure chance). Nor would we necessarily know about the people with high cholesterol despite being on the drug unless we had recruited them to our case group. Consequently, we can't complete the risk calculations because we don't know the true incidence of hypercholesterolaemia. Odds and ORs, on the other hand, simply compare the event rate between groups; there is no requirement for knowledge of the incidence. The OR is constructed in the same way as an RR but it is important to realize that the denominator in calculating the odds to go into that ratio is different:

$$\text{Risk} = \frac{\text{Events}}{(\text{Events} + \text{Non-events})}$$

$$\text{Odds} = \frac{\text{Events}}{\text{Non-events}}$$

This does mean that for very rare events, (events + non-events) is almost numerically equivalent to non-events and so, in those settings, the calculated values of risk and odds are similar.

For our statin trial, the odds and OR for hypercholesterolaemia is:

$$\text{Odds for treatment group} = \frac{15}{85} = 0.18$$

$$\text{Odds for placebo group} = \frac{40}{60} = 0.67$$

$$\text{OR} = \frac{0.18}{0.67} = 0.27$$

Even though these ratios both derive from the same data, they give the impression of a significantly different scale of the treatment effect; 0.27 vs. 0.38. We must always view the choice of OR and RR with a critical eye when reviewing research: as mentioned, the OR tends to exaggerate the association between intervention and effect. If the RR is <1.0, the OR tends to be further away from 1.0 and similarly, when the RR is >1.0 the OR is higher still. Researchers may inadvertently (or even deliberately!) select a ratio which misrepresents the significance of whatever treatment effect they describe in their study.

Finally, we need to consider the hazard ratio (HR). As with risk, hazard does not necessarily refer to a negative outcome – we can talk about the hazard of cure or the risk of treatment success; these are statistical terms which differ from the lay use of the words. The key difference between hazard and risk is that hazard accounts for the progression of time since the start of the experiment. The HR is the incidence rate of the event in one group at one specific time divided by the incidence rate of the same event in another group. Conventionally, this is used to describe survival phenomena on a Kaplan–Meier chart (Figure 1.10). The RR describes the likelihood of surviving, the HR describes the difference in survival rates between the groups at any given time point – i.e. how far apart the lines are on the Kaplan–Meier chart. The problem with the HR is that it is time-dependent. The Kaplan–Meier chart for endovascular vs. open aneurysm repair (see Figure 1.10) demonstrates an initial survival advantage at 1 year (with a favourable HR of 0.92) but, in the long term, we know there is currently no survival advantage between the two approaches. The lines on the chart converge and meet (the HR reduces towards 1.0 by 1.5 years). An aneurysm surgery study with only short follow-up may quote a single HR and mislead us as to the true mortality benefits between the treatments. Of course, using the Kaplan–Meier chart also helps illustrate this effect better – we can see the lines converging and diverging with time. We effectively see multiple HRs represented rather than the typical, single end-of-study HR quoted in most research. Figure 1.10 demonstrates that, in fact, by 4 years post-surgery, open repair has a survival benefit (HR 1.22) and that once again, by around 5.5 years, there is no difference between the two techniques.

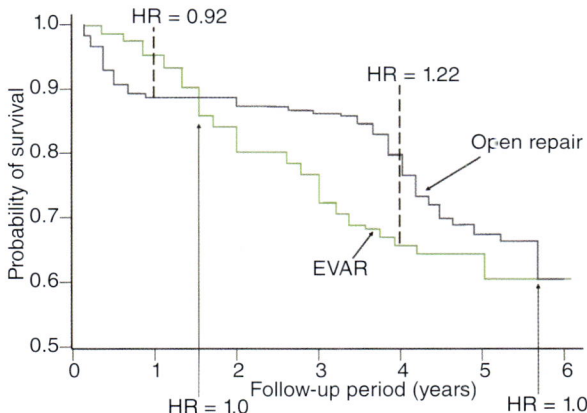

Figure 1.10 A Kaplan–Meier chart for survival after open or endovascular aneurysm repair

Confidence Intervals

Confidence intervals (CIs) are an exercise in describing the relationship between experimental data and the true population parameter in terms of probability. Depending on the sample size and other factors, the confidence *level* is determined ahead of the study by the research team. Typically, research is conducted at the 95% confidence level. Study statistics are calculated and CIs are then constructed to describe the probability relationship between the statistic and the corresponding population parameter, e.g. sample mean and population mean. The true meaning of the CI is often misunderstood. It doesn't mean that 95% of the data fall within the range (compared to standard deviation), nor does it mean that there is a 95% chance of the true parameter lying within that range (probably the most common misconception). The fact behind this latter idea is that, once a study has been conducted, the data collated and the CI determined, the true value for the population parameter has either been included or not.

What the interval does tell us is that, if we repeat our experiment multiple times, we would be confident that the true parameter would lie within the CI range in 95% of our repeat experiments. Or – perhaps a more straightforward way to define it on similar lines – there is a 95% chance that the data of a future experiment will contain the true population parameter within the range defined by the CI. Both are subtly different from the usual misconceived definition (95% chance the true value lies within the CI range) because they are an expression of probability about a future repeat experiment.

CIs are often reported with respect to the ratios we have discussed earlier. When such an interval includes 1.0 this suggests the results are statistically non-significant. To take our earlier example of the new statin, you will remember that an RR <1.0 implies the statin reduces the risk of developing hypercholesterolaemia whilst a RR >1.0 implies the statin leads to an increased risk of developing the condition. So, if the researchers reported the results as 'RR 0.6 (95% CI 0.4–1.2)' this would mean there was a 95% probability that, in the next study of this drug, we could expect the true risk of hypercholesterolaemia to be somewhere between 60% reduced and 20% increased. Clearly this is nonsense. A CI such as this tells us the study is inconclusive. Again, a critical eye is required; even a very convincing RR, even 0.1, must be completely disregarded if the CI includes 1.0.

> The fragility index is a measure of how robust the results of a study are with regard to considering the effect of changing the non-events to events. It denotes the size of this change that will render the overall result of the trial non-significant. In the example study of a new statin drug, 11 additional events would be required to raise the *p*-value to >0.05; i.e. there would need to be 26, rather than 15, patients in the treatment group with cholesterol >5.0. This fragility index of 11 is quite high; few studies in critical care medicine, for example, have an index outside single figures.

Hypothesis Testing

The process for hypothesis testing involves defining a *null hypothesis* (denoted H_0) in respect of the chosen outcome. The null hypothesis usually stipulates that there is no relationship between the dependent and independent variable. In everyday research, that equates to meaning the H_0 proposes the treatment or intervention does not have any effect (the *alternative hypothesis*, that there is a treatment effect being the one the researchers seek to promote). The basis of hypothesis testing is to perform a study which allows us to gather data to reject the null hypothesis and so imply truth to the alternative hypothesis (note, that's not quite the same as proving the alternative hypothesis is correct).

Of course, there is always scope for 'error' which refers to statistical error rather than a slip of the pen. Statistical errors fall into two categories: type 1 and type 2 errors.

Type 1 error is incorrect rejection of the H_0 or, in other words, concluding that there is an effect where there is not (a false positive). By definition, the probability of a test making a type 1 error is quantified by alpha (α).

Type 2 error is the converse of type 1 error. It is an incorrect failure to reject the H_0, i.e. reaching the conclusion that there is no treatment effect when, in fact, there is (a false negative). The probability of a type 2 error occurring is denoted by the value of beta (β).

Power Calculation

The power of a test is a measure of its capacity to correctly reject a false null hypothesis (i.e. detecting a treatment effect). Power is equal to $1 - \beta$. An acceptable value for β is commonly taken to be 0.2. Power is therefore usually 0.8. This means that if there is an effect there would be an 80% chance of detecting it.

Power is affected by:

- Sample size
  - an increased sample size is better able to detect an effect if present
- Variability of observations
  - a decreased standard deviation enhances the power of a study
- Effect size
  - the power of a study is greater if the magnitude of the effect being investigated is large
- Significance level
  - taking a larger value for α, e.g. 0.05 rather than 0.01 (but with it, accepting a greater risk of a type 1 error), yields greater power

This process involves setting a significance level (α) (usually 0.05 or less) and making a prediction about the likely size of the treatment effect. The latter might be based on prior research or a pilot study. For example, let's say a pilot study demonstrated that our new statin reduced the risk of hypercholesterolaemia from 12% to 10%. The research team statistician would take this and the selected significance level and perform the calculation.

The key result of the power calculation is to tell the researchers what sample size they are likely to require to prove the treatment effect. A larger treatment effect or a lower significance level (e.g. 0.05 rather than 0.02) will require a smaller sample to prove the effect.

The *p*-value quoted for a statistical test is a measure of the strength of the evidence against the null hypothesis but, importantly, not the probability of its truthfulness. A smaller *p*-value indicates that it is less probable the outcome was due to chance. In other words, in conjunction with the significance threshold set at the study-design phase, it tells us whether or not we should reject the null hypothesis. If the *p*-value is greater than the selected significance threshold, then the null hypothesis is accepted, as there is not sufficient evidence to reject it (which may be because the treatment is ineffective but may just reflect an inadequate sample size). It is key to realize that this is an all-or-nothing phenomenon because it refers to the probability of the outcome being due to chance, not the strength of association between variables. This actually makes *p*-value interpretation quite straightforward: the result is either statistically significant (*p*-value less than α) or it is not (*p*-value greater than α). A *p*-value of 0.06 against an α value of 0.05 is no more relevant than a *p*-value of 0.8; the result is still inconclusive.

This is all Sherlock Holmes stuff – *reductio ad absurdum*. We accept the alternative hypothesis on the basis of rejecting the null hypothesis. But what about the 'however improbable' part? Hypothesis testing assumes the alternative hypothesis is plausible and fair – we only actually statistically test the null hypothesis. We must, therefore, always think about the plausibility of our alternative hypothesis in determining the null hypothesis. In statistics, the 'Neptune story' is sometimes used to illustrate this. Astronomers had two choices when they noted the odd wobble to the orbit of Uranus in 1846; there was another planet creating a gravity influence on Uranus or else Newton's laws of gravity were wrong. If, rather than question their own experimental methods or the plausibility of the idea that Newton's laws were in error, they simply carried on observing the wobbling orbit, a strange thing would have happened. The evidence of a strange gravitational anomaly undermining Newton would have accumulated to such an extent that, by chance, the alternative hypothesis (Newton is wrong) would have been accepted.

The Hypothesis Tests

Now we understand the *p*-value, we need to determine how we will generate it. This comes down to the choice of statistical testing we use. There is a very long list of peculiarly named tests. We will focus on the common ones. It is helpful to subdivide the tests into those which apply to parametric data and those for non-parametric data (Table 1.5). Using the wrong test for the type of data will lead to an erroneous result.

The key tests to grasp are the t-test and the chi-squared test so we will discuss these in a little more detail than the others.

The mathematics of the t-test is complex but, in essence, it is used to test if there is a significant difference between two means (means, because it's used for parametric data). It comes in three forms. The one sample t-test compares a sample mean to a comparison. For example, we could analyze the anaesthetic machine log data to determine if the average MAC of sevoflurane delivered in that theatre was 1.0. There are two other forms of t-test which create a little confusion: the two-sample test and the paired test. Both compare the means between two groups of data but one (the paired test) tests the means within the same group at two separate points. For example, we could compare the average mark at the FRCA for two groups of trainees from different deaneries using a two-sample test, as the groups (we assume) are independent of one another. What about trainees who were unsuccessful at the first attempt? We could send them all on a revision course and then use a paired t-test to compare their pre-course and post-course FRCA score. This would give us an idea as to the effectiveness of the course. The difference in the statistical philosophy behind the paired and two-sample test is that the null hypothesis for the paired test states there is no difference between the means in a pairwise comparison whereas a two-sample null hypothesis states there is no difference in the means between the groups.

Table 1.5 Appropriate hypothesis tests by type of data

Parametric tests	Non-parametric tests
Student's t-test	Chi-squared test
ANOVA	Mann–Whitney U test
	Wilcoxon signed rank test

The chi-squared (X^2) test of independence, to give it its full name, tests if any relationship exists between two groups of categorical data. The X^2 distribution has other statistical applications, particularly the X^2 goodness-of-fit test, which tests how a sample distribution matches that of a population. We are focusing on the former, however. The test compares the expected values against the observed values in an experiment and this usually involves construction of a so-called contingency table (Table 1.6). We could use this to test the hypothesis that our FRCA revision course improves the performance of trainees in the exam but, to use the test, we need categorical data not continuous data so, rather than compare scores, we compare numbers of passes and failures:

This is a two-by-two table as there are two groups and two outcomes. It is possible to use the X^2 test to compare more categories and groups. We could add another category for those who score full marks in the structured oral exam. This alters a quantity called the degrees of freedom, something we need to know when interpreting the final value for X^2. The degrees of freedom can be calculated as:

(Number of rows − 1) × (Total for the column − 1)

The expected values are calculated by assuming the null hypothesis – that there is no difference in outcome across the groups. Mathematically, this equates, for each cell in the table, to:

$$= \frac{\text{(Total for the row} \times \text{Total for the column)}}{\text{Grand total}}$$

Table 1.7 adds the values for row- and column-totals from the original contingency table and uses them to calculate the *expected values*:

All this information is combined in the X^2 calculation to give a value for X^2. Reference tables allow cross-referencing of the degrees of freedom and X^2 value to determine whether or not the result is significant at a given threshold. The calculation is:

$$X^2 = \sum \frac{(Observed - Expected)^2}{Expected}$$

In case you are interested, our example gives a value for X^2 of 7.88 which, for 1 degree of freedom, corresponds to a *p*-value of 0.005; it seems probable our exam revision course is a good thing.

Small numbers in the study groups need an alternative version of the chi-squared test: Fisher's exact test. Ronald Fisher also devised the analysis of variance – ANOVA. This test can be thought of as the application of multiple two-sample t-tests and allows testing of three or more means.

The Mann–Whitney U and Wilcoxon signed rank sum tests apply to non-parametric data. While these tests can also actually be used for parametric data, parametric tests cannot be used for non-parametric data. The crux of these tests is that, rather than means, they rely on medians. This protects the outcome from the effect of skew and outliers, hence their application for non-normally distributed data. The Mann–Whitney U test is the non-parametric equivalent of the independent t-test and the Wilcoxon signed rank sum test is the equivalent of the paired t-test.

Beware: Wilcoxon had a hand in the evolution of the Mann–Whitney test and this sometimes goes by the name of the Mann–Whitney–Wilcoxon (MWW) or even the Wilcoxon rank sum test; don't confuse these with the Wilcoxon signed rank sum test.

Table 1.6 Example contingency table as a precursor to a X^2 analysis

	Exam passed	Exam failed
Attended course	15	3
Did not attend course	20	25

Table 1.7 Expected and observed values

	Exam passed	Exam failed	Row totals
Attended course	(18 × 35)/63 = 10	(18 × 28)/63 = 8	18
Did not attend course	(45 × 35)/63 = 25	(45 × 28)/63 = 20	45
Column totals	35	28	63

Application to Clinical Practice

Systematic Review

This is the process of searching for all relevant studies that satisfy predefined inclusion and exclusion criteria. This results in a list of studies which then each provide a value for the specified outcome measure.

The advantages of systematic review include the distillation of existing information on a given topic into a manageable summary. This in itself may strengthen the power of the existing evidence – particularly if quantitative analysis is carried out, i.e. as a meta-analysis.

Meta-analysis

This is the process of combining separate studies to produce one overarching study with its own numerical results. The combination of the results may be done with the Mantel–Haenszel procedure if the studies are sufficiently homogeneous. There are specific methods to test for heterogeneity of studies. These include the Cochrane Q test and the I^2 statistic. For the latter, a value from 0 to 100 is obtained, with homogeneity (similarity) indicated with values of <50.

To present the findings, it can be helpful to construct a Forest plot. An example is shown in Figure 1.11.

The RR (or OR) can be displayed for each study graphically, with CIs depicted as horizontal lines extending either side. A vertical line represents no effect of the intervention. From glancing at a Forest plot, we can swiftly note:

- individual study outcomes
- CI widths (likely to be wider with smaller studies)
- CIs which overlap the line of no effect
- significance of effect overall

Publication Bias

We should remain vigilant for bias in the context of systematic reviews and meta-analyses. This may stem from inclusion bias (inclusion/exclusion criteria affecting included studies), or publication bias (a problem that stems from journals, authors or language, e.g. restricting studies to those in English).

A funnel plot can go some way to indicating whether publication bias may be a problem. By plotting a scatter diagram with a measure of study precision (e.g. sample size or standard error) on the y-axis

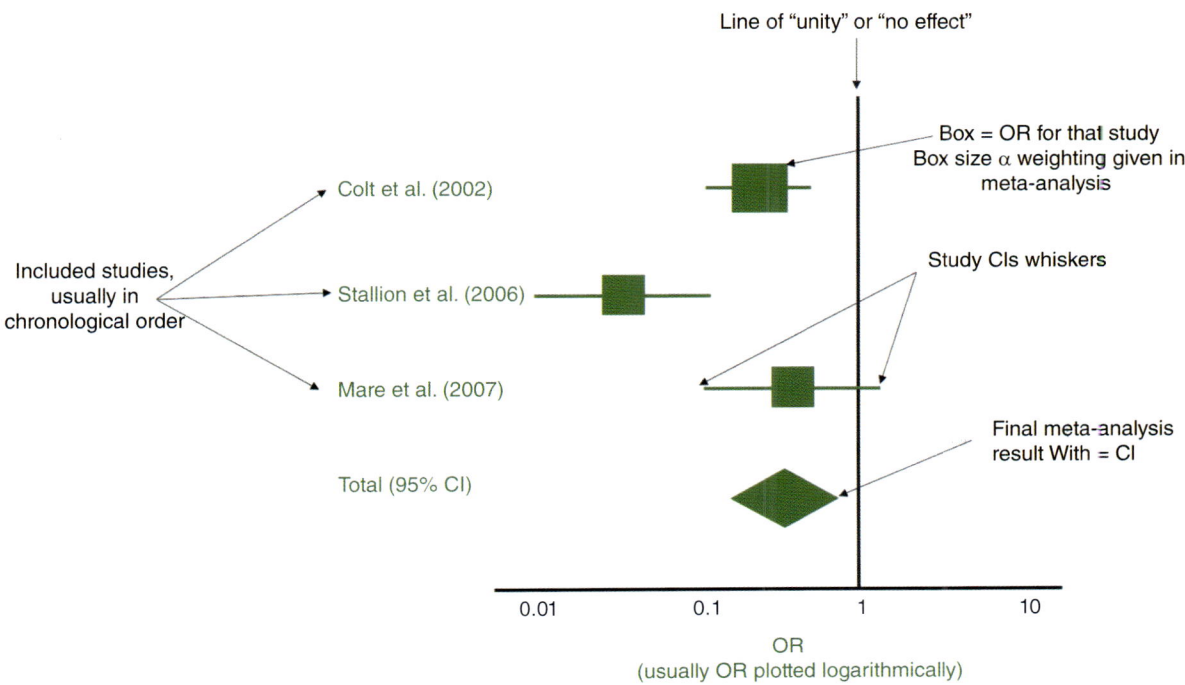

Figure 1.11 A Forest plot as a graphical depiction of the conclusion of a meta-analysis

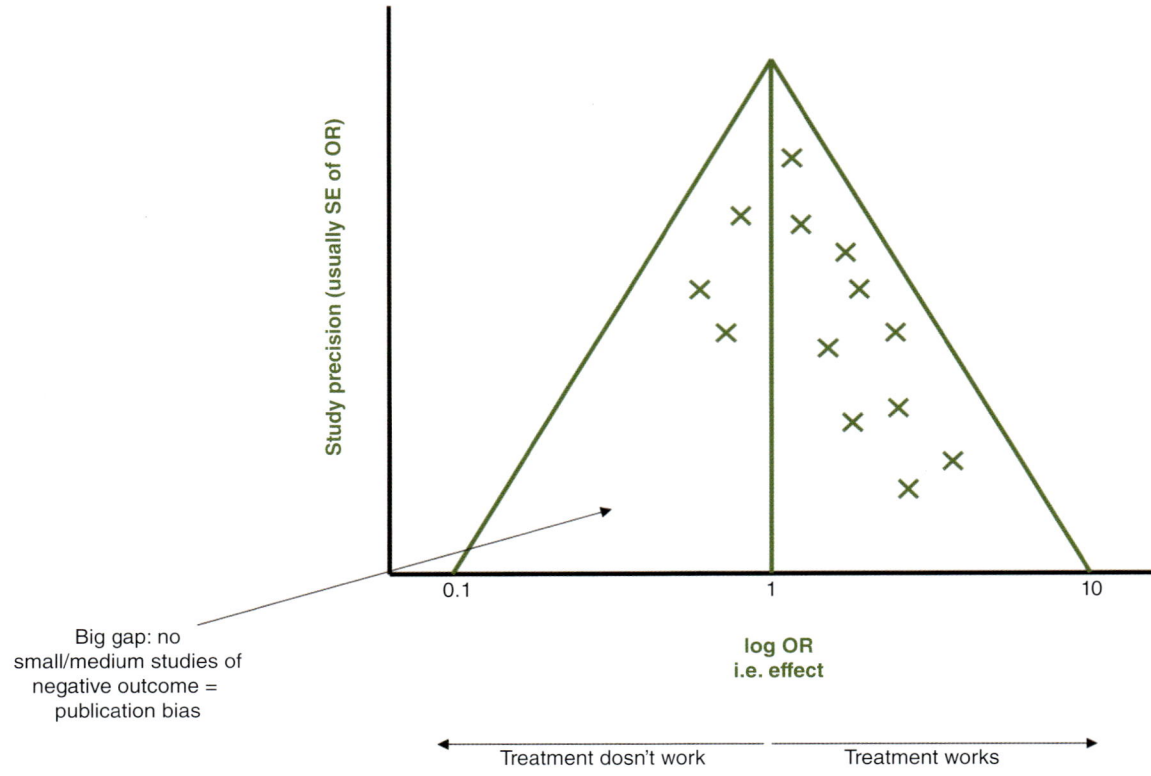

Figure 1.12 Funnel plot, illustrating the effects of publication bias within a meta-analysis

and effect size on the x-axis (e.g. log OR), we can assess the shape of the funnel. Asymmetry is indicative of publication bias, as in Figure 1.12.

Evidence-Based Medicine

Evidence-based medicine describes the process of using critically appraised medical literature to guide decisions regarding management of individual patients or particular conditions and disease processes.

A five-step approach to this process was originally described in 1992 by Cook *et al.*, in the context of examining the literature for a monoclonal antibody therapy [4]:

(1) Translation of uncertainty to an answerable question including critical questioning, study design and levels of evidence
(2) Systematic retrieval of the best evidence available
(3) Critical appraisal of evidence for internal validity, clinical relevance and applicability
(4) Application of results in practice
(5) Evaluation of performance

In essence, we should be able to define the specific question we want to answer and be able to seek out the evidence pertaining to that. Having done so, we need then to be able to assess this evidence, deciding what is important, sensible and relates to our initial enquiry. Having put into practice what we have determined it remains important to reflect on the process in order to improve future evidence-based practice.

Summary

We can now approach our initial scenario by constructing a PICO question to structure our search of the literature: for total knee replacement surgery is femoral nerve block superior to local infiltration in reducing post-operative pain scores and opiate consumption? An appropriate search will likely return a mixture of clinical trials and systematic reviews or meta-analyses. We should carefully sift these for ones which directly answer our required outcome, i.e. ignoring those which look at length of stay, wound infection, etc.

As has been discussed throughout this chapter, the essence of a good trial lies in its preparation. Therefore, we should pay attention to the Methods section of the study, looking in particular to see that the study has been set up in such a way as to answer the question posed in a valid way. Have appropriate data been collected and tested, have sources of bias and confounding variables been excluded?

Ultimately, the trials we turn up may prove inadequate to answer the question and we have discussed how we could then design our own study. We need to review our PICO question and construct a study which is practical, ethical and overcomes the weaknesses of the work in the published literature. For reasons we have covered, this perfect study is rarely possible to conduct!

Questions

MCQs – select true or false for each response

1. With regard to appropriate measures of central tendency for different types of data:
   (a) The mode is appropriate for quantitative discrete data
   (b) The mode is appropriate for quantitative continuous data
   (c) The mean is not an appropriate measure for quantitative discrete data
   (d) The median is not an appropriate measure for ordinal data
   (e) The mean is appropriate for ordinal data
2. Consider the following statements, and mark them as true or false:
   (a) The incorrect rejection of a true null hypothesis is known as a type 1 error
   (b) The ability of a test to correctly identify a positive outcome where one exists is specificity
   (c) A test with 80% sensitivity will have a false positive rate of 20%
   (d) The alpha (α) error is the probability of accepting a false positive statement
   (e) The null hypothesis is commonly rejected when the p-value is <0.5

SBAs – select the single *best answer* to each stem

3. Which of the following methods will increase the power of a study most easily?
   (a) Increase α
   (b) Increase sample size
   (c) Increase effect size
   (d) Reduce error
   (e) Repeat the study
4. You encounter a graph with the depicted appearance in a study you are reading. Which of the following options best describes it?

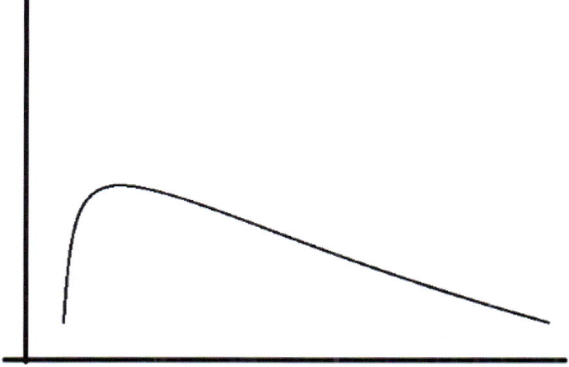

   (a) Normal distribution
   (b) Positive skew
   (c) Negative skew
   (d) Bimodal distribution
   (e) Histogram

Answers

1. TFFFF
   Continuous data, such as weight, will rarely have one data point exactly the same as another, as such they have no mode. Ordinal data, such as ASA grade, cannot be assessed by the mean but the median is suitable.
2. TFFTF
   Specificity is the ability to correctly identify negative outcomes, sensitivity is the ability to correctly identify positive outcomes. An 80% sensitivity therefore implies a 20% false negative rate. The α error rate corresponds to the level of probability at which

the null hypothesis is rejected and is typically set at 0.05, not 0.5.

3. (a)

Increasing α will very easily increase the power but at the expense of a risk of type I error (note the question asks for the easiest not the best way to increase power!). Increasing sample size is the best way but rarely the easiest. Effect size is not under direct control. Reduction in error would also be effective although the stem isn't sufficiently specific; beta (β) error needs to be reduced, whereas reducing α error would reduce power. Repeating the study won't make any difference to power unless the methodology is improved.

4. (b)

This is a positive skew because the outliers have a higher (positive) x-axis value. By definition, it is therefore neither normal nor negatively skewed. There is only one mode so it is not bimodal. A histogram is a frequency depiction of continuous data but within 'bins'.

References

1. K. F. Schulz, D. G. Altman, D. Moher. CONSORT 2010 Statement: updated guidelines for reporting parallel group randomised trials. *British Medical Journal* 340, 2010; c332.
2. P. B. Hjortrup, N. Haase, J. Wetterslev, A. Perner. Gone fishing in a fluid trial. *Critical Care and Resuscitation Journal*, 18(1), 2016; 55–58.
3. A. Bradford Hill. The environment and disease: association or causation? *Proceedings of The Royal Society of Medicine*, 58(5), 1965; 295–300.
4. D. J. Cook, R. Jaeschke, G. H. Guyatt. Critical appraisal of therapeutic interventions in the intensive care unit: human monoclonal antibody treatment in sepsis. Journal Club of the Hamilton Regional Critical Care Group. *Journal of Intensive Care Medicine*, 7(6), 1992; 275–282.

Chapter 2

Basic Physics and Electronics

Emma Foster and Hozefa Ebrahim

Learning Objectives

- To be able to describe the relevance to anaesthesia and clinical measurement of the SI system and recall which units are among the base units, and which are derived
- To develop an understanding of the simple laws of mechanics in terms of the basic mathematical relationships between mass, force, work, power and energy
- To describe, in simple terms, the physical concepts underpinning electricity, magnetism and electromagnetism
- To develop an understanding of the fundamentals of electronic circuits in relation to medical devices: parallel vs. series circuits, current, resistance, impedance, capacitance and inductance

Chapter Content

- Dimensions and International System of Units
- Basic electricity – voltage, current and resistance
- Simple circuits
- Capacitance, reactance, impedance and inductance
- Energy, work and power
- Mechanics
- Magnetism
- Electromagnets, motors and dynamos

Scenario

Whilst on a busy on-call in ICU, you are called to a cardiac arrest on the ward. There has been a power cut and, when you arrive, you see the patient still suspended in a hoist where they suffered their collapse. The staff are trying to administer CPR but, with every chest compression, the hoist sags with the effort. The battery is flat on the hoist.

You wonder how effective the compressions really can be in the hoist; what relevance does Newton's third law of motion have here? How does Newton's second law of motion have a bearing when it comes to the manual handling of the patient onto a firm surface? The patient is morbidly obese: how might this affect the efficacy of the defibrillator? Can the defibrillator function in the absence of mains power?

Introduction

Basic physics and electronics underpin all of our daily activities. A healthy understanding of these principles can make our lives much easier. We use terms of measurement to quantify everything from the home to work, and beyond. We use these terms to describe how fast we should perform cardiac compressions, and quantify the charge used to defibrillate our patients. There are simple circuits lighting our wards, and more complex circuits running our defibrillators and clinical measurement devices. This chapter aims to explain these concepts in the context of everyday life, and how knowledge of this will make the treatment of patients better.

Dimensions and International System of Units

The International System of Units (SI) is the international authority for all measurements. It is important for everyone in their day-to-day lives from allowing us to tell a friend how long it will be until we meet them (time), to accurately following a recipe (mass, temperature). The system that we use today initially started its development in France during the French Revolution in the 1790s. Before this there was no universal convention on measurement. This meant that everyone measured objects and amounts differently. For example, in Britain alone, there have been at least six different 'pounds' ranging from 350 g (Tower pound) to 500 g (metric pound). The currency, a 'pound sterling', was originally derived from the value of a mass: a Tower pound of silver. This made it difficult for, in particular, the wealthy members of the population to measure and quantify their goods, leading to errors in transactions and fraud. It was as a result of this that the committee of the Académie des Sciences was convened by Louis XVI of France and his national assembly, to develop a unified form of measurement. This resulted in the production of the units of length (metres) and mass (kilogram) that were quantified and standardized.

The metre is a simple, well-known form of measurement, but actually originated from some rather complicated mathematics. The committee defined a metre as the ten-millionth part of one-quarter of the terrestrial meridian (where the distance from the north pole to the equator is a quarter meridian). It then took the committee a further 7 years to work out the distance from the north pole to the equator! They meanwhile defined mass in kilograms, leading to the first two base SI units.

The next step in the development of the system was the measurement of time in seconds, in the course of Carl Friedrich Gauss's work in quantifying the Earth's magnetic field. Perhaps somewhat ironically, further development of the system then slowed somewhat. In the 1860s, the British Association for Advancement of Science realized the requirement for a system of base units and derived units. It is upon this that all other measurements are based. Originally, as length and mass were established by the French, other countries that adopted the metre and kilogram were reliant on France for exact copies. This caused a few problems, as some international relationships, for example between Britain and France, have had a turbulent history. This led to the formation of the Bureau International des Poids et Mesures (BIPM) in 1875, which provided prototypes of the metre and kilogram, bringing the metric system to a wider global audience.

Electricity was considered in the 1860s as a possibility for another base unit although it took until 1900 for Giorgi to provide this base unit as the ampere, a measure of electrical current. The base units for temperature (kelvin) and luminescence (candela) were developed more recently, in 1954, just prior to the establishment of the currently known SI system in 1960. Temperature is measured in kelvin and 1 K is defined as 1/273.16 of the thermodynamic triple point of water (see Chapter 3). Candela measures the intensity of luminescence. The word itself derives from the original definition: the light produced by a 'standard candle'. This had a particular specification in terms of the weight, type of wax and speed of burn.

The final addition to this system of seven base units was the amount of substance (mole), introduced in 1971. This is important for a number of concepts in both chemistry and physics; for example, Avogadro's hypothesis. Table 2.1 lists the SI base units and their definitions. Note that the written name of a unit is in lower case, even when named after an individual. Such eponymous units, however, have a capitalized symbol. Thus, the unit of temperature is the kelvin, symbol K.

Table 2.1 SI base units

Quantity name	Unit symbol	Unit name	Specific definitions
Length	m	metre	Distance travelled by light in a vacuum in 1/299,792,458 s
Mass	kg	kilogram	Defined by linking the definitions of the metre and the second through the value of Plank's constant ($6.626070150 \times 10^{-34}$ kg m^2 s^{-1})
Time	s	second	Based on a frequency of radiation emitted from caesium-133
Electric current	A	ampere	Constant current which is maintained in two straight parallel conductors of infinite length of negligible circular cross section, placed 1 m apart in a vacuum that would produce a force equal to 2×10^{-7} N
Thermodynamic temperature	K	kelvin	1/273.16 of the thermodynamic temperature of the triple point of water
Intensity of luminescence	Cd	candela	Luminous intensity in a given direction of a source that emits monochromatic radiation of frequency 540×10^{12} Hz and that has a radiant intensity in that direction of 1/683 W sr^{-1}
Amount of substance	mol	mole	Amount of substance of a system which contains as many elementary entities as there are atoms in 0.012 kg of carbon-12

Table 2.2 Common derived units

Name	Symbol	Quantity	In terms of SI units	In terms of SI base units
Newton	N	Force, weight	–	$kg\ m\ s^{-2}$
Pascal	Pa	Pressure	$N\ m^{-2}$	$kg\ m^{-1}\ s^{-2}$
Joule	J	Energy, work, heat	$N\ m$	$kg\ m^2\ s^{-2}$
Watt	W	Power	$J\ s^{-1}$	$kg\ m^2\ s^{-3}$
Coulomb	C	Charge	–	$s\ A$
Volt	V	Voltage, potential difference	$W\ A^{-1}$	$kg\ m^2\ s^{-3}\ A^{-1}$
Farad	F	Capacitance	$C\ V^{-1}$	$kg^{-1}\ m^{-2}\ s^4\ A^2$
Ohm	Ω	Electric resistance	$V\ A^{-1}$	$kg\ m^2\ s^{-3}\ A^{-2}$
Siemens	S	Conductance	$A\ V^{-1}$	$kg^{-1}\ m^{-2}\ s^3\ A^2$
Weber	Wb	Magnetic flux	$V\ s$	$kg\ m^2\ s^{-2}\ A^{-1}$
Tesla	T	Magnetic field strength	$Wb\ m^{-2}$	$kg\ s^{-2}\ A^{-1}$
Henry	H	Inductance	$Wb\ A^{-1}$	$kg\ m^2\ s^{-2}\ A^{-2}$
Degree Celsius	°C	Temperature relative to K	–	K

The kilogram is the only SI unit which includes an SI prefix ('kilo'). It is also the only unit which, until very recently, was still defined by the properties of an artefact (a cylinder of platinum–iridium alloy, kept under three glass bell jars, locked in a vault in Paris) rather than as a measurement that can be replicated in any laboratory. That changed in November 2018, when metrologists agreed a new definition based on Plank's constant, $6.626070150 \times 10^{-34}\ kg\ m^2\ s^{-1}$. Until that point, it had been impossible to measure the constant with sufficient accuracy (20 parts per billion). This has now been achieved (to 13 parts per billion), allowing the new definition to be introduced.

The derived units are forms of measurement that have been developed from the base units described above and help to allow us to quantify other phenomena more easily. There are 22 derived units, which are defined in terms of the base units. For example, voltage is actually watts per ampere or, in its base unit dimensions, $kg\ m^2\ s^{-3}\ A^{-1}$. Table 2.2 above demonstrates 13 of the commonly used derived units.

Most medical journals and reference texts follow a relatively strict convention on the way in which scientific units are reported. The main feature of this is that most follow the system used in Table 2.2 whereby the solidus, or 'forward slash', is avoided in favour of negative exponents to denote the division of units. In this system, any unit which would be 'below the line' is instead raised to a negative exponent, i.e. $^{-1}$. Then, if a unit would normally be squared or cubed but would also be 'below the line', it would be notated as $^{-2}$ or $^{-3}$ respectively. Separation of the units often depends on an individual publisher's style; some use a space (such as in this book), others a middle dot or a full-stop. If we use the example of the units for acceleration, metres per second per second, there are several correct ways in which this can be indicated:

$$m/s^2$$

or, as more commonly favoured by most publishers:

$$m\ s^{-2}\ (or\ m \cdot s^{-2}\ or\ m.s^{-2})$$

Note that multiple uses of a solidus are not acceptable notation in any setting, e.g. m/s/s.

There are a few other points of correctness worth considering.
- Unit symbols do not have a plural form, i.e. '70 cms' is incorrect, it is '70 cm'.
- Whilst unit symbols are typically an abbreviation (cm for centimetre, for example), they are not followed by a full-stop except at the end of a sentence, i.e. '150 cm tall', not '150 cm. tall'.

- Values should always be specified numerically and with symbols for units, i.e. '15 A', not 'fifteen amps', 'fifteen A' or '15 amps'.
- There should always be a space between the value and the unit with the exception of angles. Therefore, even though the symbol is the same, be careful with degrees; a temperature is 15 °C (not 15°C) but an angle is 45°, not 45 °.

Basic Electricity: Voltage, Current and Resistance

The word 'electricity' is derived from the Greek word for amber – *elektron*. This was initially used in the seventeenth century as a result of the Greeks noting that when rods of amber were rubbed against certain materials, they could then be used to attract other substances. This was the first recorded observation of static electricity. Although this was the initial usage of the word electricity, the earliest records of electricity itself actually date back to the Ancient Egyptians, who recorded that certain Nile fish were able to shock wading fishermen.

Electricity is a set of physical features that are associated with the presence and flow of charge. The importance of electricity to modern, everyday life is self-evident. Electricity is the movement of electrons through conducting materials of which the most obvious group are metals, e.g. copper and aluminium. Protons, found in the nucleus of atoms, are fixed in position in metals; however, the electrons in these conductors are free to move. It is this movement of electrons which gives rise to their conducting properties, essential for electricity. The SI unit in respect of electricity is the ampere. This defines electrical current: the flow of electric charge from one point to another. Electrical current is directly analogous to current in a fluid, the water molecules in a river equating to electrons in a copper wire. The faster the flow of water, the stronger the current. Similarly, the faster the movement of electrons down the wire, the higher the electrical current. This can be measured with a galvanometer. A galvanometer is any instrument which transduces current into a mechanical movement, the most common application being the ammeter, which is used to quantify current. Other applications of galvanometers include steering mechanisms for lasers, e.g. barcode scanners. One ampere is equal to one coulomb of charge passing a fixed point in one second:

Electrical current = Flow of electric charge, measured in amperes

To understand resistance, imagine a river containing boulders and tree roots. As the water encounters these obstructions, the current is opposed by the resistance posed by these objects. The same can be said of electrical current moving through a circuit. The resistance introduced, both by the wires themselves and also components in the circuit, can be quantified; the unit is the ohm. The resistance introduced by the wires themselves is proportional to their length and inversely proportional to the cross-sectional area of the wire and the conductivity of the material from which it is made.

One further factor is the potential difference in the circuit. This can be considered as the difference in height between the source of the river and the estuary. This is quantified as the voltage; the electrical potential to drive an electrical current of one ampere through a resistance of one ohm is one volt:

The potential difference (or voltage) between two points in a circuit is the amount of work done in moving a unit of charge between those two points

Electrical current, potential difference and resistance are all interrelated and explained by Ohm's law, which states that the potential difference between two points is the product of the resistance and the current flowing:

Voltage = Current × Resistance

Voltage, Current and Resistance in Simple Circuits

A simple circuit involves a wire that connects to a cell and another component, for example a lamp (or other point of resistance). The water analogy can be extended. The cell is a pump generating constant pressure (potential difference), resulting in flow of water (current). Constrictions, or perhaps an impeller in the pipe, offer resistance to flow in much the same way that a resistor or motor in a circuit alters the current in an electrical circuit.

There are two basic ways in which circuits can be connected: series and parallel. Each of these will be discussed in turn. The easiest way to describe the relationships of components in series is via the use of resistors.

Chapter 2: Basic Physics and Electronics

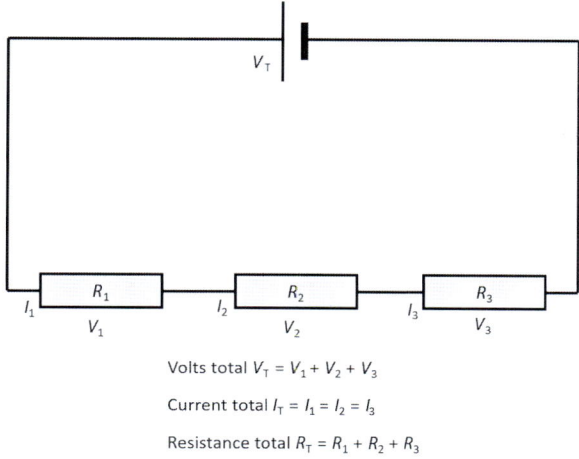

Volts total $V_T = V_1 + V_2 + V_3$

Current total $I_T = I_1 = I_2 = I_3$

Resistance total $R_T = R_1 + R_2 + R_3$

Figure 2.1 Resistors arranged in series

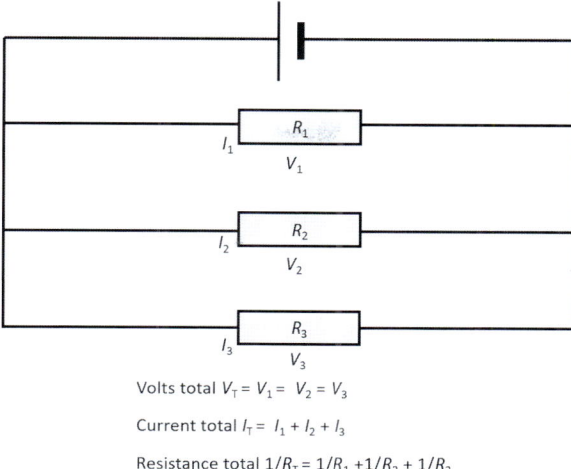

Volts total $V_T = V_1 = V_2 = V_3$

Current total $I_T = I_1 + I_2 + I_3$

Resistance total $1/R_T = 1/R_1 + 1/R_2 + 1/R_3$

Figure 2.2 Resistors arranged in parallel

In a *series* circuit, the components follow one after another. As the flow of electrons must encounter all three resistors in the path from the negative to the positive terminal of the cell, the magnitude of the current is a property of the whole circuit. It is a constant, regardless of where it is measured in this simple series circuit. The voltage is, similarly, a constant property (dictated by the rating of the cell) but, through application of Ohm's law, it can be seen that the voltage across each resistor is in direct proportionality to its resistance (see Figure 2.1)

Figure 2.2, by contrast, demonstrates a circuit connected in *parallel*. In this arrangement, the flow of electrons is shared between each of the branches of the circuit. As the flow only encounters the resistor in its own branch of the circuit before reaching the positive terminal, the current in each branch varies depending on the resistance of that branch only: I_1, I_2 and I_3. As each branch is, in effect, directly and separately connected to the terminals of the cell, each branch receives the same potential difference – that rated on the cell. So now, in contrast to a series circuit, the voltage is the constant, not the current. The currents through each branch are added to determine the current in the whole circuit. Again, by application of Ohm's law, we can understand how to combine the resistances; their reciprocals are summed (see Figure 2.2):

$$\frac{1}{R_T} = \frac{1}{R_1} + \frac{1}{R_2} + \frac{1}{R_3}$$

In the river analogy, consider the course as it encounters an island and splits into two branches either side of the island, each as broad as the original stream. The greater the number of paths (and therefore the total width of the river), the lower the resistance to flow. Therefore, the overall volume of the water passing downstream is greater.

Capacitance, Reactance, Impedance and Inductance

Simple circuits have been discussed above; however, there are a number of further components that can be added into circuits that make them more complex and capable. The symbols for and function of these components are shown in Figure 2.3.

The behaviour of a number of the components varies depending on the type of current which is passed through them – direct current (DC) or alternating current (AC). DC passes solely in one direction around a circuit whilst alternating current fluctuates rapidly, in a forward and backwards direction, best described by a sinusoidal waveform from a mathematical standpoint. DC is produced by cells (chemical or photovoltaic). It was in this form that commercial electricity was first transmitted by Thomas Edison, who is often credited with the invention of the light bulb. AC is now, however, the most commonly transmitted form of mains electricity. High-voltage (up to 400 kV), low-current

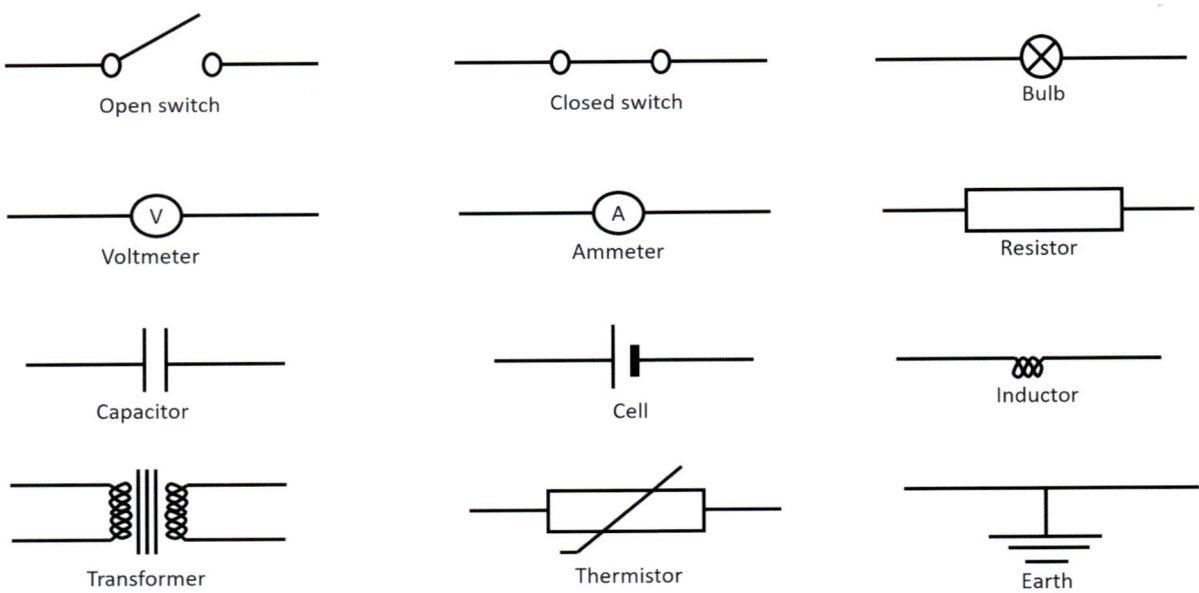

Figure 2.3 Symbols of common electrical components

transmission is best suited to provide transmission over long distances without significant losses in overhead cables. The high-voltage mains supply then requires transformers to enable the voltage to be stepped down to normal operating levels.

> Due to capacitive losses, subterranean cables carrying AC become inefficient after around 50 miles. There are a number of submarine cables linking the UK to Ireland and Europe and, to overcome this problem, they carry high-voltage DC instead. These cables have to run in opposing pairs, however, otherwise the magnetic field from a single high-voltage DC cable is enough to disturb navigation aids of ships sailing above them.

Impedance is a property of circuits and components that describes the total opposition to the flow of current. It is comprised of resistance and reactance. Only resistive effects (as described by Ohm's law) are relevant in DC circuits. For AC circuits, however, the oscillation of the current also leads to inductive and capacitive effects, which together oppose the current. These effects are collectively quantified as the reactance (again measured in ohms but denoted X). Reactance decreases as the current frequency increases. For an AC circuit, total opposition to current flow (impedance) is therefore the sum of reactance and resistance.

Capacitance, as mentioned above, is the ability to store electrical charge. It is equal to charge per unit voltage. This is given by the equation:

$$C = \frac{Q}{V}$$

Charge (Q) is measured in coulombs where one coulomb is the number of electrons passing a point when a current of one ampere flows for one second. Capacitance is measured in farads or, more commonly in practical applications, microfarads.

A capacitor consists of a pair of conducting plates that are separated by a dielectric (insulating) material; usually air, porcelain, glass or plastic. The amount of charge that is able to be stored is dependent on the size of the plates and the thickness and type of the dielectric material used. Capacitors block DC as they have a high resistance but allow AC to pass as they have a low reactance. Capacitors only charge using DC. They are the fundamental component of defibrillators and this will be discussed in more detail in Chapter 13.

Inductance describes the tendency of a conductor to generate an electromotive force (EMF) that opposes the current change (a so-called 'back-EMF'). In simple terms, it resists a change in the flow of electrons. Inductance is measured in henrys (H). An inductor is best constructed of a wire coiled multiple times around a ferrous core, although even a straight wire will exhibit some inductance. As current starts to flow through the coil, it generates a magnetic field which opposes instantaneous flow of current. Similarly, if the power source is disconnected, the magnetic field begins to collapse and this changing field generates a further EMF, which prevents instantaneous cessation of current flow. This can be likened to the inertia and momentum of a water wheel. Initially, it takes a lot of water to start the wheel turning as the inertia resists the flow of water in the channel. However, once it is turning, it will keep going and requires a smaller force to continue. Reducing flow of water into the channel will not easily reduce flow out as the momentum in the water wheel will tend to keep it spinning and it will draw water through as it slows.

Inductors are affected by DC and AC in the opposite way to capacitors. Inductors block AC due to high reactance but pass DC as they have low resistance. The magnetic field enables inductors to induce a current in neighbouring conductors. This is known as mutual inductance and is the underlying principle of transformers. A transformer is an arrangement of two coils of wire on separate circuits but wrapped on the same ferrous core. Connecting a power source to the first coil causes it to produce a magnetic field. This field induces a current in the neighbouring coil. The magnitude of the current induced in the second coil is dependent on the ratio of the number of turns of wire in each of the two coils. Where the primary coil has more windings than the secondary coil, as in Figure 2.4, this constitutes a step-down transformer. In the example shown in Figure 2.4, ten primary windings and five secondary windings is a ratio of 2:1 and so the output voltage of the transformer will be half that of the input. If the primary coil has fewer windings than the secondary coil, the transformer is a step-up device. This form of construction is also the principle behind floating circuits that are used to isolate patients in theatre from the mains supply. This is discussed in greater depth in Chapter 10.

> Capacitance – ability to store charge, measured in farads (F)
> Inductance – ability to induce a magnetic field, measured in henrys (H)

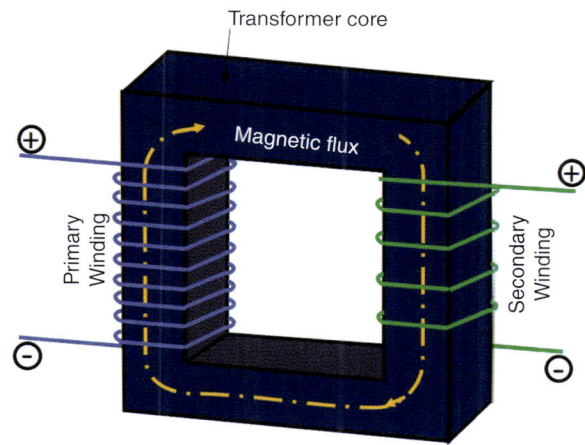

Figure 2.4 A transformer, in this case a step-down transformer

Energy, Work and Power

The term *energy* derives initially from the Ancient Greek term, *energeia*, meaning activity or operation. It is thought it appeared for the first time in the work of Aristotle in the fourth century but it is very different from what we consider as energy today. Aristotle, being a philosopher, talked of energy as a concept that included happiness. It was far later in history that energy was defined in a format that is recognizable today. This came through the work of Gottfried Leibniz and Isaac Newton in the late seventeenth century, originally dubbed *vis viva* (the Latin for 'living force'). Energies in the form of kinetic and potential energy were then documented in the early 1800s.

Energy is interrelated with work via the first law of thermodynamics. This states that the total energy of an isolated system is constant and that energy can be transformed from one form to another but it can never be created or destroyed. Energy itself is then defined as the capacity for doing work. It is measured in joules. As suggested, there are a number of different forms of energy. These are included in Table 2.3.

> First law of thermodynamics – Energy can be transformed from one form to another but never created or destroyed

Work done (joules) is equal to the product of the force acting on an object (newtons) multiplied by the displacement it causes (metres).

> Work = Force × Displacement

Table 2.3 Different forms of energy

Form of energy	Description
Kinetic energy	Energy an object has due to its movement
Electromagnetic energy	Energy radiated as electromagnetic waves from an object. Examples include light, microwaves, infrared and many others across the electromagnetic spectrum
Potential energy	Stored energy, e.g. gravitational (due to vertical displacement), electrical or chemical
Thermal energy	Internal energy of an object due to the kinetic energy of vibration of atoms or molecules
Sound energy	Energy associated with elastic oscillation of atoms or molecules within a medium

Work, as a physics concept, was originally described in 1826 by Gaspard-Gustave Coriolis, a French mathematician. His research looked at weights lifted to a height via the use of mining steam engines. The SI unit of measurement for work is the joule.

Kinetic energy is the energy an object possesses as a consequence of its movement. Work is required to accelerate an object of a given mass from a rest state to a given velocity. Consider the example of a firework rocket. At rest on the ground, the rocket possesses potential energy in the chemical bonds of the gunpowder. When lit, the rocket ignites and energy is converted to many other forms. For example, kinetic energy as it propels into the sky, electromagnetic energy in the colourful light seen, and also thermal and sound energy. Some is also converted to gravitational potential energy: the rocket case and stick will later fall back to earth as a result. No energy is lost, only converted to other forms – the concept of conservation of energy.

$$\text{Kinetic energy} = \tfrac{1}{2}\text{Mass} \times \text{Velocity}^2$$

Potential energy is stored energy (see Table 2.3). This can occur in a number of different forms: electrical energy (capacitors), chemical energy (chemical bonds in food sources, batteries or fuels), elastic energy and gravitational potential energy. The ability to store energy is essential to life. It allows us to store the energy from the food we eat and release it slowly as required to complete our everyday activities.

Power is the rate at which energy is used per unit time. This can be calculated by work done divided by time taken. It is measured in watts, which equate to joules per second. A powerful machine is one that is able to give high energy or work per unit time. For example, consider two versions of the same car, one having a higher specification engine. The power of modern engines is usually given in the brochure (in kW). Of course, the more intuitive measure we often use to compare cars is the 0–60 miles per hour (mph) time; the mass of the cars is the same (same model) as is final velocity (60 mph) so the kinetic energy is identical. The more powerful engine will deliver this in a shorter time (as per the relationship between power, time and energy) resulting in faster acceleration.

$$\text{Power} = \text{Energy expended per unit time}$$

Mechanics

The inception of mechanics as a mathematical discipline is largely attributed to Sir Isaac Newton. Born in 1642, he was an English physicist, mathematician and natural philosopher. In his work, *Philosophiæ Naturalis Principia Mathematica* (or often just *Principia*) published in 1687, he described three universal laws of motion that were the basis for modern mechanics [1]. These laws of motion explain the relationships between force, velocity and acceleration and will subsequently be discussed along with their definitions. The inspiration for these theories is the stuff of legend; they are said to have been developed by Sir Isaac following the pivotal moment when he saw an apple fall from a tree in the garden of the family home at Woolsthorpe Manor in Lincolnshire. (There is no evidence that it hit him on the head, as per popular myth!) It is reported that this led him to consider why apples always fall perpendicular to the ground. So was born modern mechanics.

The principal variables involved in the laws of motion, as mentioned above, are force, velocity, acceleration and pressure:

(1) Force is an interaction which, if unopposed, will result in a change in state of motion of an object (newtons, N)
(2) Velocity is the speed at which an object moves in a specific direction (m s^{-1})
(3) Acceleration is the rate of change of the velocity of an object (m s^{-2})
(4) Pressure is force per unit area (pascal, Pa, N m^{-2})

Force, velocity and, therefore, acceleration, all have a directional component as well as a magnitude. They are therefore vector quantities. For example, the force of thrust (forward direction) must have greater magnitude than the forces of drag (backwards direction) otherwise the object will not accelerate forwards. Similarly, consider a car driving continuously around a roundabout; the indicated speed on the speedometer may remain the same but the velocity changes continuously because the direction varies. Acceleration is related to velocity. It is the change of velocity with respect to time. In fact, the car on the roundabout is accelerating as the direction is changing around a central point. This is a particular form of acceleration called centripetal acceleration. The reaction to this (see Newton's third law, below) gives rise to the so-called, 'lateral-G' – the sensation that you are sliding towards the outside of your seat as the car goes around the corner.

Newton's first law of motion states that, in the absence of external forces, an object will remain at rest or at a constant velocity (technically, a state of rest is a constant velocity: zero!). To take an example, an object moving over a frictionless surface in a vacuum will continue to move in a straight line at a constant velocity. Perhaps the closest real-world analogy is an ice-hockey rink. The ice and air resistance inevitably induce some drag on a puck once it is struck but, unless it meets the barrier or another stick, it will continue on its path at a relatively constant velocity. As an extension of his first law, Newton also described the terms momentum and inertia. Inertia is the resistance to change in state of motion as a consequence of its mass. The concept links the first law to a property of the object. Momentum is a quantity of motion derived as the product of mass and velocity. All objects have momentum if they are moving. Momentum has direction as it derived from velocity:

$$\text{Momentum} = \text{Mass} \times \text{Velocity}$$

The concepts of mass and momentum are unified in Newton's second law which states that the acceleration of an object is proportional to the net force applied and inversely proportional to the mass. This rearranges to the familiar equation:

$$\text{Force} = \text{Mass} \times \text{Acceleration}$$

Acceleration is rate of change of velocity and therefore it can be seen that the above equation also states that force equals rate of change of momentum. The ice-hockey puck will accelerate more rapidly if more force is applied with the stick (the mass is a property of the puck). Of course, if we substituted a lead puck without the players knowing it (increasing the mass), they would get frustrated by the lack of acceleration they could impart to it with the same effort.

Following on from the term mass is that of weight. In everyday parlance, these terms are used interchangeably. However, in physics they have specific meanings. Weight is the mass of the object multiplied by the acceleration due to gravity. On Earth acceleration due to gravity is 9.81 m s^{-2}. However, this would be different on the Moon. As a result, the weight of an individual would be different if they were standing on Earth as opposed to the Moon even though their mass remains the same in both places.

Finally, Newton's third law of motion states that for every action there is an equal and opposite reaction. This considers the forces present on objects as a whole. Two of our ice-hockey players, equally matched in size, come to a disagreement. When both are pushing against each other on the ice, neither moves as each exerts an equal force in the opposite direction. By extension, consider this: when you walk across the ground, do you move forwards or do you stay still and push the ground backwards, reducing the Earth's rate of rotation by an infinitesimally small amount in the process? Both are in fact true, it depends simply on what Newtonian mechanics refers to as the frame of reference.

The final aspect of basic mechanics is pressure. This is the force that is applied to an object per unit surface area. A clinically important example of this relationship is that of different-sized syringes, all pressed with the same thumb. In a 20-ml syringe, the plunger has a large area so the force of the thumb effort is widely distributed, resulting in a relatively low pressure at the syringe tip. However, if we compare this to a 2-ml syringe with a smaller plunger area for the same force, there is a higher pressure created (see Chapter 4).

$$\text{Pressure} = \text{Force applied per units area } (\text{N m}^{-2})$$

Magnetism

There is a myth behind the discovery of magnets. An elderly Cretan shepherd was herding his sheep in Magnesia in northern Greece. He noticed that the nails in his shoes had become stuck to a black rock on which he was walking. In order for him to find out why this occurred, he dug up the earth underneath and found that deposits of a natural iron oxide were causing the effect.

A magnet is any object or material that is able to produce a magnetic field. Magnetism is a physical characteristic that occurs as a result of forces between magnets that lead to magnetic fields, which either attract or repel other objects.

An early invention to employ magnetism was the compass. William Gilbert, in the 1600s, was the first person to realize that the Earth generates a magnetic field, and that magnets could be made. This breakthrough led to further research and, in 1820, Hans Christian Ørsted demonstrated the principles of electromagnets that are used in many everyday objects, including televisions, telephones and MRI scanners.

The material of the magnet and the object being affected are two of the main determinants of the strength of the interaction. The strongest of all the interactions are from permanent magnets. These consist of ferrous materials, such as iron. The effects of a single magnet are demonstrated using iron filings and a magnet from the classic school experiment (see Figure 2.5). It is the effect of magnets on other objects that gives rise to their useful nature in MRI scanners and televisions. A magnetic field is a consequence of attributes of the electrons in the magnet (specifically, their quantum mechanical properties). All magnetic fields are inherently dipolar, having a north and a south pole. With regard to these poles, opposite poles attract and like poles repel each other (see Figure 2.6).

A magnet produces a magnetic field surrounding itself. This field is expressed in both direction and magnitude in three-dimensional space: this is referred to as a *vector field*. Understanding this three-dimensional construct helps us to predict how other ferromagnetic objects will behave when they interact with this field. Paramagnetism is the term given when objects are *attracted* by a magnetic field and diamagnetism is the term when materials are *repelled* by a magnetic field.

The strength of a magnetic field is complex to define and this can be done in a number of ways: it depends, for example, on whether we are discussing the field's influence on another magnet or a charged particle, whether in a vacuum or not. In basic terms, the number of field lines encountered at any given point within the field is proportional to the magnitude of the field and this is measured in webers (Wb). Practically, if you move a wire through a magnetic field, crossing the field lines, a uniform 1-Wb field will induce a 1-V EMF if it crosses the field in 1 s. If it crosses the field twice as quickly, it will induce a 2-V EMF: This is quantified by Faraday's law of electromagnetic induction. The magnetic flux density is the density of the field lines per unit surface area. Hence, it is measured in the magnetic flux per unit area, the tesla (T; 1 T = 1 Wb m^{-2}). The difference between webers and teslas is a little like the difference between heat capacity and specific heat capacity – for T and specific heat capacity, the denominator is specified in each case: 1 m^2 and 1 kg, respectively (see Chapter 3 for more on specific heat capacity).

The Earth itself is a form of permanent magnet as a result of the motion of its molten ferrous core. The resulting magnetic field protects the atmosphere from the destructive effects of the solar wind and cosmic rays. The other consequence of the motion of the core is that the magnetic north pole of Earth can also move over time and, in fact, reverses altogether every few hundred thousand years. The magnetic field currently emerges from the Earth at the geographic south pole and returns to the ground at the geographic north pole due to this phenomenon (Figure 2.7).

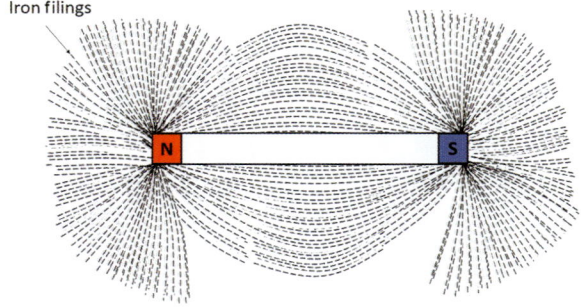

Figure 2.5 Effect of a magnet on iron filings

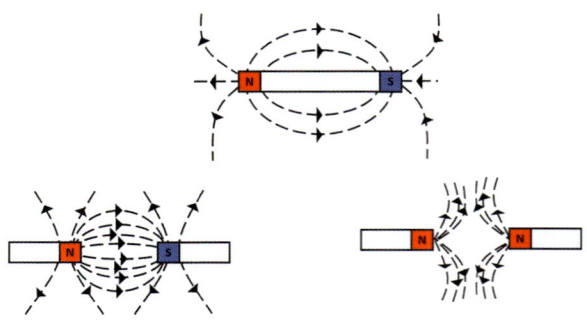

Figure 2.6 Attractive and repellent forces of magnets

Electromagnets, Motors and Dynamos

One of the important applications of magnetism is in electromagnets. You will recall from above that, when an electrical current passes through a wire, it creates a magnetic field that surrounds that wire. This can be enhanced by repeatedly coiling the wire, adding an iron core, or increasing the current. Each of these steps increases the strength of the magnetic field. This is the central principle on which a transformer relies (see above). The difference between electromagnets and permanent magnets is that the electromagnets only work as a magnet when there is a current flowing, therefore they can be switched on and off.

Electromagnetism is the principle behind electrical motors. Michael Faraday was a British scientist, building on the earlier work of Hans Christian Øersted. Faraday's initial work involved a permanent magnet with a dish of mercury surrounding it and a freely moving wire hanging above the mercury so that the tip dipped into the liquid metal. He then connected a battery to the mercury to complete the circuit. This caused the current-carrying wire to circle around the magnet.

The development of the electric motor was firstly via the DC motor which involves a loop of wire suspended between a permanent magnet and connected to a power source. As the current flows through the wire it generates an electromagnetic field, which repels the permanent magnet, causing the loop to move. After half a turn, the wire stops moving as the electromagnetic field is now aligned to that of the permanent magnet. However, the coil is electrified via a commutator, an arrangement which causes the current to switch directions every half turn of the loop. This means the wire continues to turn in the same direction, as the magnetic field continually reverses its polarity to stay out of alignment with that of the permanent magnet. See Figure 2.8 for a diagram of this.

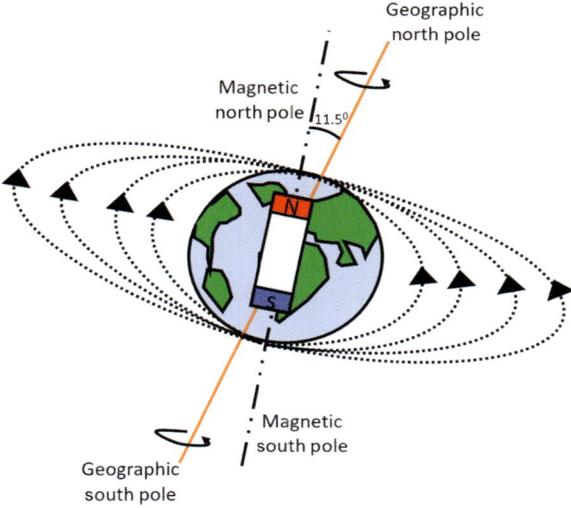

Figure 2.7 Earth's magnetic and geographic poles

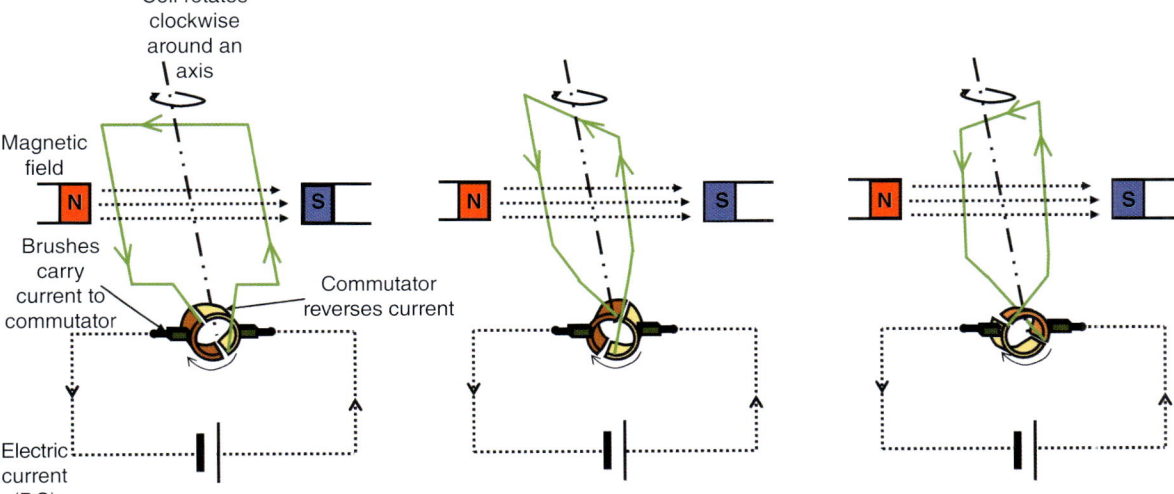

Figure 2.8 Electric DC motor

The importance of electric motors cannot be overstated. Meanwhile, the dynamo uses the same principles of electromagnetism, but in reverse: it converts mechanical energy into electrical energy. The construction is nearly identical; mechanical energy is applied to the spindle to rotate the wires in the field of a permanent magnet. This induces a current in the coils. This underpins power generation for mains supply but the principle can also be used as a transducer to convert a mechanical effort into an electrical signal for measurement.

Summary

As you have read, basic physics and electronics are fundamental to many of our simplest daily actions. A sound understanding of these principles will positively impact on our practice. For example, performing cardiac compressions on a patient in a hoist, swinging like a pendulum, is not as effective as treating them on their bed. Using Newton's teachings, we can see that upon each compression, rather than depressing the chest wall and subsequently the heart, we will instead push the patient further away. Our defibrillators use up electrical energy. They contain cells (batteries) that allow us to perform defibrillation away from a mains source, but this is only if the machine has been charged previously.

Questions

MCQs – select true or false for each response

1. The following statements are correct:
   (a) Pressure = Area/Force
   (b) Force = Mass × Acceleration
   (c) Voltage = Current/Resistance
   (d) Power = Work × Time
   (e) Capacitance = Charge/Voltage
2. The following statements are true:
   (a) Current is measured in amperes
   (b) Voltage is flow of electrons
   (c) In a circuit with three resistors connected in series, the total current is the sum of the current across each resistor
   (d) In a circuit with three resistors connected in parallel the total voltage is the sum of the voltage across each resistor
   (e) Resistance is voltage divided by current
3. The following statements regarding capacitance and impedance are true:
   (a) Impedance is the sum of reactance and resistance
   (b) Capacitance is measured in henrys
   (c) Dielectric material separates the plates of a capacitor
   (d) Capacitors block alternating current (AC) as they have a high reactance but allow direct current (DC) to pass as they have a low resistance
   (e) A defibrillator is based on the principle of an inductor
4. Regarding Newton's laws of motion, the following are true:
   (a) One newton is the force required to increase the velocity of a 1-kg mass by 1 m s^{-1}
   (b) Newton's second law of motion states that for every action there is an equal and opposite reaction
   (c) Acceleration is measured in metres per second
   (d) Newton's first law of motion states that in the absence of external forces an object in motion continues to move
   (e) Newton's third law of motion states that the acceleration of an object is inversely proportional to the mass of an object
5. The statements regarding magnetism below are either true or false:
   (a) Two south poles of a magnet will attract
   (b) Diamagnetism is the term given when objects are attracted by a magnetic field
   (c) Iron is a permanent magnet
   (d) Magnetic flux is measured in webers
   (e) The magnetic and geographical north pole seen on maps of the world are found at the same place

1. FTFFT
   Pressure is force divided by area, voltage is current multiplied by resistance and power is work divided by time. All these relationships contain terms which do relate to each other but the maths as given in some of the questions is incorrect!
2. TFFFT
   Voltage, or potential difference, is the work done in moving unit charge a specified distance between two points. In a series circuit, current across each

resistance is the same as the total current of the circuit. For a parallel circuit, the voltage is the same at all points in the circuit.

3. TFTFF

Capacitance is measured in farads. As capacitors have low reactance, they allow AC to pass but their high resistance tends to block DC. A defibrillator contains a number of components, including inductors, but the key element is a capacitor to store the large charge required.

4. TFFTF

Newton's second law states that acceleration is proportional to the force applied and inversely proportional to the mass of an object. Newton's third law states that every action has an equal and opposite reaction. Velocity is quantified in metres per second and acceleration describes the change in velocity with time so is quantified as metres per second-squared.

5. FFTTF

Like poles will repel as will objects in a magnetic field which are diamagnetic. Iron is a permanent magnet but that doesn't mean all pieces of iron are magnets: a permanently magnetic substance means it can be magnetized by application of a magnetic field and that this magnetism is maintained after removal of the external field. The geographic and magnetic polar axes of the Earth are slightly inclined from one another so the poles are not co-located and, in fact, the magnetic axis is currently inverted. In other words, the magnetic north pole (near the geographic north pole) actually repels the south pole of a magnet.

References

1. I. Newton. *Philosophiæ Naturalis Principia Mathematica*, 1687.

Chapter 3
Heat, Temperature and Humidity

Hozefa Ebrahim and Sean Chadwick

Learning Objectives

- To understand the concept of heat and temperature
- To appreciate the clinical importance of temperature measurement, and how this is performed
- To understand how heat can be transferred: conduction, convection, radiation, but also how respiratory and evaporative heat losses are important in clinical practice
- To understand the importance of measuring humidity
- To explain how gases are humidified

Chapter Content

- Laws of thermodynamics
- Heat
- Temperature
- Humidity

Scenario

A 12-year-old child has been listed for change of dressings following severe burns. The procedure will be under general anaesthetic in the operating theatre and is scheduled to last one hour. The heating in the operating theatre has been adjusted and the ambient temperature reads 30 °C.

Consider the following questions as you read this chapter. Why does a burns patient suffer significant heat loss during his in-patient stay, and what can be done to prevent this? What is the difference between heat and temperature? What is meant by 'absolute zero'? Define the laws of thermodynamics. What are the different methods of temperature and humidity measurement, and where do we use them?

Introduction

The concept of heat and temperature can be confusing. Heat is a term for energy and is measured in joules. Temperature, on the other hand, represents the effect of kinetic energy on its medium. It is a quantification of how hot or cold a subject is.

Consider two items which can produce heat; a candle and a forced-warm-air blanket system. A candle has the ability to burn us while a warming blanket wrapped around us will be quite comfortable. Even though the candle flame does so much more damage to us, it only has a fraction of the energy that the warming blanket provides. More of this will be explained in the heat section.

Thermodynamics is a branch of physics that connects temperature with energy.

The Laws of Thermodynamics

There are four laws of thermodynamics, zeroth to third.

- The zeroth law of thermodynamics states that if two systems are in thermal equilibrium with a third system, they must all be in thermal equilibrium with each other.
- The first law of thermodynamics states that the total energy of a closed system remains constant; energy cannot be created or destroyed (energy can, however, be converted from one form to another).
- The second law of thermodynamics states that entropy (the measure of disorder within a system) of the universe increases over time. It also explains that heat cannot flow from a colder location to a hotter location.
- The third law of thermodynamics describes entropy at absolute zero (0 K or –273.15 °C). In a perfectly crystalline compound, entropy is zero at absolute zero temperature, i.e. no thermal energy exists.

The concept of absolute zero will be explained in the temperature section.

Heat

'The distinction between hot bodies and cold ones is familiar to all and is associated in our minds with the difference of the sensations which we experience in touching various objects, according as they are hot or cold.'
James Clerk Maxwell, *Scottish physicist* [1]

Consider this question: what possesses more thermal energy, an ice-cold lake or a red-hot poker? Potentially counterintuitive as the answer may be, the ice-cold lake actually possesses more thermal energy. To increase the temperature of the lake from absolute zero (−273.15 °C) to 0 °C requires far greater energy compared to that required to increase the temperature of a poker to the red-hot temperature of around 700 °C. This is simply because of the huge volume of water within a lake compared to the 2 kg of iron forming the poker.

Energy is defined as the capacity for doing work. Work is done when a constant force is applied to an object in the direction of the applied force. The SI unit for energy is the joule. Energy may take the form of kinetic, potential, gravitational, electric, chemical, magnetic, elastic or thermal. Energy cannot be destroyed, only changed from one form to another.

Heat is the specific term given to thermal energy. It is transferred naturally down a temperature gradient (from a hotter substance to a colder substance) until both substances reach equal temperature. No energy is lost.

Heat Transfer

The temperature of a substance will increase as heat energy is added to increase the kinetic energy of the molecules. Heat may be transferred from one substance to another by conduction, convection or radiation (Figure 3.1). Conduction and convection involve movement of molecules. Radiation involves electromagnetic waves. Combinations of these three mechanisms also exist, such as evaporation and respiration. Evaporative losses from the gut mucosa and the respiratory tract of are of particular clinical relevance.

- **Conduction:** transfer of heat energy through a substance or between two substances in contact with each other from a hot surface to a cooler surface. Heat energy is transferred from one molecule to another by an increase in kinetic energy of these molecules. An example would be the exposure of a warm body to the cold operating table.
- **Convection:** transfer of heat energy by movement of molecules from a hot environment to a cooler environment. The molecules of air above a warm body are heated by conduction. The air expands and becomes less dense as it is heated and then rises and moves to cooler areas and is in turn replaced by cooler air creating a convection current. This in turn causes more heat energy to be transferred from the warm surface to the new, cool air replacing the warmed air. This is how an exposed patient gets cold in a cold operating theatre.

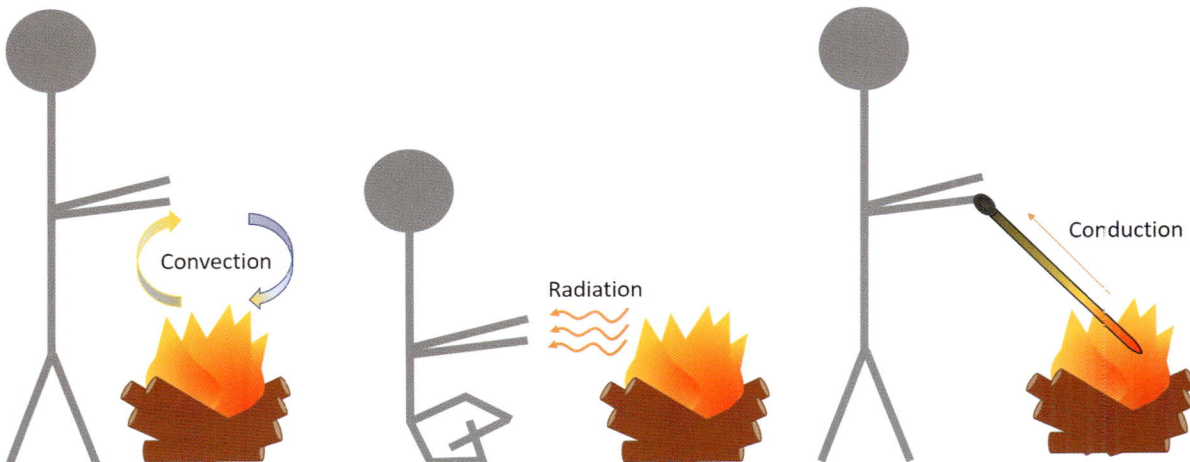

Figure 3.1 Convection, radiation and conduction

- **Radiation:** all substances emit and absorb heat in the form of thermal radiation, a form of non-ionizing radiation. No molecules are involved, unlike conduction and convection. Instead, radiation involves electromagnetic waves over a spectrum of wavelengths, primarily in the infrared region. The hotter a substance is, the more infrared radiation it emits. This means heat energy can be transferred by radiation in a vacuum and without substances being in contact with one another.

Various materials have different conductive properties, otherwise known as conduction coefficients. The materials are given numbers that depend on their relative rates of conduction. Materials are compared to silver (coefficient of heat conduction of 100). Examples of the coefficient of some other substances include copper (92), iron (11), snow (0.16), water (0.12), wood (0.03). A perfect vacuum has a conduction coefficient of zero.

Materials that are poor conductors of heat are good insulators. Air is an excellent insulator when it is locked in an enclosed space. It has a conduction coefficient of 0.006. The air locked in-between feathers, hair and fibres is what allows those materials to keep us so warm. The Inuit traditionally make good use of natural insulative properties in keeping themselves warm with animal fur and building igloos from snow which, incidentally, has the same insulating properties as bricks.

Ionizing radiation refers to the type of radiation that carries enough energy to liberate electrons from atoms and molecules. It consists of highly energetic sub-atomic particles or electromagnetic waves. These atoms and molecules that have been stripped of an electron or two become charged (ionized). Not all of the electromagnetic spectrum is considered ionizing. Gamma waves, X-rays and the higher part of the ultra-violet spectrum possess ionizing capacity whereas visible light, infrared, radio waves and microwaves do not.

The discovery of infrared radiation is ascribed to William Herschel, the astronomer. Herschel used a prism to refract light from the Sun and detected the infrared wave through an increase in the temperature recorded by a thermometer.

Clinical Heat Loss

Heat is also lost from the body when water liquid is transformed into water vapour. The amount of energy transferred can be calculated through the concept of latent heat of vaporization, which we will discuss below. The amount of heat lost in this way will depend on the body surface area exposed. For example, a patient undergoing a laparotomy has a large area of wet tissue exposed to the environment. As the water on the surface of the bowel evaporates, the energy required to turn it from liquid to vapour comes from the body tissues. Similarly, if an individual wears wet clothes, some of the energy required to dry those clothes comes from the person themselves.

Another form of heat loss is through respiration as a combination of the concepts explained above. Water liquid on the internal surface of the airways is converted to water vapour. This results in energy loss, equating to the latent heat of vaporization of that moisture. The water vapour is subsequently expelled through the airways into the environment through a convective process or, more specifically, through bulk flow. A heat and moisture exchanger in the anaesthetic breathing system will decrease heat loss through respiration.

Clinical heat loss is via a combination of the methods described above. No two situations are the same, and the proportions of heat lost through these different methods vary from one patient to another. For example, a burns patient will lose a significant amount of energy from evaporation. Anaesthetized

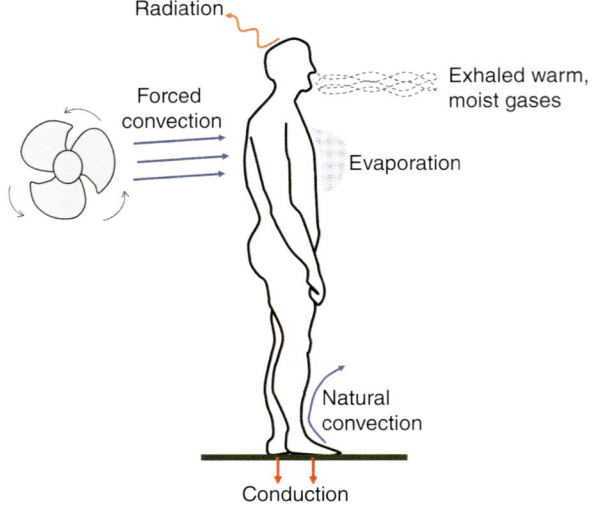

Figure 3.2 Heat loss from the body

patients lose a significant amount of heat through radiation due to the increased peripheral vasodilatation caused by anaesthetic agents. Generally speaking, however, it is accepted that the largest amount of energy is lost through radiation (40%), followed by convection (30%), evaporation from the skin (20%), whereas respiration accounts for approximately 10%. In clinical practice, heat lost through conduction is minimal. These figures are not fixed, and when evaluating potential sources of heat loss in the clinical setting, one should take the context into consideration.

Heat Capacity

Heat capacity is the thermal energy required to increase the temperature of a given object by one kelvin, and has the unit J K^{-1}. In the example of the lake mentioned earlier, the thermal energy required to increase the temperature of millions of cubic metres of water from absolute zero to the freezing point of water would be phenomenal because the heat capacity of such a large mass of water is enormous. In comparison, heating the poker that only weighs 2 kg to 700 °C would take less energy, even though the temperature increase is significantly greater (973 K as opposed to 273 K).

Specific heat capacity (SHC) is the thermal energy required to increase the temperature of 1 kg of a substance by 1 K, without changing its state of matter. It has the units J kg^{-1} K^{-1}. The word 'specific' denotes that the quantity of the substance is specified in the definition, i.e. 1 kg. The molar heat capacity is the thermal energy required to increase the temperature of one mole of a substance by 1 K without changing the state of matter. It has the units J mol^{-1} K^{-1}. Solids and liquids usually have a higher specific heat capacity than gases.

The SHC of water is approximately 4.2 kJ kg^{-1} K^{-1}, whereas that of copper is only 0.38 kJ kg^{-1} K^{-1}, and iron is 0.45 kJ kg^{-1} K^{-1}. Copper is used as the heat sink in many modern vaporizers due to its high thermal conductivity (nearly 100 times that of water) and its relatively high SHC compared to other good conductors of heat. For further details see Chapter 8.

Latent Heat of Fusion and Vaporization

Intermolecular and interatomic forces exist between all particles. In solids, these forces are relatively strong, slightly weaker in liquids and much smaller in gases. In order to change the phase of matter, some energy will be required to overcome these forces.

The energy required to change this state of matter is known as latent heat. Alternatively, latent heat can be explained as the heat energy required to change the state of matter without changing its temperature. Latent heat of fusion is the thermal energy required to change a solid to a liquid without changing its temperature. The latent heat of vaporization is the thermal energy required to change a liquid to gas without changing its temperature.

Specific latent heat is the thermal energy required to convert 1 kg of a substance from one phase (state) to another at a given temperature. Clearly, hotter substances will require less thermal energy to change the object's phase as it will already have a higher energy content. As the temperature of the substance increases until it reaches the critical temperature of that substance, the specific latent heat will decrease such that, at the critical temperature, no further energy will be required to change the state of that substance and the specific latent heat will be zero.

More about latent heat of fusion and vaporization can be found in Chapter 8.

Temperature

Temperature is a measurable physical property and is the quantification of the average kinetic energy of the molecules within a substance. It is an expression of how hot or cold a substance is. Substances with a higher temperature will contain molecules with a higher average kinetic energy. Objects of a higher temperature will transfer thermal energy to objects of a lower temperature. The SI unit for temperature is the kelvin. One kelvin is defined as 1/273.16 of the thermodynamic temperature of the triple point of water. Temperature is also measured via the Celsius and Fahrenheit scales. One degree Celsius is equal to one kelvin in magnitude.

Absolute Zero

Absolute zero is a calculated, theoretical temperature at which the thermal kinetic energy of all known matter will be zero. It is denoted as 0 K on the kelvin scale which equates to –273.15 °C on the Celsius scale.

Triple Point of Water

The triple point of a pure substance is the temperature and pressure at which that substance can exist in equilibrium in all three phases (solid, liquid and gaseous states).

Chapter 3: Heat, Temperature and Humidity

The triple point of water is 0.01 °C (273.16 K), at 611.7 Pa. This figure is fixed by definition rather than measured; indeed, it is the definition upon which kelvin is based. The concept of the triple point was initially described by James Thomson in 1873. James Thomson was the brother of Lord Kelvin.

Thermometric Properties

All thermometers are based upon utilizing particular physical properties. The properties of many substances change with temperature and when this change is predictable and measurable, the property may be utilized in the design of a temperature-measuring device. The science behind measuring properties associated with temperature changes is known as **thermometry**. Thermometric properties used in thermometers include:

- liquid expansion
- changes in the size and shape of solids
- Charles's law
- changes in electromagnetic wave properties
- changes in electrical resistance
- Seebeck effect
- thermal radiation
- thermochromism

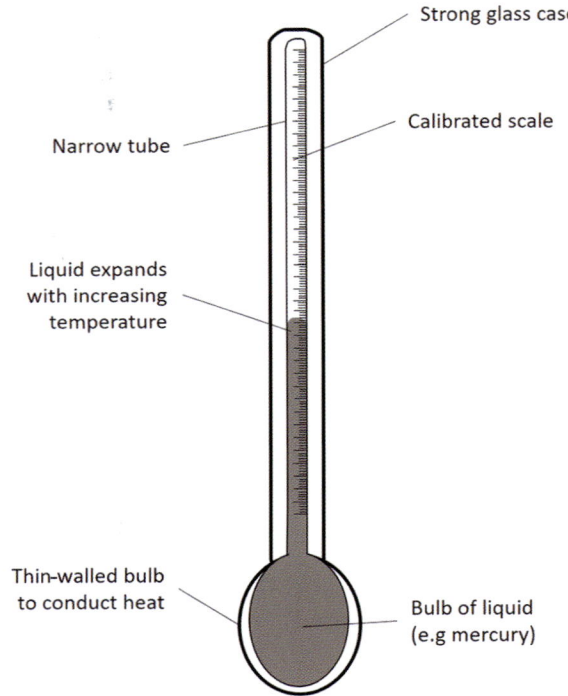

Figure 3.3 Mercury thermometer

Temperature Measurement

Thermometers can be broadly classified into electrical and non-electrical devices:

Non-electrical thermometers

- Liquid (mercury and alcohol)
- Bourdon gauge
- Bimetallic strip
- Liquid-crystal

Electrical devices

- Infrared thermometers and thermopiles
- Resistance wire thermometers
- Thermistors
- Thermocouples
- Fibre-optic thermometry

Non-electrical thermometers

Liquid thermometers are historically the most well-known thermometers. They are based on the thermometric principle of fluid expansion. As the temperature of a liquid increases, so does the volume. The

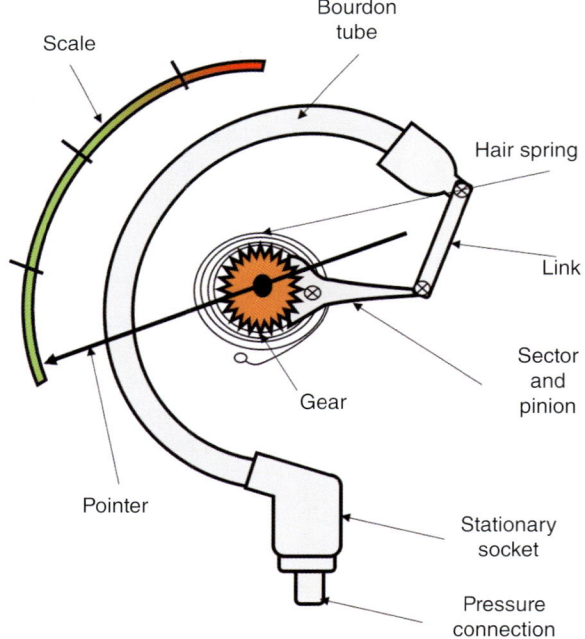

Figure 3.4 Bourdon gauge thermometer

most common examples are mercury and alcohol thermometers (Figure 3.3). These devices are simple, cheap, reusable, and no power supply is needed. However, they have a slow response time, are easily broken, dangerous if broken and have a potential for cross-infection. They are no longer used in clinical practice.

The **Bourdon gauge thermometer** works on a similar principle (Figure 3.4). A temperature-sensing bulb contains a fluid. As the temperature increases, the fluid expands. Unlike the mercury thermometer however, this fluid expansion causes a hollow spiral metal tube to unwind. This in turn moves a pointer on a calibrated scale. This is another example of a cheap, simple and robust instrument though it is relatively inaccurate.

The **bimetallic-strip thermometer** is another example utilizing the thermal expansion principle – this time, in metals. Two metals, usually copper and steel, are fixed together as in Figure 3.5. Copper and steel have slightly different thermal expansion coefficients – they expand by differing amounts in response to any given increase in temperature. Due to the fact that they are attached to each other, there is a resulting bending movement, since one expands more than the other. This predictable movement can be read against a calibrated scale and hence used to measure temperature change. This method is also cheap, simple and does not require any power source. It has a slow response time, however.

Liquid-crystal thermometers are based upon thermochromism – the physical property of colour change in response to changes in temperature. The principle has many commercial uses: telling us when water has reached boiling point by the colour of the kettle, and when milk is safe to give our babies when the bottle has reached the right colour. It can also be used against a calibrated temperature scale. The technology is relatively cheap and simple, but each crystal has a limited temperature range. In practical terms in theatre, this limits its use. They are useful for home thermometers for measuring a child's temperature with a forehead strip or for a simple display of the temperature within the room.

Electrical devices

Blackbody radiation is the thermal energy radiated from any object above absolute zero. It does not include reflected electromagnetic radiation. An assumption is made that the object is opaque and non-reflective. Hence the term, *blackbody*. The amount of radiation is dependent on its temperature. At room temperature, most of the thermal radiation is in the infrared spectrum, but the frequency increases with temperature. The spectrum of wavelengths is dependent on the temperature. **Infrared thermometers** measure radiation emitted from a hot body. Common clinical applications include the tympanic-membrane infrared thermometer. Radiation emitted from the eardrum is sensed by a thermopile, an electronic device that converts thermal energy into an electrical signal. A **thermopile** is actually composed of several thermocouples connected in series; see below for more detail on thermocouples. The tympanic membrane closely approximates the blood supply of the hypothalamus, and therefore gives an accurate indication of core temperature. However, if anything obstructs the direct line of sight from the eardrum to the thermopile (earwax or soft tissue), the sensor will sense radiation from the surrounding tissue instead. This is a source of error. Tympanic-membrane thermometers are more expensive than most non-electrical devices, although they are quick and portable.

There are two types of thermometer that detect a change in electrical resistance in response to a temperature change. The first is a **platinum resistance thermometer**. Resistance and temperature have a reliable, linear relationship over a large temperature

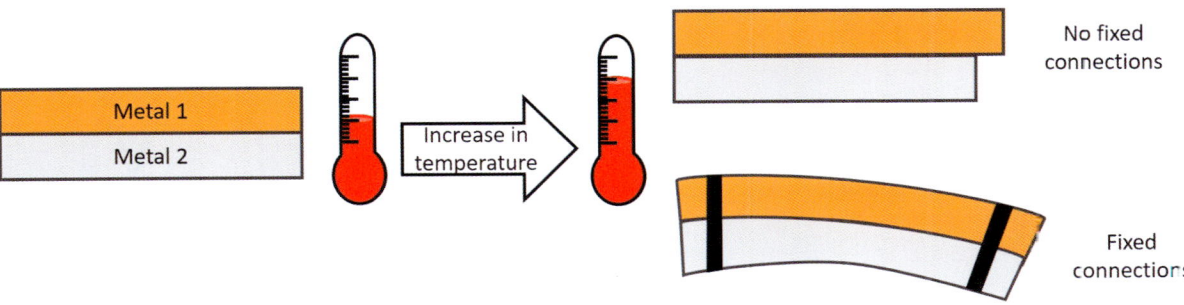

Figure 3.5 Bimetallic-strip thermometer

range. Electrons in a platinum wire are usually free to flow in response to a potential difference. However, with increasing temperature, the increased agitation of the molecules impedes the flow of electrons. The change in resistance is detected using a Wheatstone bridge. This change in resistance is calibrated against temperature. Platinum wire resistors are cheap, simple, quick, accurate and not prone to drift (gradual loss of accurate calibration).

Thermistors also use the physical property of a change in resistance in response to temperature. However, these are constructed using a semiconductor material. Unlike platinum wires, not all electrons in a semiconductor are in free flow. Increasing the temperature increases the proportion of free electrons available to conduct electricity, and hence decreases the resistance.

As seen in Figure 3.6, the relationship between temperature and resistance is that they are inversely proportional to each other. When calibrating thermometers, the materials are carefully chosen to provide a reliably predictable relationship.

Thermocouples rely on a physical concept known as the Seebeck effect. When two dissimilar metals form a junction, a potential difference develops between the two metals. This potential difference varies reliably with temperature. In the example shown in Figure 3.7, there are in fact two junctions: one for sensing and another as a reference at a known temperature. The example shows the reference junction placed in an ice bath at 0 °C. In practical devices, however, the reference junction employs a thermistor thermometer and a Wheatstone bridge to calculate the exact temperature of the reference junction. The benefits of a thermocouple are that it is cheap, very fast at detecting temperature changes, can be made very small and can measure a wide range of temperatures. Cheap devices, however, can be inaccurate.

Fibre-optic thermometers are used in environments that have high electromagnetic wave interference, such as MRI scanners and the electrical switchgear room. In such environments, standard electrical devices may prove inaccurate. A completely non-metallic fibre-optic tube has a gallium–arsenic (GaAs) semiconductor crystal mounted at its tip. Light is shone at the crystal through the fibre-optic

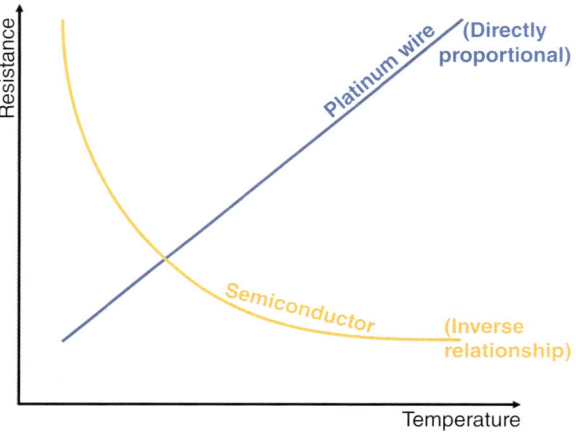

Figure 3.6 Relationship between resistance and temperature for platinum wires and semiconductors

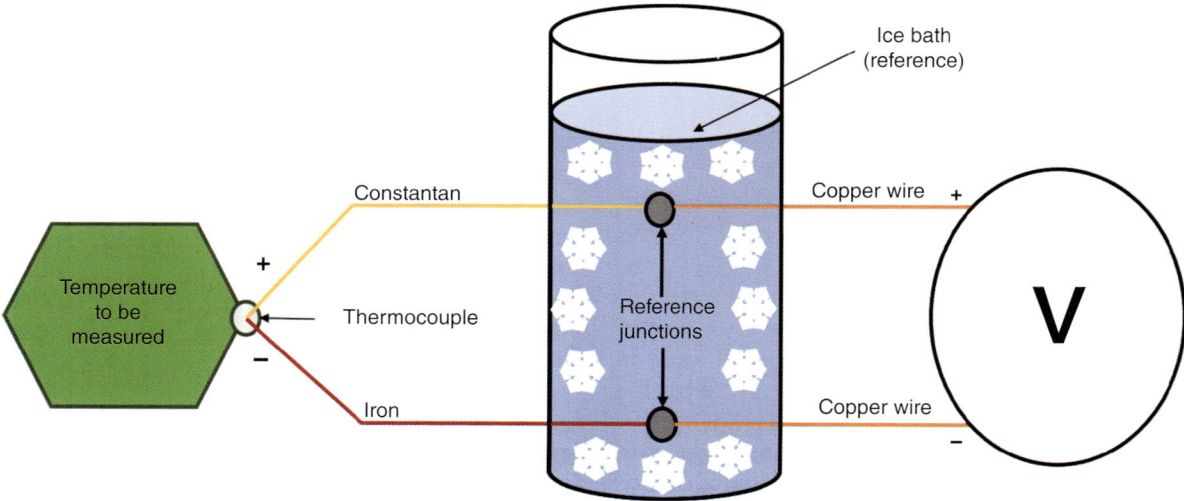

Figure 3.7 A thermocouple

tube, a proportion of which is absorbed by the crystal, and then the reflected light is detected by a photosensor. The exact spectrum of light absorbed by the crystal will depend on its temperature, and shifts by approximately 0.4 nm K^{-1}. This spectrum shift is used to measure temperature. They are not used much in the anaesthetic environment.

Other techniques to measure temperature also exist, which are mentioned for the sake of completeness. They do not have any practical use in the modern theatre. Examples include the Galilean thermometer and phosphor thermometry.

Humidity

Over the last 100 years there have been 32 serious reported explosions in theatres in England and Wales resulting in four deaths. The most common cause is a static spark and the second most common is diathermy. Two of the known incidents were related to the anaesthetist smoking in theatre! The last reported death due to an explosion was in 1954 and happened as a circuit of cyclopropane was being changed on a cold, dry, winter's day,

Fortunately, it is now many decades since that last fatal accident. This is due to our better understanding of the relationship between temperature and humidity and their interaction with the equipment, drugs and environment in which we work. Humidification is also of relevance to the patient to protect the airway from drying out as well as reducing heat loss during mechanical ventilation.

Humidity is defined as the amount of water vapour in the air and can be expressed in three different ways:

- Absolute humidity
- Relative humidity
- Specific humidity

Absolute humidity is the mass of water vapour present in a given volume of air. This is expressed as mg l^{-1} or g m^{-3} (which are numerically equivalent). The maximum amount of water vapour that a given volume of air can hold is dependent on the temperature of that volume of air and is known as the saturation point. As the temperature of the specific volume of air increases, so the capacity to contain water in the form of vapour increases. Simply put: the hotter the air, the more water it can hold.

Relative humidity (RH) is the ratio of the mass of water vapour in a given volume of air to the mass needed to fully saturate that given volume of air at that specified temperature. This is expressed as a percentage. When we talk about humidity we usually refer to relative humidity. For example, at atmospheric pressure of 760 mmHg, 1 m^3 of 100%-saturated air at 20 °C contains 17 g of water. If this same volume of air were to be warmed to 37 °C, the mass of water vapour, and therefore absolute humidity, will remain the same but the relative humidity will drop to 39%. This is because at 37 °C, 1 m^3 of air contains 44 g water when fully saturated and the ratio of 17 to 44 is 39%.

Relative humidity may also be expressed as a ratio of vapour pressures.

$$RH = \frac{\text{Partial pressure of water vapour}}{\text{Saturated vapour pressure}} \times 100$$

Specific humidity is the ratio of water vapour to dry air in a particular mass and is sometimes referred to as humidity ratio.

The dew point is the temperature at which the prevailing absolute humidity would result in 100% relative humidity. It is expressed in degrees Celsius. When the ambient temperature matches the dew point, condensation will form as the air cannot hold that mass of vapour water at that temperature – we call this dew. On a practical note, the dew point tells us at what temperature to store a gas to prevent condensation. The concept of the dew point can be used to measure humidity.

The difference between the dew point and surface temperature can be used to predict the cloud base. It's a rough rule of thumb because it assumes a linear relationship between temperature and altitude and homogeneous absolute humidity within the atmosphere. With that in mind, however, for every 1 °C difference between temperature and dew point, you would expect a 400 feet increase in cloud base: on a 9 °C day with a 4 °C dew point (5 °C degree 'split'), the clouds will be roughly at 2,000 feet. If the temperature is 9 °C with a 9 °C dew point, the cloud base is zero feet – fog!

Measurement of Humidity

There are many methods of measuring humidity. Some methods are discussed here for academic purposes only. To the anaesthetist, many of these methods are now of historical value only. Instruments include;

- Regnault's hygrometer
- hair hygrometer
- psychrometer (wet/dry bulb hygrometer)
- chilled mirror hygrometer
- capacitive hygrometer
- resistive hygrometer
- humidity transducers
- gravimetric (mass) hygrometer
- colour-change crystal hygrometer

Regnault's hygrometer measures relative humidity from the dew point (Figure 3.8a). Sample air is blown through a silver tube of ether (diethyl ether), cooling it to a point at which condensation or misting appears on the outer surface of the tube. This temperature is recorded as the dew point. Saturated vapour pressures are obtained from tables, and the absolute humidity of the measured air can be calculated from these tables. They are accurate from below freezing point to 100 °C.

The **hair hygrometer** measures relative humidity directly (Figure 3.8b). The device employs a strand of hair (human or horse) under tension. The length of the hair is highly dependent on humidity. The change of the length of hair is used to move a pointer along a calibrated scale. Devices are accurate between 30% and 90% relative humidity.

The **wet and dry bulb hygrometer** measures relative humidity using a set of tables (Figure 3.8c). Also known as a **psychrometer**, this device is based on the temperature difference related to evaporation of water and the resulting cooling effect of latent heat of vaporization. There are two glass mercury thermometers: one measuring ambient temperature (dry bulb) and the other, the cooling effect of evaporating water from the cloth or sock surrounding its bulb (wet bulb). The evaporation reduces the temperature in the wet-bulb side compared to the dry thermometer and the rate of evaporation is dependent on the ambient humidity. The device is accurate between 0 and 100% ± 2% relative humidity down to freezing point.

The **chilled mirror hygrometer** measures relative humidity using dew point and a photodetector (Figure 3.8d). It is a development on the wet and dry bulb hygrometer. A chilled silver or copper mirror at constant temperature is used. There is constant electronic feedback to detect condensation, which results in a capacitive or resistive change, as described below. It is regarded as accurate from below freezing point to 100 °C, although it needs frequent calibration and cleaning.

Capacitive hygrometers rely on the change in electrical characteristics of a capacitor, caused by the presence of water vapour (Figure 3.8e). Water vapour is absorbed by the dielectric material between the conducting plates, in this case usually a polymer or metal oxide. This results in a change in the capacitance, which can be measured and correlated to a calibration table of capacitance versus humidity. These devices are accurate between 5% and 95% relative humidity. They can operate below freezing up to 200 °C. They are relatively less accurate but cost-effective so are easily incorporated into everyday electronics.

Resistive hygrometers measure relative humidity due to a change in resistance occurring as a result of changes in humidity (Figure 3.8f). Metal contacts are arranged in a comb-like manner. They are surrounded by hygroscopic salts (cobalt/lithium), whose resistance changes in response to their water content. As humidity increases, the resistance of the salts decreases, and hence the current flow increases. They measure relative humidity. These instruments are accurate between 5% and 95% but are less sensitive than a capacitive hygrometer. They are small and robust, and therefore easily incorporated into everyday electronics.

The **gravimetric hygrometer** is regarded as one of the most accurate direct measurement methods. It directly measures the mass of a fixed volume of air, and compares this to the mass of dry air. The difference represents the mass of water vapour. It is cumbersome and expensive, however, and its use is limited to the calibration of other devices.

Colour-change crystal hygrometers are based on the physical property that some crystals change colour when they come in contact with water. This can be utilized in a simple visual indicator of humidity. Typical examples include the baby-comfort cards placed in a child's room. These devices are cheap and simple, though not precise enough for use in clinical environments.

Relationship of Humidity to Temperature and Heat

The temperature as we actually perceive it, known as the apparent temperature, is affected by the relative humidity of the surrounding environment, amongst other factors. In the hot operating theatre, as in the reference scenario, the body's ability to perspire and

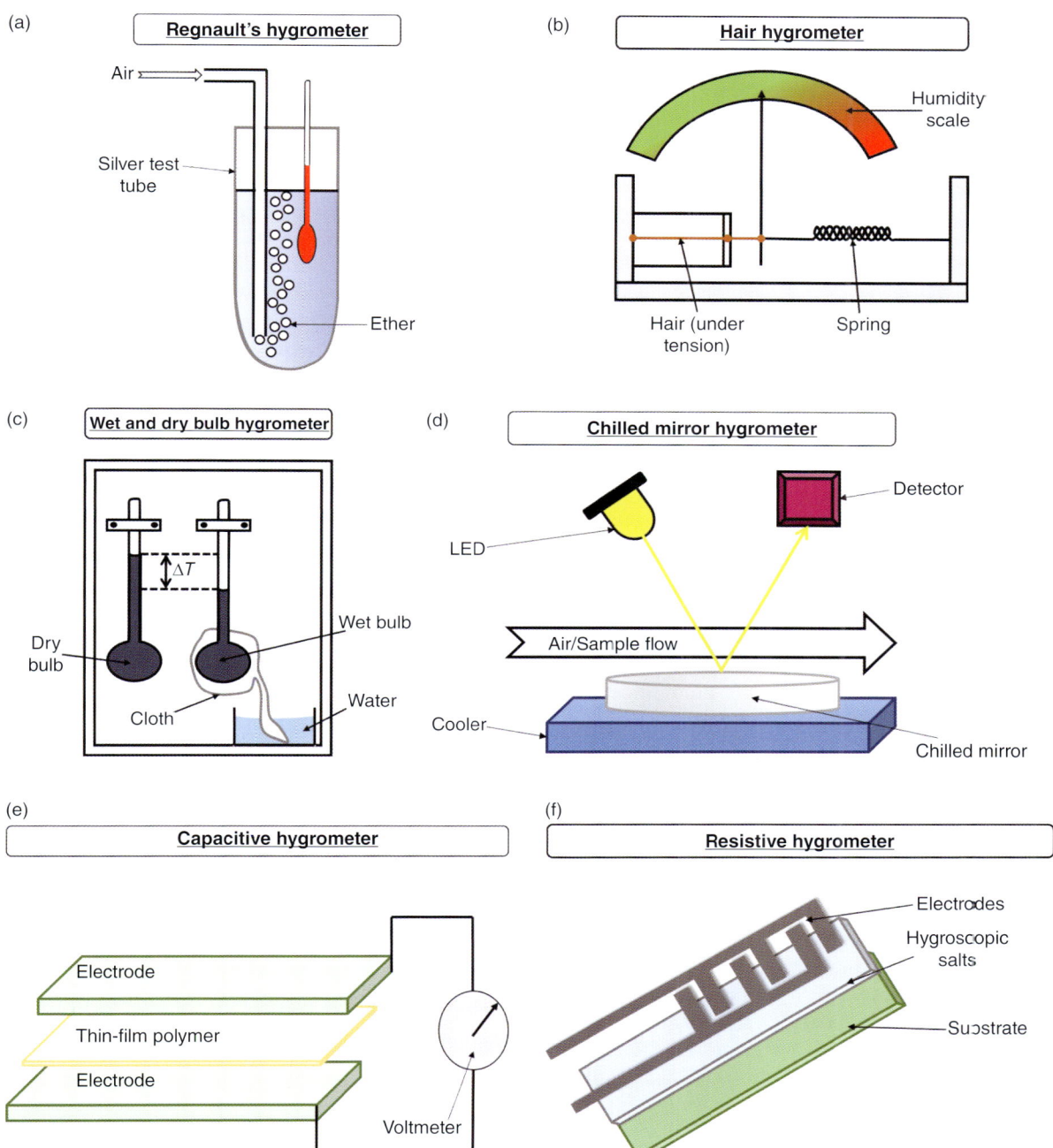

Figure 3.8 Hygrometers: (a) Regnault's, (b) hair, (c) psychrometer, (d) chilled mirror, (e) capacitive and (f) resistive

consequently lose heat is reduced. As a result, both patient and practitioners feel warmer.

In our case, the child will lose less heat and water to the environment during their dressing change due to reduced sweat production and latent heat of vaporization. In the extreme case of heat illness, this can lead not only to a change in the apparent temperature but the actual temperature of the body.

If the heat load exceeds the body's ability to lose heat, body temperature can rise to dangerous levels.

The apparent temperature calculation was devised in 1984 by Robert Steadman and it allows the ambient temperature to be corrected to account for how the human body would perceive it after the effects of humidity, wind speed and solar radiation are accounted for. This is useful in forecasting the risk of heat illness epidemics from a public health perspective.

$$\text{Apparent temperature} = T_d + e - W + \left(\frac{Q}{W}\right)$$

where T_d is the dry bulb temperature, e is the water vapour pressure, W is the windspeed at 10 m elevation and Q is the net solar radiation absorbed per square metre).

Humidification in Clinical Practice

Humidification is relevant to both the anaesthetist and other members of the operating theatre. For patients who have had their upper airways bypassed by endotracheal intubation or tracheostomy, humidification is important to preserve normal mucosal function and reduce heat loss. Under normal conditions, air entering the trachea has been warmed and humidified on its journey through the upper airways and is almost fully saturated – about 90% relative humidity and still not fully up to body temperature (typically 34 °C and therefore 90% relative humidity equates, conveniently for memorizing, to 34 g m^{-3}). By the time it reaches the alveoli, it is at body temperature and fully saturated. At 37 °C, 100% relative humidity is an absolute humidity of 44 g m^{-3}. Dry gases supplementing spontaneous or mechanical ventilation reduce mucosal ciliary function, which may lead to tenacious secretions with increased susceptibility to infection, and mucus plugs obstructing the airways. Exposure to dry gases over a long period of time will lead to mucosal ciliary wasting and keratinization.

Humidification of the theatre environment is beneficial to the patient as well as to the staff. Optimal relative humidity at room temperature of 22 °C to 24 °C for humans to feel comfortable is generally accepted to be between 45% and 50%. When the relative humidity falls below 35%, staff in theatre may develop dry eyes, dry mouth and respiratory problems and will also be at risk of electric shocks.

Electric shock is a result of the build-up of static electricity in theatre and subsequent earthing of that static charge by flow through a conducting body to ground. In the presence of flammable materials and an oxygen-enriched environment, this can lead to a risk of explosion. Simply increasing the humidity in theatre will make the air more conductive and avoid the build-up and subsequent discharge of static electricity. For this reason, the relative humidity is kept between 50% and 70% in the operating theatre, a compromise between safety and comfort (see Chapter 10).

The lightning bolt is simply a scaled-up version of the sparks seen in domestic occurrences of static discharge. The flash occurs because the air in the discharge channel is heated to such a high temperature (~28,000 K) that it is converted into plasma and emits light by incandescence. The clap of thunder is the result of the shock wave created as the superheated air expands explosively.

Methods of Humidification

Air can be humidified actively or passively.

Passive methods include:

- Heat and moisture exchanger

Active methods include:

- Hot- and cold-water bath humidifiers
- Nebulizers

Heat and moisture exchangers (HMEs) are simple, inexpensive, enclosed units contained with an inlet and outlet. The materials enclosed may include ceramic, paper, cellulose, fine steel or aluminium fibres in a hygroscopic medium such as calcium chloride, lithium chloride or silica gel. Warm, humidified, expired gas passes from the patient, through the HME. The water vapour condenses within the cooler, hygroscopic medium and is then re-used for humidification of the next cycle of inspired gas. Under optimum conditions, up to 25 g m^{-3} of water vapour or a relative humidity of 60% to 70% may be achieved. The efficacy will be reduced in warmer environments due to reduced condensation.

The HME is simultaneously warmed by the latent heat of water condensing within it. This heat is also released during subsequent inspiratory cycles and may reach temperatures of between 29 °C and 34 °C. Some HME devices have microbial filtering properties (HME filters) with efficiencies of more than 99.99%. These microbial filtering properties are due to direct particle barrier as well as electrostatic forces within the HME filter (Figure 3.9). Note that not all HME devices include a filtration capability so an additional filter may be required to protect non-disposable elements of the anaesthetic equipment.

Water-bath humidifiers can employ either hot or cold water. **Cold-water-bath humidifiers** direct the gas flow through water, which then carries water vapour as it bubbles through it. It is relatively inefficient as the bubbles produced are large and the loss of heat from the latent heat of vaporization reduces the capacity to humidify more gas yet further.

Hot-water-bath humidifiers are more effective but require a heating element. The maximum humidity achievable is increased by warming the water using an electric heater and incorporating a thermostat to maintain an operating temperature of 40 °C to 45 °C. The gas is not at this temperature by the time it reaches the patient – this avoids the risk of airway burns but also results in an increase in relative humidity with the slight drop in temperature. Inspired gas arrives at the patient at around 37 °C at almost 100% relative humidity. This helps prevent heat loss, mucosal damage and subsequent ventilator-associated infections in long-term mechanical respiratory support. A thermistor positioned at the patient end of the circuit will allow real-time adjustment to achieve the desired humidity and temperature of inspired gas. This will avoid the risk of burns and provide a more accurate control of humidity than if just the water reservoir temperature was monitored. The problem of large gas bubbles is also alleviated as there is no need to bubble gas through the water to achieve humidification; the dry gas simply passes over the water's surface in the reservoir to become saturated with water vapour. A further refinement may include passing inspired gas through a perforated screen, causing a foam of water and gas to form. A water trap is placed between the humidifier and the patient at a level below the patient. This reduces the risk of airflow obstruction through condensation forming in the circuit and helps avoid inadvertent delivery of hot water into the patient's airway.

Nebulizers humidify air by creating an aerosol of water droplets, suspended in the air. They do not convert water into a vapour or gas. The resultant droplet size is required to be 2–5 μm in diameter to ensure they penetrate deeply into the lungs without simply settling out in the larger airways. Nebulization occurs in different ways. A jet nebulizer utilizes the Venturi effect (Figure 3.10). A high-pressure jet of air is forced through a small orifice. This creates a pressure differential, which causes the liquid to be sucked into the gas stream and split into tiny fragments. An ultrasonic nebulizer produces a high frequency 'shaking effect', causing the water droplets to be formed. A disc nebulizer draws water onto a spinning disc, and the resultant centrifugal force on the water creates microscopic water droplets.

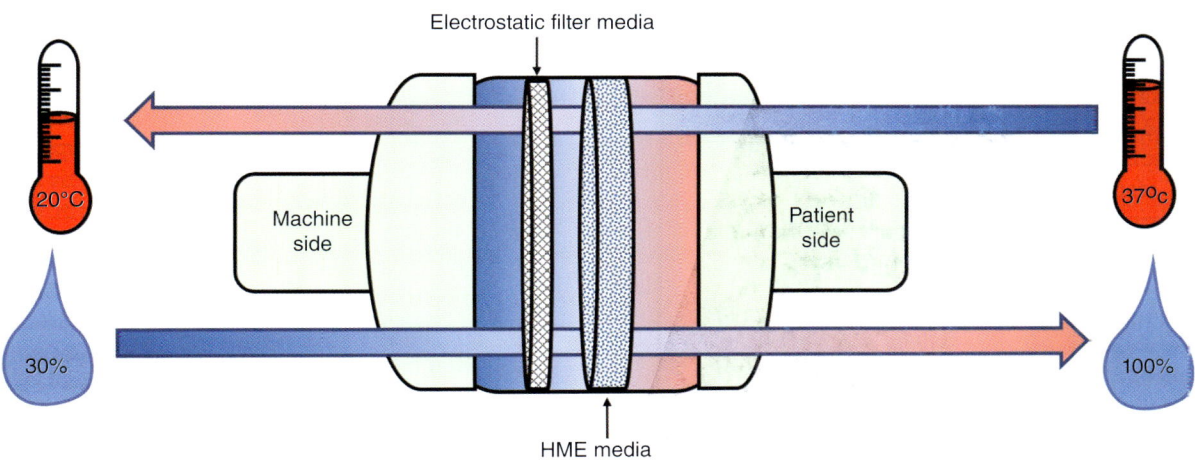

Figure 3.9 An HME filter

Chapter 3: Heat, Temperature and Humidity

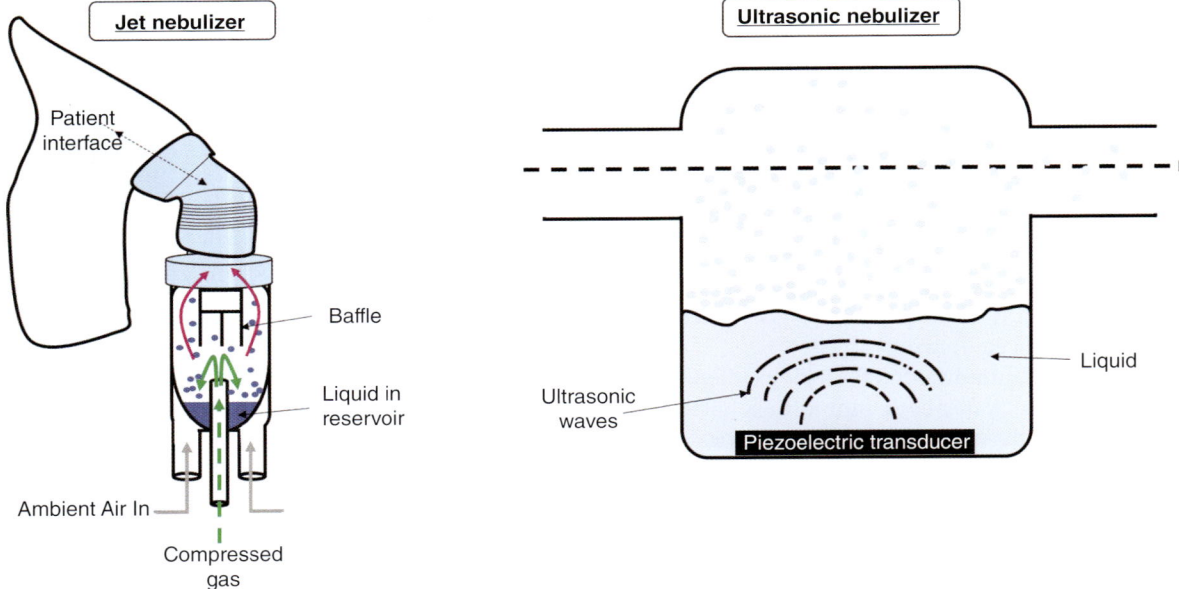

Figure 3.10 Conventional jet and ultrasonic nebulizers

Summary

The concepts of temperature, heat and humidity are fundamental to the practice of anaesthesia and intensive care medicine. These concepts are governed by the laws of thermodynamics. Energy cannot be destroyed, but often changes from one form to another. Heat is a form of energy. Heat energy can flow from one place to another and is dependent on temperature gradients. Measurement of temperature has evolved over the years, and we can employ various different tools depending on the environment and requirement. These various tools are described here.

Humidity is a construct of water in the air. This can be described in both absolute and relative terms, as above. Measurement of humidity is important for both safety and comfort, and various humidity-measuring devices employ different physical principles. Indeed, we often adapt the humidity of our environment to suit our requirement.

Questions

MCQs – select true or false for each response

1. Regarding heat and temperature:
   (a) A kelvin is defined as 1/273.16 of the thermodynamic temperature of the triple point of water
   (b) The triple point of water is the temperature and pressure at which its three different phases are in equilibrium
   (c) The triple point of water occurs at 100 °C
   (d) Temperature (K) is equal to temperature (°C) + 273.16
   (e) Heat capacity is defined as the quantity of heat required to raise the temperature of an object by 1/273.16 K

2. There are many different ways to measure temperature in anaesthetic practice. Which of the following concerning mercury thermometers are true?
   (a) They have a fast response time
   (b) They are used to measure temperatures up to 300 °C
   (c) They rely on the principle of liquid expansion
   (d) They require a power supply
   (e) They are expensive, therefore limiting their use

3. Regarding heat capacity, latent heat and temperature:
   (a) The difference between specific heat capacity and heat capacity relates to the mass of substance involved

(b) Heat is a form of kinetic energy which can be transferred from a colder substance to a hotter substance
(c) Temperature is the property of a substance that determines whether an object will receive heat or give heat to another object
(d) An example of latent heat of fusion is the heat associated with a solid dissolving into a liquid at a constant temperature
(e) A clinical example of latent heat is in the use of ethyl chloride spray for topical anaesthesia

4. Absolute humidity
   (a) Decreases as a gas is heated
   (b) Will vary with the temperature of the air
   (c) In the alveoli is 34 g m^{-3} when fully saturated at 37 °C
   (d) Is the mass of water vapour present in a given volume of air
   (e) Has the units, grams per cubic metre (g m^{-3}) or kilograms per cubic metre (kg m^{-3})

5. Regarding humidifiers:
   (a) Water overload is a danger if using ultrasonic nebulizers
   (b) Ideal droplet size in a nebulizer humidifier is between 2 μm and 5 μm
   (c) A heat and moisture exchanger is more efficient than a heated water bath
   (d) A hot-water-bath humidifier is more effective than a cold-water-bath humidification system
   (e) Heat and moisture exchangers are active humidifiers

6. Which of the following are correct regarding the physical processes involved when a substance is kept in a closed system or sealed environment?
   (a) The substance in its gaseous state and above its critical temperature is classed as a vapour
   (b) Kinetic energy of molecules increases with temperature
   (c) Saturated vapour pressure is not affected by changes in temperature
   (d) Saturated vapour pressure is independent of ambient pressure
   (e) Heat energy is absorbed from the environment during the transition from the liquid to the gaseous phase

Answers

1. TTFFF

   This question is worded to ensure candidates truly understand the concept of the kelvin. The first two statements are the correct definitions. The triple point occurs at 273.16 K, which is 0.01 °C. The term °C is a derived unit. The freezing point of water, which is 0 °C, is 273.15 K. Heat capacity is the amount of heat (a form of energy, measured in joules) required to raise the temperature of an **object** by 1 K, so its unit would be J K^{-1}. Specific heat capacity is the amount of energy required to raise the temperature of 1 kg of a substance by 1 K.

2. FFTFF

   Mercury thermometers are liquid-expansion devices. Their response time is slow (measured in minutes) and they have a relatively narrow temperature range. Special devices are required for low and high temperatures. They do not require a power supply and are cheap although concerns around the safety of mercury-containing devices and the contamination due to breakage now limit their use (mercury in glass sphygmomanometers is similarly now only used occasionally).

3. TTTFT

   Heat cannot be created or destroyed. Heat is energy and is subject to the law of conservation of energy. Temperature is a description of the average kinetic energy of the molecules in a substance. It is possible, for example, for 1 l of water to be colder than 1 g of iron even though it might contain significantly more heat energy. This is due to the higher specific heat capacity of water (it requires more heat to raise the temperature of 1 kg of water by 1 °C than it does to raise the temperature of 1 kg of iron by 1 °C) and the fact that there is 1,000 times as much water as there is iron in this example.

   If the temperature of a given object increases then there must be more heat per molecule on average and, therefore, more heat in total.

   If heat is added to a solid substance, such as water ice, its temperature will increase until it reaches the melting point of the substance. At this point, further heat will cause more melting until the whole amount is liquid. Then the temperature will begin to rise again until the boiling point is reached. Here, further heat will cause evaporation until the whole amount is converted to vapour. Then the temperature will begin to rise again. The energy used in melting is the latent heat of fusion and the energy used in evaporation is the latent heat of vaporization. The heat can be reclaimed if the substance is condensed and then frozen.

4. FFFTT

Absolute humidity is the mass of water in a given unit of gas. This does not change with temperature. Relative humidity is this same quantity expressed as a proportion of the total amount of water that the gas can hold. As the amount a gas can hold increases with temperature, relative humidity falls as a gas is heated. In the alveoli, fully saturated air has an absolute humidity of 44 g m^{-3}. The figure of 34 g m^{-3} is for the upper trachea at 34 °C.

5. TTFTF

Water overload is a risk with ultrasonic nebulizers. Droplets of greater than 5 μm will be deposited in the trachea and bronchi. Those less than 2 μm may impair gas exchange. Heat and moisture exchangers (HMEs) are passive systems, less efficient than water baths.

6. FTFTT

In order for a liquid to change to a gas, thermal energy is required, termed the latent heat of vaporization; heat energy is utilized as kinetic energy to aid the change of phase. Saturated vapour pressure therefore is affected by changes in temperature due to the relationship between heat and kinetic energy; the higher the temperature the greater the saturated vapour pressure and kinetic energy. Ambient pressure, however, causes no such change. A vapour exists when a gaseous substance is below its critical temperature; above this point it can only be a gas.

References

1. J. Clerk Maxwell. *Theory of Heat*, 3rd edn (Longmans, Green and Co., 1872).

Chapter 4

Behaviour of Fluids

Hozefa Ebrahim, Sunita Balla and James Rudge

Learning Objectives

- To understand the definition and behaviour of fluids, with specific attention to the variables that influence flow
- To understand the difference between Newtonian and non-Newtonian fluids, and what factors influence whether fluids flow in a laminar or turbulent fashion.
- To understand how fluids mix – including the principles behind Brownian motion, diffusion and osmosis
- To understand the relationship between energy, pressure and flow of fluids
- To understand the definition and origins of the gas laws

Chapter Content

- Viscosity
- Newtonian fluids
- Non-Newtonian fluids
- Movement and mixing of fluids
- Fluid mechanics
- Gas laws

Scenario

Consider a normal day working as an anaesthetist. There are various phenomena that we may take for granted. These may range from the force we may exert when injecting through a syringe, the time it takes to pour honey into our porridge or the temperature of our bicycle tyre after a 60-minute cycle. The physical principles behind these phenomena make for interesting reading.

Why does it feel easier to inject fluid out of a 2-ml syringe than a 20-ml syringe? Why does one get the feeling of shortness of breath on the top of Mount Everest? Why is it harder to pour honey than milk? Why does my bicycle tyre feel hot after I've inflated it? How does an aeroplane lift off the ground?

Introduction

What is a fluid? A fluid is a substance that is capable of flowing and changes its shape at a steady rate when acted upon by a force. Fluids possess no rigidity and change their shape to fill the container into which they are poured.

Fluids are conventionally classified as either liquids or gases. The most important difference between these two types of fluid lies in their relative compressibility: gases can be compressed much more easily than liquids. Consequently, any intervention that involves significant pressure variations is generally accompanied by much larger changes in density in the case of a gas than in the case of a liquid.

The similar physical behaviours of gases and liquids in motion have led to the development of the science of fluid mechanics.

Fluid mechanics is premised on three major assumptions:

1. Fluids are *isotropic* media: i.e. the physical properties are independent of direction through the fluid.
2. Fluids are regarded as *Newtonian*: i.e. there is a linear relationship between the local rate of change of the shape of a body and the force applied to it, as first postulated by Newton. In reality, many of the common 'fluids' we use on a daily basis do not follow these assumptions and are described as non-Newtonian.
3. The macroscopic motion of ordinary fluids is well described by Newtonian dynamics; the effects dictated by quantum mechanics and general relativity can be safely ignored.

Chapter 4: Behaviour of Fluids

Table 4.1 The viscosity of some common fluids at room temperature

Material	Viscosity (centipoise)
Water	1
Diethyl ether	0.23
Benzene	0.65
Mercury	1.5
Milk	3
Motor oil	Approximately 500
Honey	Approximately 10,000
Ketchup	Approximately 50,000
Peanut butter	Approximately 250,000

Are powders fluids? A powder is a substance that can flow, made up of microscopic grains. A traditional fluid can also be considered to have (sub-)microscopic grains. However, the larger the grain, the greater the propensity to flow in a non-linear manner, thus not behaving like an ideal fluid.

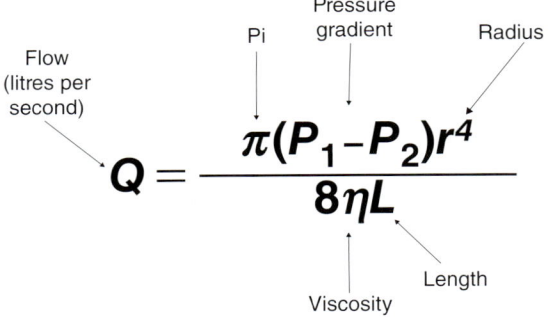

Figure 4.1 The Hagen–Poiseuille equation

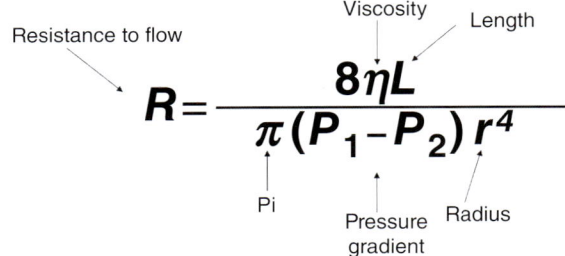

Figure 4.2 Resistance to flow

Viscosity

Viscosity is the property of a fluid that causes it to resist flow; it refers to the *stickiness* of a fluid. When comparing the flow of water through a tube with a more viscous substance such as honey, water flows faster. The velocities of the adjacent layers of the fluid differ, and a 'slip' occurs between parallel layers as a result of the shear forces acting between them. Flow is dependent on the intermolecular forces. At higher temperatures, the molecules have more kinetic energy and, therefore, it is easier to break the intermolecular bonds and thus viscosity decreases. For any given force applied, the flow will then increase as viscosity decreases. This relationship is explained in more detail below – see the Hagen–Poiseuille equation.

Table 4.1 shows the viscosities of different materials at room temperature. Viscosity is measured in centipoise. One centipoise equals one millipascal second (mPa s)

Newtonian Fluids

Newtonian fluids are those in which viscosity, η, is constant, regardless of the velocity gradients produced during flow. Indeed, viscosity defines whether a fluid is Newtonian – a fluid in which the viscous stress arising from its movement is directly proportional to the rate of change of its deformation. Importantly, the viscosity does not depend on the rate of flow of the fluid. While no real fluid fits the definition perfectly, many common liquids and gases, such as water and air, are often assumed to be Newtonian for practical calculations. Some fluids, however, do not behave in this way. These are consequently referred to as non-Newtonian fluids (see below). The viscosity of a Newtonian fluid decreases with rising temperature. Hence flow increases with temperature.

All gases obey Newton's law and are Newtonian fluids. Mineral oils and blends of mineral oils are also generally Newtonian in flow behaviour. The viscosity of a Newtonian fluid, at a given temperature and pressure, can be determined with a single measurement at any shear rate.

The Hagen–Poiseuille Equation

Laminar flow in Newtonian fluids (fluids with constant viscosities) is governed by Poiseuille's law and the Hagen–Poiseuille equation (Figure 4.1).

Rearranging this equation, we can highlight the important variables that determine resistance to this flow (Figure 4.2).

Chapter 4: Behaviour of Fluids

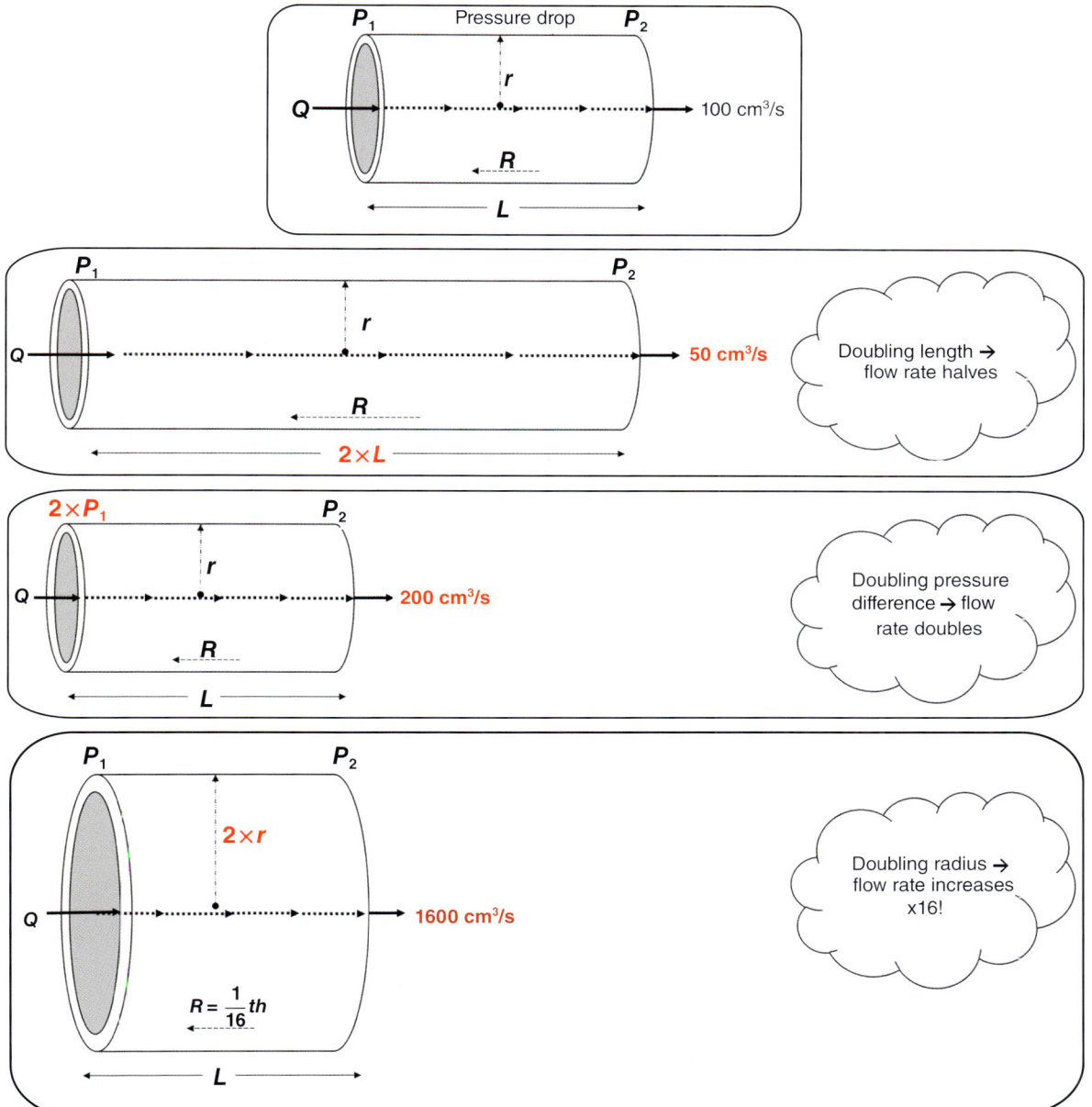

Figure 4.3 Variables influencing the flow of a fluid through a tube

It therefore follows that flow is directly proportional to the pressure difference, and to the fourth power of the radius (Figure 4.3). Note, therefore, that the flow increases markedly as the radius increases. This explains why a 1-mm airway narrowing in a child, whose airway may only be 5 mm at the outset, results in such a drastic reduction in air flow.

Turbulent Flow

Viscosity is an important variable in laminar flow. Density of a fluid, however, comes into play when flow is turbulent; flow of fluid is inversely proportional to its density under these conditions. For this reason, a mixture of helium in oxygen can be used in airway obstructive conditions such as stridor or severe bronchospasm. The lower density of helium reduces the resistance to flow when it is turbulent and so improves the efficiency of respiration. Of course, viscosity is still important as well; its effect on the Reynolds number predisposes to laminar flow, which is preferable in this situation.

Reynolds Number

Reynolds number is a dimensionless number which determines the probability of transition between laminar and turbulent flow. It is influenced by variables concerning both the fluid and the system within which the system flows. It can be applied to any system; for example, blood flowing through a vessel, or air flowing down the airways.

Laminar flow occurs at low Reynolds numbers, when flow is influenced more by viscosity, and is characterized by a smooth, efficient motion. Turbulent flow, however, occurs at higher values of Reynolds number. The flow tends to be erratic and inefficient, being characterized by eddies and vortices.

To calculate the Reynolds number, we use the following equation:

$$Re = \frac{\rho u L}{\mu} = \frac{uL}{\nu}$$

where

- ρ = the density of the fluid (kg m^{-3})
- u = fluid velocity (m s^{-1})
- L = length of the tube (m)
- ν = kinematic viscosity of the fluid (m^2 s^{-1})
- μ = dynamic viscosity of the fluid (N s m^{-2})

A calculated figure above 2,000 generally suggests that flow will be turbulent. However, it must be remembered that this is not an exact prediction. Small anomalies on the surface and shape of the vessel through which the fluid flows will have a significant effect on flow dynamics. Nevertheless, understanding the factors that induce turbulence is an important aspect of clinical care.

The dynamic viscosity is that quantity colloquially referred to as the viscosity. The kinematic velocity is the ratio of dynamic viscosity to density of the fluid – hence the slightly peculiar units of m^2 s^{-1}. The unit practically used for kinematic velocity is the stoke (St): 1 St = 1 cm^2 s^{-1}.

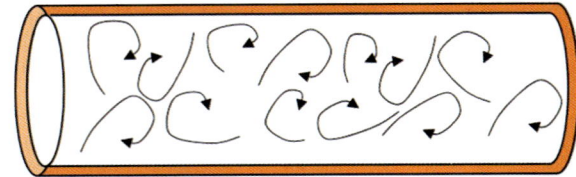

Turbulent flow

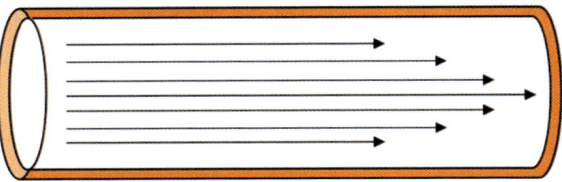

Laminar flow

Figure 4.4 Laminar and turbulent flow

The length of the arrows in the diagram of laminar flow (Figure 4.4) represents the speed of flow in different regions of the fluid. To minimize complexity, just consider the smooth-sided tube which is illustrated (curving or ridged tubes are more complicated!). Frictional interactions between the fluid and tube side-wall mean the outer layer travels slowest. The fluid adjacent to this is slowed slightly by its interaction with the outer layer. The next layer is affected a little less and so on. The central stream is least affected and travels fastest. This diagrammatic representation is called the velocity profile. The layers are otherwise known as laminae, hence laminar flow. As the figure also shows, turbulent flow lacks this level of organization and flow is much more chaotic.

Non-Newtonian Fluids

Unfortunately, most fluids do not follow the convenient rules of Newtonian behaviour. For these non-Newtonian fluids, the viscosity is not linearly related to the shear rate (or rate of relative movement). Similarly, the shear stress is not linearly related to the shear rate. In other words, the viscosity changes depending on how the fluid is moving.

Non-Newtonian fluids can be subclassified according to how their behaviour deviates from Newtonian models. Shear-thinning fluids, such as blood, become less viscous as the shear rate between the layers increases. An important clinical consequence

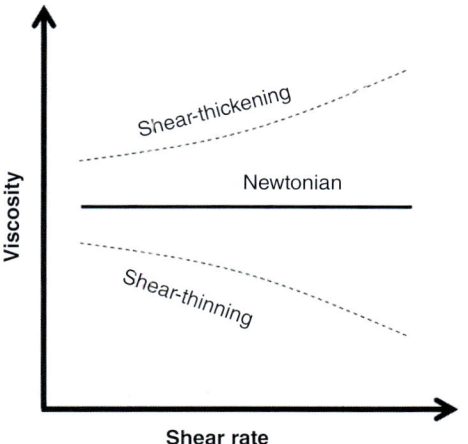 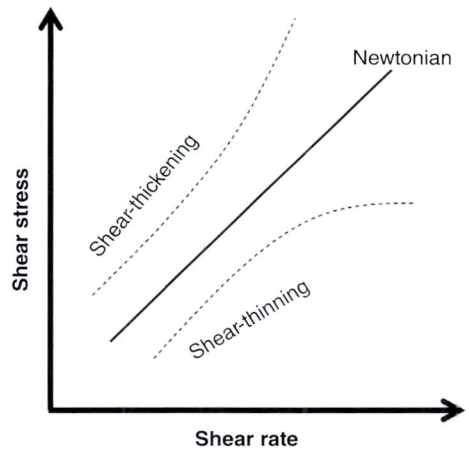

Figure 4.5 Comparison between Newtonian and non-Newtonian fluids

of this is that slower blood flow means more viscous blood which, in turn, alters microvascular flow as the viscosity changes. Meanwhile, shear-thickening fluids such as the cornflour–water mix, Oobleck, become more viscous as they are agitated. Some fluids change their viscosity according to the duration over which the shear force is applied; rheopectic fluids, such as synovial fluid, thicken with time whereas thixotropic fluids become thinner the longer they are agitated, for example ketchup, non-drip paint and cytoplasm. The study of these concepts is known as *rheology*.

Blood is a non-Newtonian fluid and its viscosity is largely dependent on haematocrit, red-cell characteristics and blood protein levels, increasing in diseases such as leukaemia. This causes a reduction in flow which can result in sludging in the pulmonary and cerebral vasculature.

It is important to realize that relationships such as the Hagen–Poiseuille equation do not accurately apply to non-Newtonian fluids (Figure 4.5). That said, for practical purposes, they are a close-enough approximation so, for example, it is reasonable to use the relationship to illustrate the importance of selecting a larger-radius cannula for rapid blood transfusion.

The Movement and Mixing of Fluids

Brownian Motion

Brownian motion describes the random movement of microscopic particles suspended in a liquid or gas. It is due to random collision with the rapidly

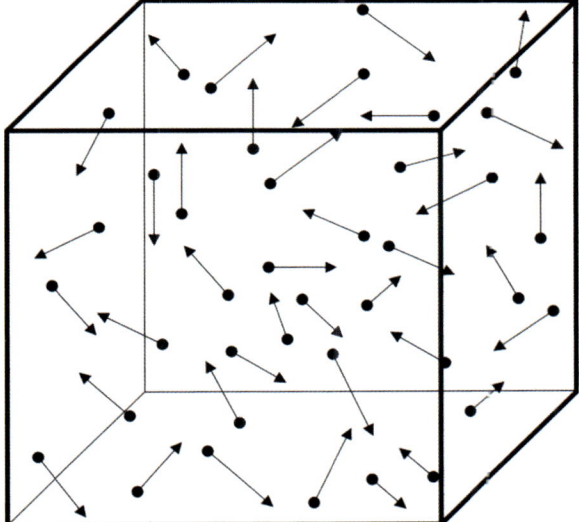

Figure 4.6 Brownian motion: the free, individual particles in the box move at random and fill the medium through which they spread

moving atoms or molecules of the fluid itself (Figure 4.6). Over a period of time, the result of this motion will be to tend to spread the particles evenly throughout the medium. For example, if a drop of food colouring is dropped into a column of water, assuming the dye is completely dissolvable in the water and has the same specific gravity, the dye will spread equally throughout the column of water. The new colour of the liquid will be uniform throughout.

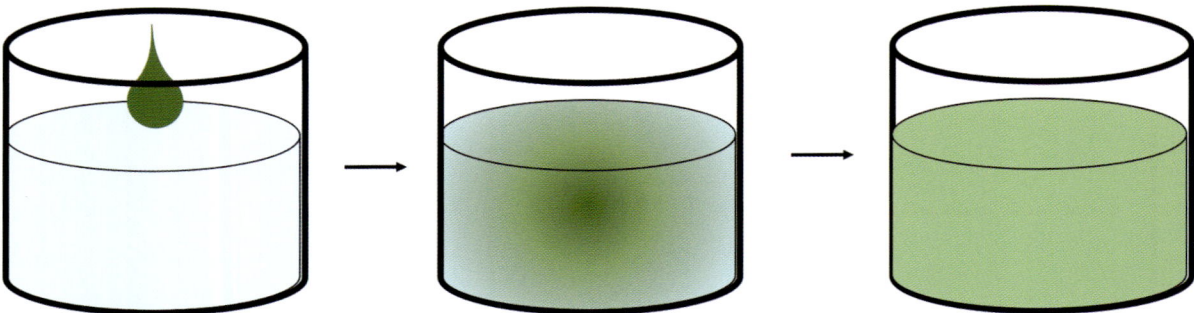

Figure 4.7 Diffusion

Diffusion

Diffusion is the term given to the physical process in which a substance tends to spread steadily from regions of high concentration to regions of lower concentration, as particles intermingle as a result of their kinetic energy.

Let us again consider the example of the drop of food colouring in a beaker of water. The droplet is a very concentrated area of solute, which eventually spreads throughout the beaker (Figure 4.7). The physical principle behind this is still Brownian motion. Dye particles will dart around, changing directions when colliding with another dye particle. The probability of changing directions is proportional to the number of particles surrounding it – otherwise known as the concentration.

Substances also diffuse more quickly at higher temperatures. In 1877, it was suggested by James Maxwell that the explanation lay in the thermal molecular energy of the particles. The idea that molecules of a liquid or gas are constantly in motion, colliding with each other and bouncing back and forth, is a prominent part of the kinetic theory of gases.

Osmosis

Osmosis describes the net movement of a solvent (usually water in biological systems) through a semi-permeable membrane so as to equalize the concentration on both sides of the membrane.

Imagine two solutions of different concentration separated by a semi-permeable membrane which is permeable to the smaller solvent molecules but not to the larger solute molecules. Over time, the solvent will tend to diffuse across the membrane from the less-concentrated to the more-concentrated solution (Figure 4.8). This is osmosis.

Osmosis is of great importance in biological processes. The transport of water across biological membranes is essential to many processes in living organisms. The tendency of this process to proceed is usually quantified in terms of osmotic pressure.

Fluid Mechanics

Fluid mechanics is a massive topic, but we are going to limit our discussion to the principles and effects that are important to anaesthesia and intensive care medicine.

Pascal's Principle

Pascal's principle is an interesting concept. A change in pressure is transmitted undiminished in an enclosed static fluid to all points throughout that fluid.

In the arrangement depicted in Figure 4.9, when a force is applied downwards on Piston A, a pressure is generated in the fluid. This change in pressure (ΔP) is constant everywhere in the fluid. This is Pascal's principle, and a physical concept of which we can make great use. The increase in pressure 'downwards' from Piston A will generate the same increase in pressure upwards on Piston B.

However, we know that pressure is equal to force (F) divided by the area (A) upon which it acts.

$$\text{Change in pressure} = \frac{\text{Force}}{\text{Area}}$$

Since we know that the pressure change will be constant throughout, we can see that:

$$\frac{\text{Force}_A}{\text{Area}_A} = \frac{\text{Force}_B}{\text{Area}_B}$$

It is clear from the equation above that if Area_B is increased, Force_B must increase by the same factor in order to balance the equation.

Chapter 4: Behaviour of Fluids

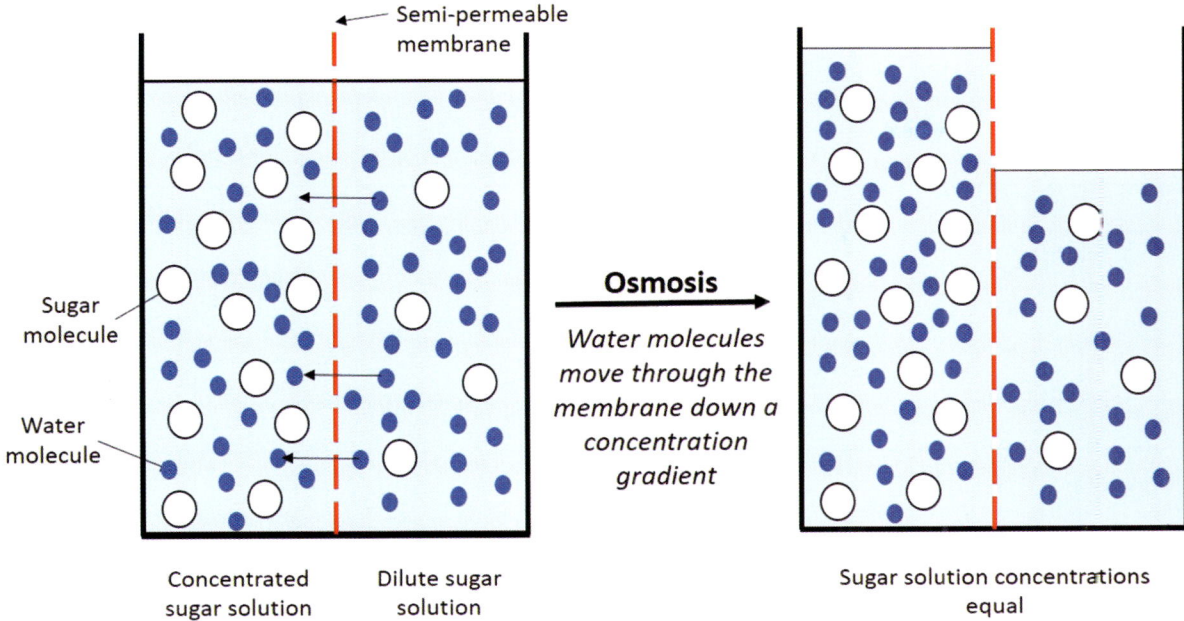

Figure 4.8 Osmosis in sugar solutions

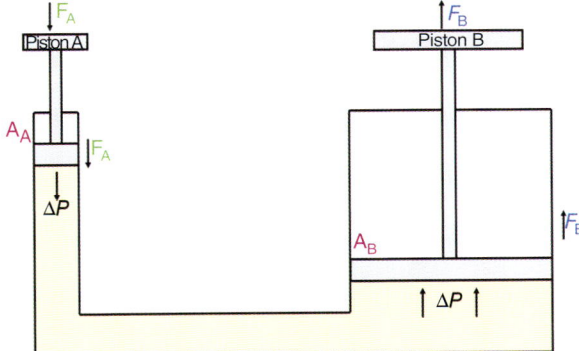

Figure 4.9 Pascal's principle

Using this principle, hydraulic pumps are used to lift very heavy weights with minimal force. There is no difference in the energy needed. Using this simple diagram, it is easier to see why one has to generate a larger force on the plunger of a 20-ml syringe than upon a 2-ml syringe, to create the same pressure.

Bernoulli Principle

Daniel Bernoulli published his work in 1738, in his book titled *Hydrodynamica* [1]. This thesis was based on the simple principle of the conservation of energy in flowing fluids.

In the equation's most simple form, designed for incompressible fluids, the principle states that the sum of all energies (potential, kinetic, internal) remains constant within a system. When applied to the flow of fluid, through a pipe for example, it explains that as the velocity of the fluid increases (and hence kinetic energy), this has to be compensated for by an equal decrease in potential and internal energy.

In the system demonstrated in Figure 4.10, on the left, flow is slow, but consequently has relatively high pressure and potential energy. As it passes through the centre narrowing, it must speed up in order to maintain flow (volume per unit time). As a result, the kinetic energy increases. However, to conserve energy, the potential energy decreases. This is manifest as a drop in pressure.

This same scenario also serves as an illustration of Newton's second law ($F = ma$). We know that pressure is related to force by the cross-sectional area of the pipe. Consequently, a pressure gradient down the pipe generates a force which, depending on the mass of fluid to which it is applied, will accelerate that fluid down the tube. The magnitude of this acceleration is quantified by Newton's equation.

The best-known example of the Bernoulli principle is that of aerodynamic lift. Due to the aerofoil shape of an aircraft wing, the speed of air above

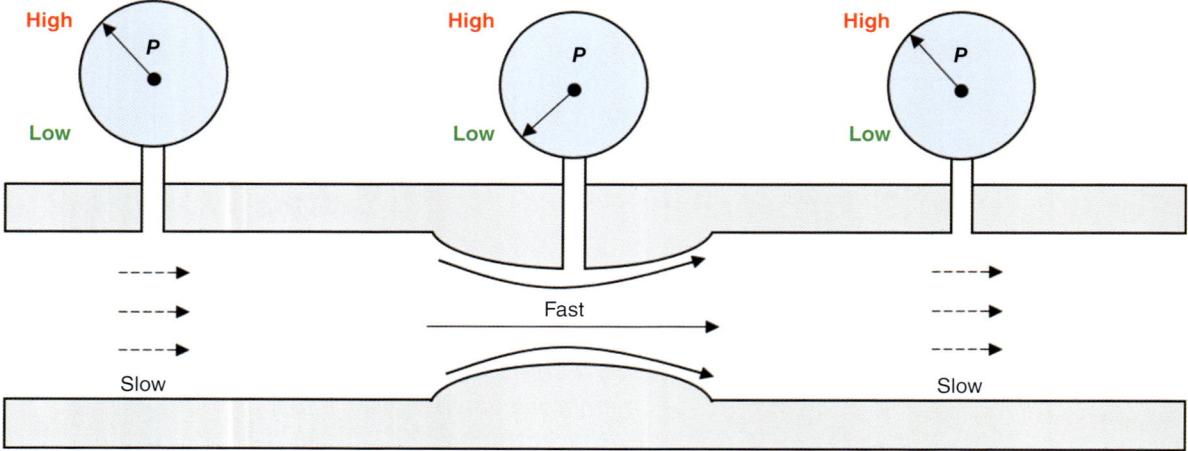

Figure 4.10 The Bernoulli principle

the wing is faster than below it. The higher speed is associated with a lower pressure, and the pressure gradient between the upper and lower surfaces of the wing causes an upward lift.

Venturi Effect

In anaesthetic practice, we rely heavily upon the Venturi effect, which in turn relies upon the Bernoulli principle. We can predict the pressure drop expected at the narrowing of a pipe, as explained by the Bernoulli principle, if the speed of the fluid and the relative sizes of the wide and narrow portions of the tube are known. If we introduce an orifice on the wall of a narrow pipe, external air will be entrained due to the pressure drop. This is known as jet entrainment.

Using this calculation, *Venturi* oxygen masks are designed to mix a predictable amount of oxygen (running through the oxygen tubing) with air (entrained through the orifice) (Figure 4.11). Presetting the oxygen flow and the diameter of the tube and orifice, Venturi oxygen masks can be manufactured to deliver a specific oxygen concentration. Because the entrainment of air and the resulting oxygen concentration is constant, these masks are referred to as fixed-performance devices. By comparison, a simple, non-Venturi face mask operates at lower oxygen flows and the entrainment of room air around the mask is much more relevant. Because the quantity of entrained air varies with the patient's respiratory effort from one breath to the next, the diluting effect of the air and the oxygen varies

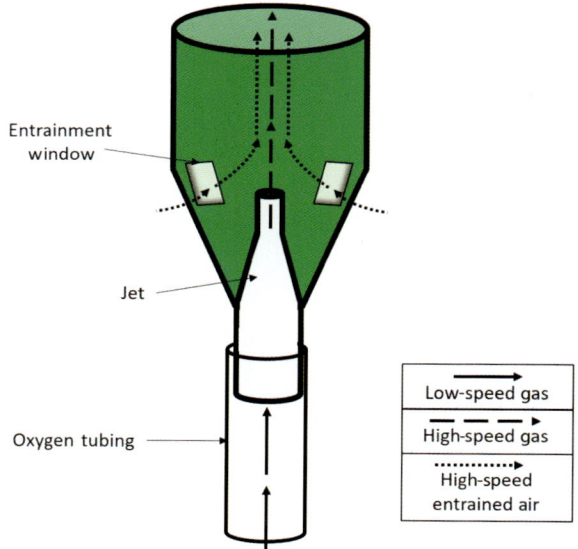

Figure 4.11 The Venturi effect

continuously. These masks (and nasal specs) are therefore referred to as variable-performance systems.

Coanda Effect

The Bernoulli principle and Venturi effect lend themselves to a further interesting phenomenon – the Coanda effect. Henri Coanda was a Romanian physicist, largely interested in aeronautics.

The Venturi effect results in a circumference of low pressure around a jet of fluid. This area of low

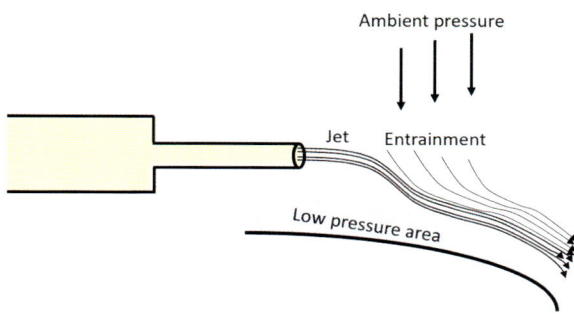

Figure 4.12 The Coanda effect

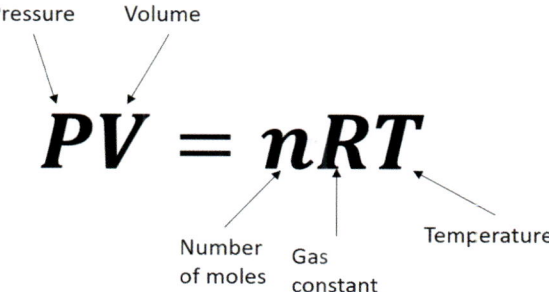

Figure 4.13 The universal gas law

pressure entrains fluid from its surroundings, and the pressure equilibrates.

However, Coanda noted that when a solid surface is placed adjacent and parallel to one side of this jet, the resulting circumferential low pressure, and subsequent 'removal' of air from this side of the jet, cannot be equilibrated as efficiently as the other 'free' side. This pressure difference causes a displacement of the jet towards the area of lower pressure; the solid surface. In effect, the low-pressure area adjacent to the solid surface can only be equilibrated by drawing gas across the stream of the jet and this creates a force on the jet stream, altering its path (Figure 4.12).

The next time you use Doppler ultrasound to visualize flow within a blood vessel, you may notice some heterogeneity within the vessel. This is, in part, due to the Coanda effect, although the reasons for this are actually multifactorial.

Some helicopters are designed without a traditional tail rotor. Yaw thrust is produced by a lengthways slit along the tail boom through which air is forced by a fan. This disrupts the downdraft from the main rotor via the Coanda effect causing the whole tail boom to act like an aerofoil. The pilot's pedals adjust airflow through the slit, allowing the nose of the aircraft to be pointed left or right.

Gas Laws

The gas laws describe the relationship between the pressure, volume and temperature of gases. By the end of the eighteenth century, scientists began to isolate pure gases which obeyed a set of laws – the ideal gas laws. The concept of an 'ideal' gas is useful as it allows predictions about how gases will behave in different clinical situations, such as altered temperature and pressure. An ideal gas has the following properties:

- The volume of the particles (atoms or molecules) relative to the volume they occupy is negligible
- The particles obey Newton's laws of motion
- The particles are so far apart that no attractive or repulsive forces exist between them

The universal gas law (Figure 4.13 above) combines all the ideal gas laws, which we'll discuss further below.

Typically, the ideal gas laws are referenced relative to 'standard temperature and pressure' (STP), i.e. 273 K (0 °C) and atmospheric pressure at sea level (101.3 kPa or 760 mmHg). Under extreme conditions, such as very low temperatures and high pressures, the gas laws are less accurate. Fortunately, the conditions of the clinical environment are close to STP and so real gases approximate well to ideal gases.

Avogadro's Law

Avogadro's law states that, under the same conditions of temperature and pressure, equal volumes of different gases will contain the same number of particles (molecules or atoms), irrespective of their chemical or physical properties. Avogadro's number is a different concept. It allows the molar mass of a substance to be related to that of the standard, carbon-12. The number of particles (carbon atoms) present in 12 g of carbon-12 (1 mol) is 6.02×10^{23} and this is Avogadro's number. Note the difference then: Avogadro's law relates the number of particles in equal volumes, Avogadro's number defines the particles in a specific amount of substance (1 mol).

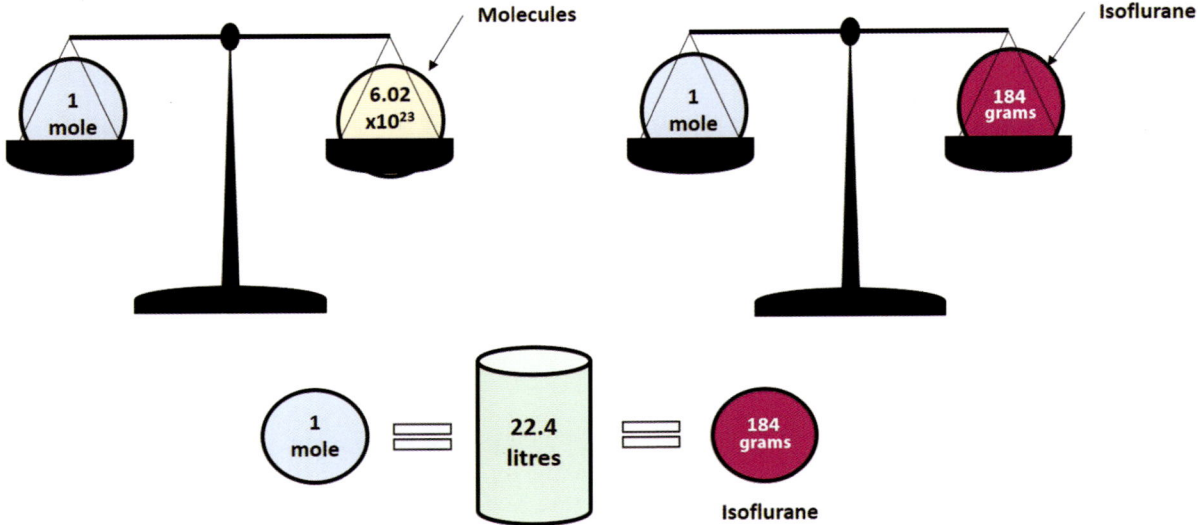

Figure 4.14. Avogadro's law and molecular mass

As seen in Figure 4.14, at STP, one mole of an ideal gas occupies 22.4 litres. If we could count the number of molecules in three balloons, each filled with 22.4 litres (i.e. 1 mole) of either carbon dioxide, hydrogen or helium, each would contain 6.02×10^{23} particles but would have differing masses.

Avogadro's equation can be summarized as:

$$\frac{V}{n} = K$$

where: V = volume of gas, n = molar amount of the gas and K = proportionality constant.

Let's consider a practical example using various anaesthetic mixtures. The molecular weight of isoflurane is 184 g mol^{-1}. Thus, 184 g of isoflurane equals 1 mole and occupies 22.4 l at STP. If a vaporizer contains 18.4 g of isoflurane, this is equal to 0.1 mol (number of moles = mass (g)/molecular mass) and will occupy 2.24 l at STP. If this volume of isoflurane is vaporized in 224 l of oxygen, the concentration will be 1% (2.24/224 = 0.01). Similarly, if this volume is vaporized into either 112 or 22.4 l of oxygen, the concentration will be 2% and 10% respectively (2.24/112 = 0.02; 2.24/22.4 = 0.1) (Figure 4.15).

Dalton's Law of Partial Pressures

Dalton's law of partial pressures states that, for a mixture of gases, the total pressure is always equal to the sum of individual partial pressures, and these pressures are related to the number of molecules and the volume they occupy.

$$P_{total} = P_{gas1} + P_{gas2}$$

where: P_{total} = total pressure, P_{gas1} = partial pressure of gas 1 and P_{gas2} = partial pressure of gas 2. Let's imagine a gas cylinder containing equal amounts (moles) of two different gases with a P_{total} of 100 kPa (P_{gas1} = 50 kPa; P_{gas2} = 50 kPa). If one gas is removed then P_{total} equals 50 kPa. Remember that the volume of the cylinder has not changed.

Clinical example: To what extent do carbon dioxide and water vapour reduce the alveolar partial pressure of oxygen (P_AO_2) when:

$F_iO_2 = 0.21$

Body temperature = 37 °C

Atmospheric pressure (P_{atm}) = 101 kPa

$P_ACO_2 = 5.0$ kPa

To calculate:

$$\begin{aligned} P_AO_2 &= FiO_2 \\ &= 0.21 \times P_{atm} \\ &= 21.2 \text{ kPa} \end{aligned}$$

In other words, the partial pressure of oxygen in the atmosphere is 21.2 kPa. Nitrogen and other gases in air take up the remaining 79.8 kPa.

Now let's see what happens in the deepest part of the lungs. Under normal conditions the partial

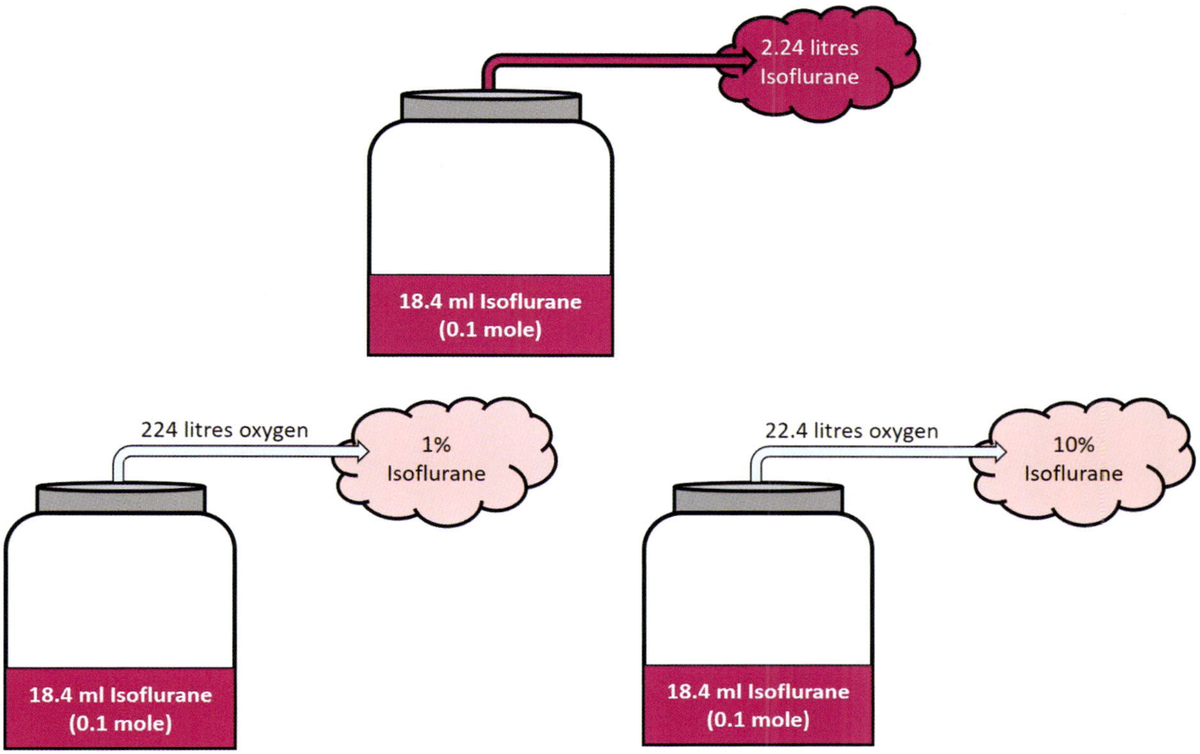

Chapter 4: Behaviour of Fluids

Figure 4.15 Avogadro's law and different concentrations

pressure of water vapour in air is 1.3 kPa. However, following humidification in the airways at 37 °C the saturated vapour pressure of water rises to 6.3 kPa. Thus:

$$P_AO_2 = FiO_2 \times (P_{total} - P_AH_2O) - P_ACO_2$$
$$= 0.21 \times (101 - 6.3) - 5.0$$
$$= 14.9 \text{ kPa}$$

This shows us that when we breathe normal 21 kPa oxygen, it becomes only 14.9 kPa by the time it reaches the depths of our lungs! This particular application of Dalton's law is the alveolar gas equation.

Boyle's Law

Boyle's law is the first ideal gas law and states that, at a constant temperature, the volume of a gas is inversely proportional to its pressure (Figure 4.16). To remember the gas laws, remember that they all relate pressure, volume and temperature in some way. There are a number of *aide memoires* to then remember which is which and, in each case, these remind you which of the three (of P, V or T) is the constant in the relationship. For Boyle's law remember that water 'Boyles' at a

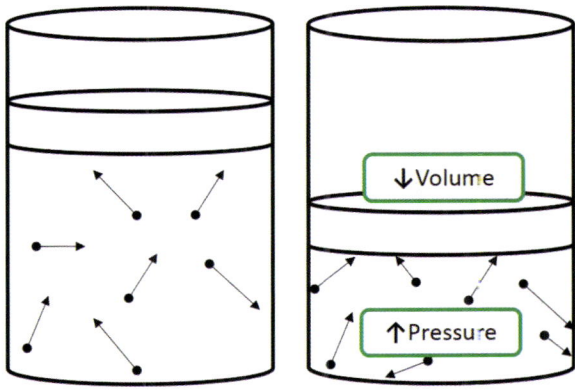

Figure 4.16 Boyle's law

'constant temperature' at sea level; therefore, Boyle's law tells you how volume and pressure are related. Mathematically, the law is given as:

$$V \propto \frac{1}{P}$$

63

Chapter 4: Behaviour of Fluids

Put another way, the product of pressure and volume is a constant:

$$PV = k$$

(P = pressure, V = volume, k = constant)

Worked example: You are about to transfer a patient who is requiring 15 l min^{-1} of oxygen. You have a full 9.4-litre oxygen cylinder (size F) with a gauge pressure of 137 bar (13,700 kPa). How long will the oxygen cylinder last?

Firstly, we need to calculate the absolute pressure in the cylinder (using SI units) and rounding atmospheric pressure from 101.325 kPa to 100 kPa for simplicity, in this example

$$P_{total} = P_{atmospheric} + P_{gauge}$$
$$= 100 + 13,700$$
$$= 13,800 \text{ kPa}$$

Next, we use Boyle's law to determine the volume of gas contained in the cylinder once it is released to atmospheric conditions:

$$P_1 \times V_1 = P_2 \times V_2$$
$$13,800 \times 9.4 = 100 \times V_2$$

Now we need to rearrange to find V_2:

$$V_2 = \frac{P_1 \times V_2}{P_2}$$
$$= \frac{13000 \times 9.4}{100}$$
$$= 1297 \, l$$

Of course, the final internal volume of the cylinder (9.4 litres) cannot discharge its contents because, at that point, the pressure will be in equilibrium with the ambient pressure. This means we need to subtract that volume from V_2 to obtain the usable volume. This gives us a final volume of 1,287 l, which, at 15 l min^{-1}, will last 85 minutes.

Charles's Law

Charles's law is the second ideal gas law and states that if the pressure of a fixed mass of gas is held constant, then the volume and temperature are proportional (Figure 4.17). It may be helpful to remember that Prince 'Charles' is under 'constant pressure' to become King:

$$V \propto T$$

or:

$$\frac{V}{T} = k$$

(V = volume, T = temperature, k = constant)

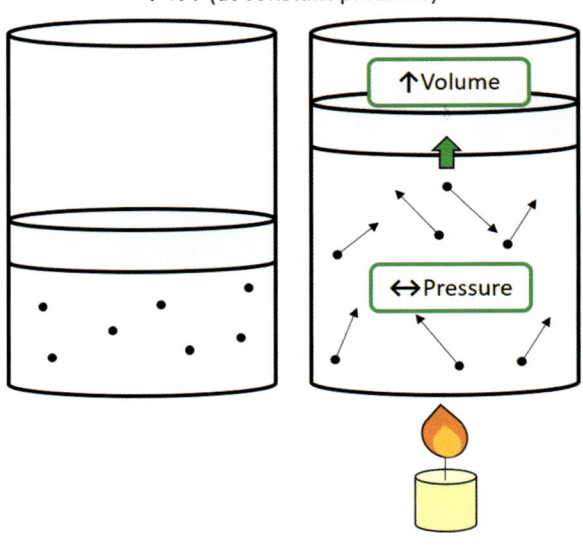

Figure 4.17 Charles's law

A very simple example of this principle is a hot air balloon: when the gas in the balloon is heated, it expands as described by Charles's law. As it expands, it becomes less dense and rises. The same principle underpins convective heat loss for an anaesthetized patient. The air is warmed by radiation and conduction from the skin. This causes the air to expand, reducing density and causing the warmed air to rise away from the patient – this is convection.

Gay-Lussac's Law

Gay-Lussac's law is the third ideal gas law and states that if the volume of a fixed mass of gas is held constant, then the pressure is proportional to temperature (Figure 4.18):

$$P \propto T$$

or:

$$\frac{P}{T} = k$$

(P = pressure, T = temperature, k = constant)

Clinical example: nitrous oxide has a low critical temperature of 36.5 °C and exists as a liquid and a vapour at room temperature. As described by Gay-Lussac's law, a rise in the ambient temperature above the critical temperature will lead to a dramatic increase in pressure within a gas cylinder of fixed volume. If this pressure exceeds the design limits of the cylinder, it could explode.

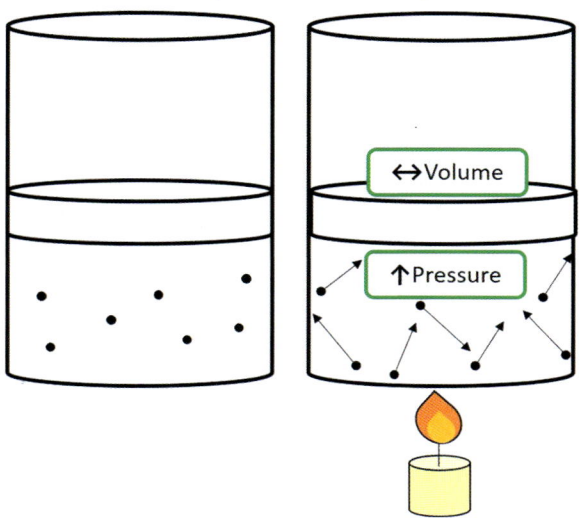

Figure 4.18 Gay-Lussac's law

Combined Gas Law

This is derived by combining the three ideal gas laws:

Boyle's law (constant temperature) : $P \times V = \text{constant}$

Charles's law (constant pressure): $\dfrac{V}{T} = \text{constant}$

Gay-Lussac's law (constant volume): $\dfrac{P}{T} = \text{constant}$

Combining all three laws:

$$\frac{PV}{T} = \text{constant}$$

The combined gas law requires that the amount of gas remain constant. We can mathematically rearrange the equation to allow quantification of the behaviour of a single quantity of gas under two different sets of conditions:

$$\frac{P_1 \times V_1}{T_1} = \frac{P_2 \times V_2}{T_2}$$

Temperature must be in kelvin whilst the values of volume and pressure can be in any units, provided they are the same on both sides of the equation.

Let's consider a clinical example. Four litres of a gas are collected at 37 °C and 760 mmHg. What is the volume of gas at standard temperature and pressure?

$P_1 = 760$ mmHg $\quad P_2 = 760$ mmHg
$V_1 = 4$ l $\quad V_2 = $ to be calculated
$T_1 = 310$ K $\quad T_2 = 273$ K

Rearranging the combined gas law for V_2:

$$V_2 = \frac{P_1 \times V_1 \times T_2}{P_2 \times T_1}$$
$$= \frac{760 \times 4 \times 273}{760 \times 310}$$
$$= 3.5 \text{ l}$$

Universal Gas Law

Remember that the combined gas law states:

$$\frac{PV}{T} = \text{constant}$$

The constant applies to a fixed amount of gas. If this amount changes, the constant will also change but the law will still hold (i.e. PV/T remains valid). The constant is directly proportional to the amount of gas in moles, n – Avogadro's law. The proportionality factor is 8.31 J K^{-1} mol^{-1}, which is the universal gas constant, R. Therefore:

$$\text{Constant} = nR$$

Applying this to the combined gas law:

$$\frac{PV}{T} = nR$$

Alternatively:

$$PV = nRT$$

Again, a clinical example. What volume would 28 g of nitrogen occupy at STP? It is important to remember that nitrogen is a gas above its critical temperature (−147 °C) and therefore cannot be liquefied at STP. Nitrogen has an atomic mass of 14 but is diatomic in its molecular form, with a molecular mass of 28. All units need to be in SI units: temperature in kelvin (273 K), pressure at sea level is 101.325 kPa (although we must use pascal as the unit of pressure in the equation, thus 101,325 Pa), and volume in cubic metres.

$$n = \frac{\text{mass of gas}}{\text{molar mass}}$$
$$= \frac{28}{28}$$
$$= 1 \text{ mol}$$

Rearranging the universal gas law for V:

$$V = \frac{nRT}{P}$$
$$= \frac{1 \times 8.31 \times 273}{101325}$$
$$= 0.0224 \; m^3 \; (\text{or } 22.4 \; l)$$

The above example neatly demonstrates how one mole of a gas occupies 22.4 l at STP.

Henry's Law of Solubility

When a liquid is placed in a closed container it exists in two phases; liquid and vapour. Over time, an equilibrium is reached between condensation and evaporation such that the amount leaving the liquid is equalled by the amount returning to the liquid. The partial pressure exerted by the vapour at equilibrium is the saturated vapour pressure (SVP). The SVP is altered by changes in temperature but not pressure. An increase in temperature pushes the equilibrium towards evaporation and increases the SVP.

Henry's law states that at a constant temperature, the amount of a given gas dissolved in a given liquid is directly proportional to the partial pressure of that gas in equilibrium with that liquid. Put simply, the greater the pressure, the more the gas dissolves.

The only factors that affect the partial pressure of a volatile agent in the blood are:
(1) The SVP of the agent
(2) Ambient temperature
(3) Alveolar concentration

If you imagine a bottle of carbonated soft drink and pour it equally between two glasses, one chilled glass and another at room temperature, which one bubbles more? The answer is the one at room temperature, because solubility is inversely proportional to temperature. As solubility falls with rising temperature, the gas bubbles out of the solution and evaporates.

Consider nitrogen; it is relatively insoluble in blood at atmospheric pressure at sea level. However, during a diving descent, the partial pressure of nitrogen increases. This causes an increase in the amount of dissolved nitrogen in the blood. If a diver ascends too quickly, dissolved nitrogen comes out of the blood and causes decompression sickness.

Graham's Law

Graham's law of diffusion states that the rate at which a gas diffuses is inversely proportional to the square root of its molecular weight.

$$\text{Rate of diffusion} \propto \frac{1}{\sqrt{\text{Molecular mass}}}$$

The larger the atom or molecule, the slower it diffuses. This explains the rates at which gases mix. For example, if the sevoflurane vaporizer is left on in the anaesthetic room with fresh gas flowing, we can use Graham's law to predict how long it will take until the vapour is smelt in the adjacent theatre (ignoring the effects of the air-conditioning system, of course). Similarly, we could use the law to compare the rate of diffusion of two different gases, based on the molecular mass. Of nitrous oxide and sevoflurane, which leak would reach our noses first?

$$\frac{\text{Rate of diffusion for nitrous oxide}}{\text{Rate of diffusion for sevoflurane}}$$

$$\propto \frac{\sqrt{\text{Molecular mass of sevoflurane}}}{\sqrt{\text{Molecular mass of nitrous oxide}}}$$

$$\propto \frac{\sqrt{200}}{\sqrt{44}}$$

$$= 2.1$$

If you were far enough away that it took 10 minutes for the sevoflurane to reach your nose, you would have been breathing the leaking nitrous oxide for more than 5 minutes already, as it would diffuse from the leaking anaesthetic machine twice as quickly.

Fick's Law

The rates of diffusion described by Graham's law do not account for transmission through biological membranes. At the risk of drifting from physics too far into physiology, it is worth mentioning Fick's law for completeness. In essence, Fick's law combines the rate of gaseous diffusion as described by Graham's law and adds parameters which account for the physical characteristics of the membrane so as to describe the amount of gas which passes through the membrane per unit of time (gas flux):

$$\text{Gas flux} = \frac{A}{T} \times D \times (P_1 - P_2)$$

where: A = surface area for diffusion, T = thickness of the membrane and P = partial pressures of the gas on either side of the membrane. The term D is the diffusion coefficient and this is where Graham's law features because D is proportional to the solubility of the gas divided by the square root of the molecular mass.

As a clinical example, the *second gas effect* is explained by Fick's law. We know from our example of Graham's law that the value of D will be 2.1 times greater for nitrous oxide than sevoflurane. As all the other terms in Fick's equation relate to the same membrane (the alveolar–capillary interface) we can see that the gas flux for both gases will be proportional to D. In other words, nitrous oxide is taken up out of the alveolus twice as quickly as sevoflurane. This concentrates the sevoflurane in the alveolus and, in turn, increases the flux of sevoflurane by increasing the partial pressure gradient for the volatile. This increases the speed of onset of anaesthesia, quite apart from the sedating influence of the nitrous oxide. This is the second gas effect.

Summary

The physics behind the behaviour of fluids is a complex yet interesting topic. As with many aspects of physics, fluid behaviour is modelled by idealistic laws but real-world characteristics depend on how closely the fluid follows these ideal Newtonian principles. Fluid flow may be laminar or turbulent in nature, and the propensity for a fluid to behave according to a laminar flow model is predicted using the Reynolds calculation. Understanding the differing characteristics of laminar and turbulent flow and having some idea as to when one is more likely than the other has significant clinical relevance.

The mixing and movement of fluids follows an ordered chaos, dictated by concepts of Brownian motion, diffusion and osmosis. These effects apply at a microscale. Fluid movement on a macroscale is described by fluid mechanics and central to this are the Pascal and Bernoulli principles which, in turn, explain the Venturi and Coanda effects. The physics behind this is employed in many of our medical devices.

The term 'fluid' includes gases and liquids but, in addition to the principles of fluid mechanics, gas behaviour is described by a further set of laws. These are Boyle's law, Charles's law and Gay-Lussac's law. These laws form the basis of the ideal gas law and are inextricably linked to Avogadro's law. These laws interweave interestingly to explain how gases behave.

Questions

MCQs – select true or false for each response

1. Which of the following are true with regards to the movement of fluids?
    (a) It is easier to inject fluid from a 20-ml syringe than a 2-ml syringe because of a larger cross-sectional area over which to exert a force
    (b) Both liquids and gases are conventionally classified as fluids
    (c) Blue motion describes the random movement of microscopic particles suspended in a liquid or gas
    (d) Graham's law of diffusion states that the rate at which gas diffuses is inversely proportional to the square root of its molecular weight
    (e) Fick's law describes the rate of passage of a gas through a membrane
2. Which of the following statements regarding laminar and turbulent flow are correct?
    (a) In laminar flow, the flow rate is inversely proportional to the fluid viscosity
    (b) In laminar flow, the flow rate is directly proportional to the fourth power of the radius
    (c) Turbulent flow will always be present if the Reynolds number is greater than 1,000
    (d) Turbulent flow will always be present if the Reynolds number is greater than 2,000
    (e) In turbulent flow, the flow rate is inversely proportional to the fluid density
3. Which of the following laws, effects and principles are accurate?
    (a) Pascal's principle describes changes in pressure adjacent to a moving fluid
    (b) The Bernoulli principle states that the sum of all energies remains constant within a closed system
    (c) The Venturi effect describes the effect upon a jet of gas when flowing adjacent to a solid surface
    (d) The Coanda effect describes the effect upon a moving jet of gas when exposed to another source of gas

(e) Henry's law is the principle behind the flight of an aeroplane
4. The gas laws describe the relationship between pressure, volume and temperature. Which of the following statements regarding the gas laws are true?
   (a) According to Boyle's law halving the volume (V) of a container will halve the absolute pressure (P) of the same mass of gas contained in that container.
   (b) At any one particular temperature, if an equilibrium exists between the rate of molecules transferring between a liquid and its vapour, the vapour above the liquid is said to be at its saturated vapour pressure (SVP)
   (c) The ideal gas law is a combination of Boyle's, Charles's, Gay-Lussac's and Avogadro's laws and states that $PV = nRT$
   (d) An adiabatic change occurs when the state of a system is altered by exchanging heat with its surroundings
   (e) Isotherms can be used to describe the relationship between temperature and volume for a substance at different pressures
5. Regarding fluid flow and pressure:
   (a) In a Venturi device, a marked fall in pressure occurs across a constriction in a tube where the cross-section gradually reduces and then increases
   (b) The Hagen–Poiseuille equation accurately predicts flow of blood within the circulation
   (c) Flow of gas within the respiratory system may be both proportional and inversely proportional to the pressure gradient
   (d) In turbulent flow, the flow through a tube is proportional to the pressure difference between the ends of a tube
   (e) In laminar flow, the resistance of a tube is a constant and can be defined as the ratio of pressure to flow

Answers

1. FTFTT
   It is actually easier to inject fluid through a smaller syringe and this principle is explained above by Pascal's principle. Brownian motion describes the random movement of microscopic particles suspended in a liquid or gas, not blue motion.

2. TTFFF
   Laminar flow is governed by the Hagen–Poiseuille equation:

   $$Q = \frac{\pi P r^4}{8 \eta L}$$

   where

   Q = flow
   P = pressure
   r = radius of tube
   η = viscosity
   L = length of tube

   Reynolds values of over 2,000 suggest a higher probability that turbulent flow will occur but this is not an exact prediction, either above or below this threshold.

3. FTFFF
   Bernoulli's principle does indeed state that the sum of all energies remains constant within a closed system. It is this principle that is utilized in Venturi masks when potential energy and kinetic energy are exchanged. Pascal's principle describes a constant pressure within the system. The Venturi and Coanda effects are similar. However, Coanda describes the effect of a jet stream when flowing beside a solid surface. The Venturi effect describes the entrainment of a gas when exposed to a moving alternative jet of gas. Henry's law describes solubility, and is not involved in the explanation of flight

4. FTTFF
   The gas laws consist of three primary laws: Boyle's law, Charles's law and the Gay-Lussac law; combined together, they make up the ideal gas law. The constant in each of the laws can be remembered by the following: Boyle = boil = temperature, (Prince) Charles = P for pressure, leaving the third law constant, which must be V, volume. For a gas to change state, heat energy must be added or taken away. However, a change of state can also occur without a gas exchanging heat energy with its environment; an adiabatic change. An isotherm is a curved line relating pressure to volume for a substance at different temperatures.

5. TFTFT
   A fall in pressure at the narrowest point of a Venturi tube is known as the Bernoulli effect and it is used in many different devices, including the Venturi oxygen mask. Due to the drop in pressure (potential energy) there is an increase in fluid velocity (kinetic energy) because the total energy of

the system must remain constant. This allows fluid or gas to be entrained at the constriction. In the Venturi mask, air is entrained, causing dilution of the oxygen to give a clinically useful concentration reaching the patient.

Fluid flow can be described as laminar or turbulent. Flow is more likely to be turbulent if the velocity increases, such as at a constriction in a tube. Reynold's number can be calculated from the velocity, diameter, density and viscosity of a fluid and is used to give a figure to show if laminar or turbulent flow is most likely to be present. In laminar flow, flow is proportional to the pressure gradient. However, in turbulent flow, the flow is proportional to the square root of the pressure gradient. Both laminar and turbulent flow exist within the respiratory tree under normal conditions, hence the relationship between pressure and flow varies. The relationship under laminar conditions is described by the Hagen–Poiseuille equation. This is a good approximation but not an accurate prediction of blood flow for two reasons. Firstly, blood is non-Newtonian and so the equation does not apply. Secondly, not all parts of the circulation are under laminar conditions, e.g. heart valves, vessel bifurcations, cardiac chambers.

References

1. D. Bernoulli. *Hydrodynamica, sive de viribus et motibus fluidorum commentarii: opus academicum ab auctore, dum Petropoli ageret, congestum* (Johannis Reinholdi Dulseckeri, 1738).

Chapter 5

Gas Measurement and Supply

Jonathan Paige

Learning Objectives
- To define pressure and be able to relate different units of pressure measurement
- To explain how pressure is measured
- To understand and describe how gas pressures are manipulated in hospitals
- To explain how gas volumes and flows can be measured
- To describe the physical principles of how medical gases are supplied to the hospital
- To explain the safety features around medical gas supplies

Chapter Content
- Measurement of pressure of gases
- Manipulation of high-pressure gases
- Gas volume measurement
- Gas flow measurement
- Supply of medical gases

Scenario
You are anaesthetizing a patient for drainage of an abscess and decide to use oxygen and nitrous oxide along with an anaesthetic vapour.

How are these gases supplied and how do we ensure accurate measures of airway pressures and tidal volumes during the procedure?

Introduction
This chapter will build upon the discussions around behaviour of gases which you will have read about in Chapter 4. Pressure and its measurement are key concepts for the anaesthetist to understand. Every day we would expect to look at and understand the relevance of blood pressure, airway pressure, gas supply pressures and even tissue pressure and its relevance to pressure injury to our patients. Pressure is the amount of force applied per unit of surface area. This is described by the equation:

$$\text{Pressure} = \frac{\text{Force}}{\text{Area}}$$

In SI units, force is measured in newtons and area in metres squared. The unit of pressure is the pascal (Pa). In reality, as the force of 1 N is small and the surface area of 1 m^2 is quite large, 1 Pa is a very small pressure so it is often more practical to use the kilopascal (kPa).

As described above, the SI unit for pressure is the pascal. However, many different units of measurement are used throughout medicine. Blood pressure is usually described in terms of millimetres of mercury (due to the historical use of the mercury sphygmomanometer), airway pressures are described in centimetres of water, piped gas supplies and cylinders can be described as atmospheres, bar or kPa. Table 5.1 gives a comparison of these units.

Table 5.1 Comparison of various pressure units

Unit	Symbol	1 kPa =	kPa unit^{-1}
Kilopascal	kPa	1	1
Millimetres of mercury	mmHg	7.5	0.133
Centimetres of water	cmH$_2$O	10.2	0.0981
Atmosphere	atm	0.0098	101.325
Bar	bar	0.01	100
Torr	torr	7.5	0.133
Pound per square inch	psi	0.145	6.89

Measurement of Pressure of Gases

When measuring pressure, the first concept to understand is that of gauge pressure versus absolute or total pressure. Gauge pressure is the pressure within a container on top of atmospheric pressure, whereas absolute pressure is the total pressure referenced against a vacuum. For example, an oxygen cylinder may have 137 atm of pressure as read on the gauge, meaning the absolute pressure is 138 atm. This is because, even when the cylinder is 'emptied' until no further gas flows out, there will still be some oxygen left within it; a volume of oxygen at 1 atm. As there is no pressure gradient between the cylinder and the environment at that point though, that final quantity of oxygen cannot be discharged.

Bourdon Gauge

The Bourdon gauge is an aneroid manometer. The term 'aneroid' derives from the Greek 'a', meaning without, and 'neros', meaning water. A Bourdon gauge relies on the principle that a flattened tube will try to return to a cylinder if the pressure within it increases. This would normally cause tiny changes in the physical dimensions of the tube. However, if the flattened tube is also coiled, as it tries to return to a cylindrical shape, this small movement will also cause the coil to straighten, amplifying the movement. A needle is attached to the end of the tube via a gear. The needle will sweep across a calibrated scale as the tube changes shape. The Bourdon gauge can be used for almost any pressure range depending on the material used to create the coil, the thickness of the wall of the tube and the gearing ratio where the needle attaches. See Chapter 3 for more details.

Manometer

A manometer works on the principle that in a tube containing fluid, a pressure applied to one end will cause the fluid to move up the tube against gravity until the force due to the pressure applied is balanced by the force acting on the fluid column due to gravity (this depends on the tube being open to the atmosphere). A typical U-tube arrangement is shown in Figure 5.1.

The pressure (P) applied over an area (A) can be calculated from the density of the fluid (ρ), volume (V) and acceleration due to gravity (g) as we know that:

$$P = \frac{F}{A}$$

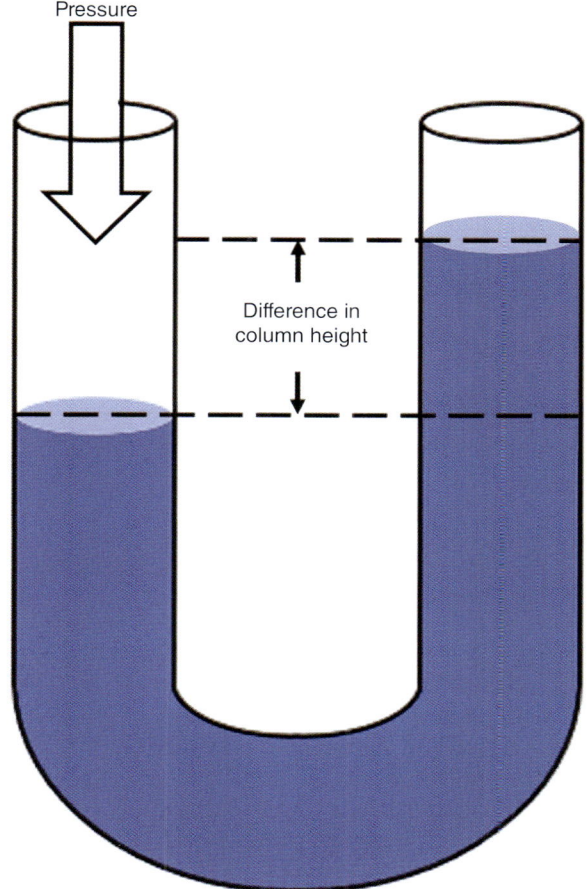

Figure 5.1 U-tube manometer

where:

$$F = ma, \quad i.e. \quad F = mg$$

and:

$$m = \rho V$$

Therefore:

$$P = \frac{mg}{A}$$
$$= \frac{\rho V g}{A}$$

As volume divided by the area gives the height (h) of the column:

$$P = \rho h g$$

This is known as the hydrostatic pressure equation and it demonstrates that the density of the fluid plays a part in determining the range of the pressure that can be measured. For higher pressure measurements like blood pressure, it is more practical to use a dense fluid (historically this was mercury); a water-based manometer would need to be nearly 3 m long to accommodate a systolic blood pressure of 200 mmHg. On the other hand, for low pressure measurements such as airway pressures, less-dense fluids, like water, give a more practical range of values.

In most instances within medicine, we simply record the pressure as the height of the column of fluids. For example, we use mmHg or cmH$_2$O rather than converting this height into pascals (the hydrostatic pressure equation would give a pressure in pascals (Pa) with appropriate SI units used for all the other terms).

A manometer can be changed into a barometer (a device which measures absolute pressure) by sealing up the end of the tube that would normally be open to the air and ensuring a vacuum exists between this sealed end and the column of fluid. This therefore means that rather than measuring a gauge pressure against atmospheric pressure, the pressure determined by the height of the column of fluid is measured against the pressure exerted by a vacuum, which is zero. Therefore, the pressure measured by this system is that of all pressures acting on the column of fluid.

The vacuum in a barometer tube is not a true vacuum. There will always be some vapour from the fluid itself within this space. It is termed a Torricellian vacuum after Italian physicist Evangelist Torricelli, who devised the mercury barometer. His name is also given to the unit of pressure which almost equates to 1 mmHg, the torr.

Manipulation of High-Pressure Gases

Pressure-Reducing Valves

Within anaesthetic practice we rely on pressure-reducing valves. They form essential components of an anaesthetic machine, allowing the high pressures of gas stores to be reduced to near-atmospheric levels so they are safe for use with patients. They also allow the circle system to function by only allowing flow in one direction, they give us control over hand ventilation via the adjustable pressure-limiting valve and they allow scavenging equipment to work.

In the pressure-reducing valve (Figure 5.2), gas from the high-pressure source forces the diaphragm up against the spring. This lifts a conical needle into the entry orifice, restricting flow into the chamber. Due to the reduced entry of gas entering the chamber, the pressure then falls. Once the gas pressure can no longer fully oppose the spring, the needle valve re-opens and pressure rises in the chamber again. In this way, provided the tension in the spring is constant, a constant downstream pressure results, even if the upstream pressure fluctuates. The degree of pressure reduction is dependent on the tension in the spring. The adjustable pressure-limiting valve in an anaesthetic circuit works by allowing the anaesthetist to adjust the tension in the valve spring. This alters the maximal pressure within the breathing circuit, which allows for artificial ventilation and positive end-expiratory pressure (PEEP) to be applied. It also protects the patient from excessive pressures generated within the circle. For more information on placement of adjustable pressure valves in breathing circuits, see Chapter 9.

Another variant of the pressure valve that is regularly used in anaesthetic practice is the two-stage Entonox valve. This is frequently found in use within the labour ward and emergency departments, allowing patients access to analgesia. The two-stage valve essentially comprises a pressure-reducing valve, connected in sequence to a demand valve (Figure 5.3). When the patient sucks on the mouthpiece, the negative pressure generated in the chamber operates a tilt valve, allowing Entonox to flow from the pressure-reducing stage. It then passes through the demand-valve portion of the apparatus and into the patient's mouth. When the patient stops inhaling, the pressure in the demand valve equilibrates to atmospheric pressure. causing the tilt valve to close and the flow of gas to cease.

Oxygen Failure Whistle

Modern anaesthetic machines use electronic sensors to detect a drop in oxygen supply pressure and alert the anaesthetist to the possibility of a hypoxic mixture of gases being delivered to the patient. Older machines, however, rely on a mechanical system such as the Ritchie whistle (Figure 5.4). This alarm is

Chapter 5: Gas Measurement and Supply

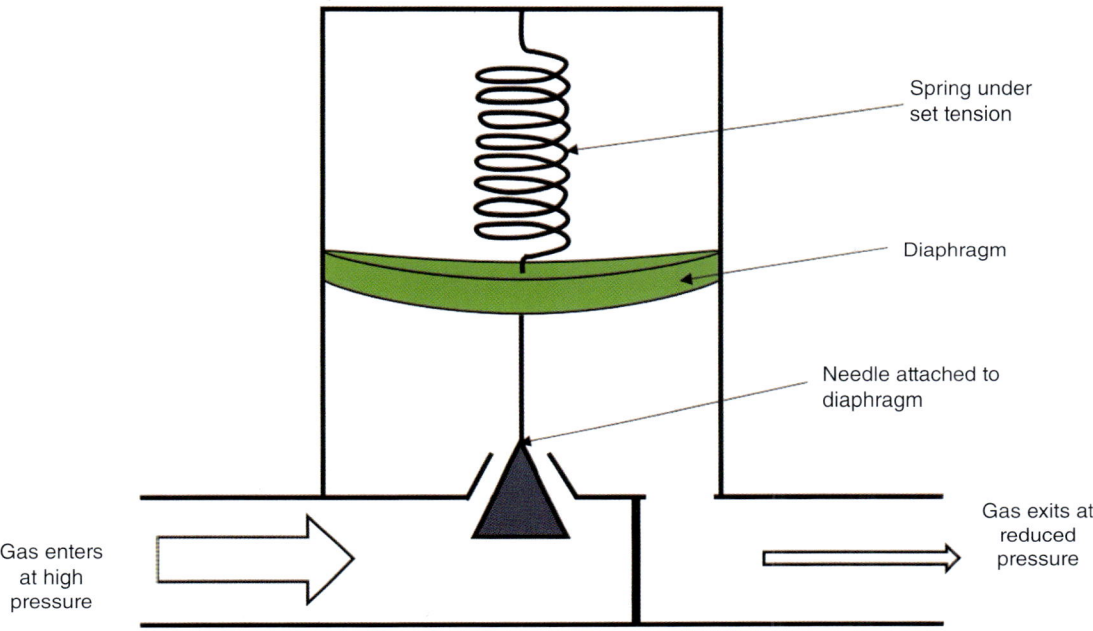

Figure 5.2 A pressure-reducing valve

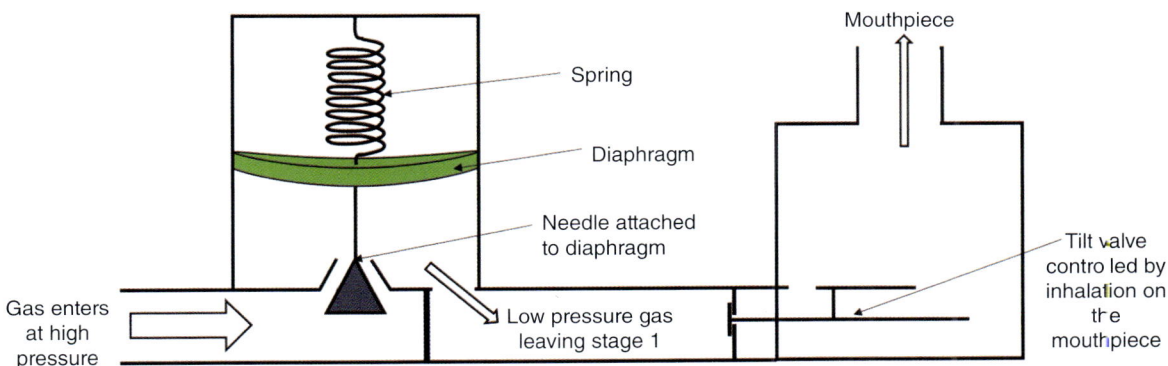

Figure 5.3 Two-stage Entonox valve

entirely pressure-driven so will continue to function in the event of electrical failure. It operates much as a pressure-reducing valve in reverse. Gas entering the main chamber applies pressure to the diaphragm against the spring. This keeps the stopper in position to occlude the exit orifice so gas cannot flow into the whistle chamber. However, as gas supply pressure falls below the set threshold, the diaphragm is not pushed up so the opening to the whistle chamber is opened and the sound is created by the rapidly diminishing flow of gas escaping via a whistle.

The simplicity of the oxygen failure whistle device was both its strength and weakness. It only relied on the pressure it was sensing in order to operate so there was no electrical or other element that could fail and cause a false-negative alarm. However, once the supply has failed the alarm can sound only as long as residual pressure remains in the system and, after that, there is no further alert. A similar device, the Bosun's whistle, also had an electrical light to cause a persisting alert after the whistle had ceased.

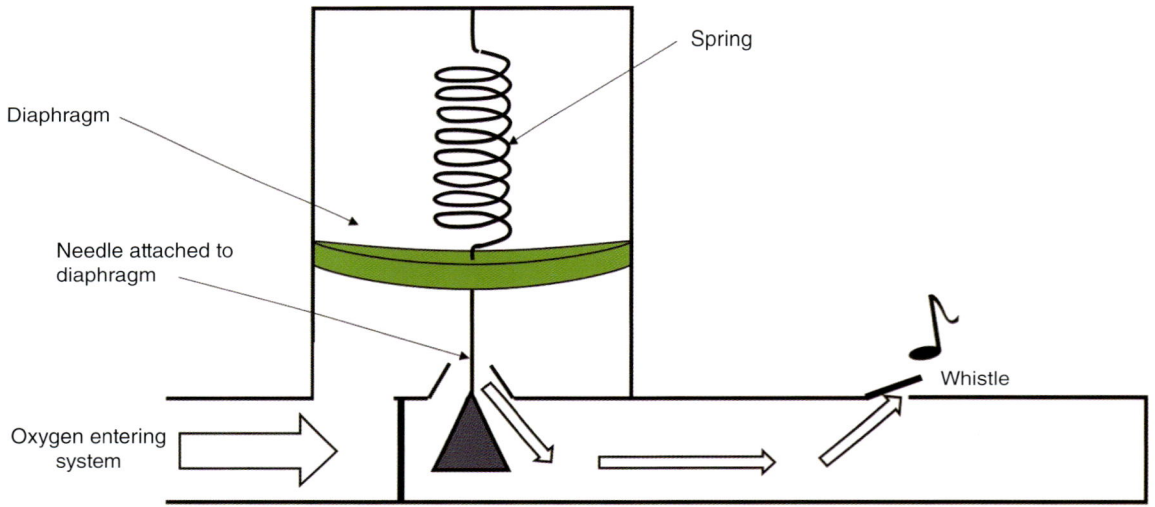

Figure 5.4 Ritchie-type oxygen failure whistle

Gas Volume Measurement

Gas volume measurement is of vital importance for the anaesthetist. During the preoperative phase, lung function can be measured through spirometry. In theatres and critical care practice, measuring tidal volumes of ventilator breaths is crucial to safe respiratory support. Quantifying the flow of gas is also important but this can be achieved very easily; flow is the volume of fluid past a point per unit time.

Benedict Roth Spirometer

The Benedict Roth spirometer was one of the first pieces of equipment used to measure volumes of gas. It consists of a mouthpiece for the patient to breathe through and a lightweight bell which acts as the collection chamber (Figure 5.5). This bell is sealed by water so it is free to move. The surface area of the water seal is kept to a minimum to reduce the amount of gas from the breaths which dissolves in the water (as this would cause inaccuracy). The bell is attached to a pencil via a system of pulleys and a rotating paper drum allows the spirometry trace to be drawn. As the patient breathes in, the bell falls due to the reduction in volume within it. This then pulls the pencil up. As the patient breathes out the reverse happens. As long as the cross-sectional area of the bell is known, the volumes of breaths drawn on the paper drum can be calculated.

Vitalograph®

The Vitalograph® is a simpler type of spirometer where the patient breathes into a set of bellows. A pencil is attached to the moving side of the bellows. A piece of calibrated paper moves along a slide, under the pencil, at a fixed speed, and this draws the spirometry trace as the patient breathes out. This is the common device found in respiratory and anaesthetic preoperative assessment clinics for obtaining values for forced vital capacity (FVC) and forced expiratory volume in 1 s (FEV_1).

Wright Respirometer

The Wright respirometer (Figure 5.6) is more usable within anaesthetic practice due to its small size when compared to the Benedict Roth spirometer or Vitalograph®. Gas enters the device and is directed so as to spin a vane mounted in the centre of the device. This is attached to a dial to give a read-out of volume. The advantage of the Wright respirometer is that a series of gears can be placed in the attachment between the vane and the dial, allowing it to be calibrated for different volume ranges. It is also light and portable,

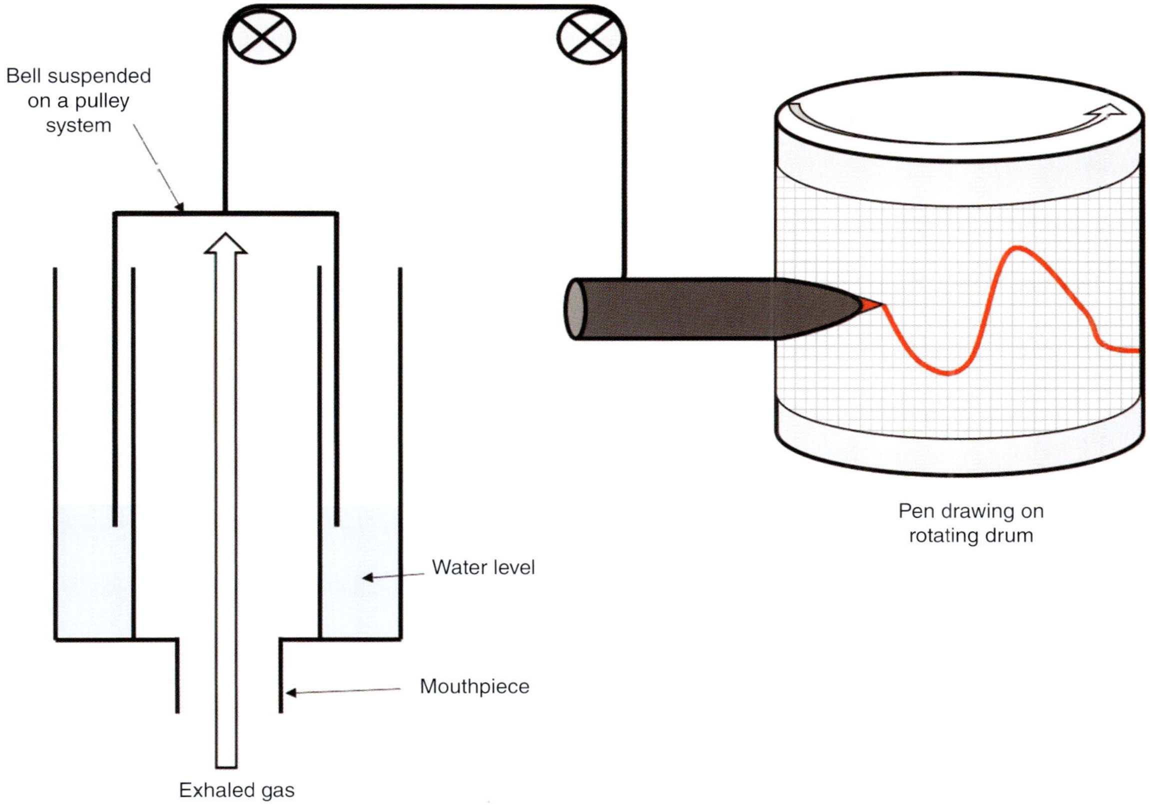

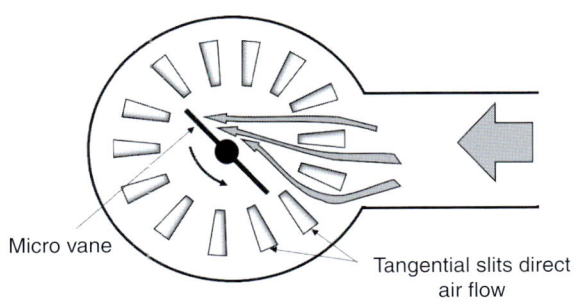

Figure 5.5 The Benedict Roth spirometer

Figure 5.6 A Wright respirometer

and requires no electrical supply. The disadvantages are that it can only measure gas flow in one direction so, to measure inspired and expired volumes, two meters need to be used. It cannot give an electrical display of the readings and it is inaccurate at high and low volumes. This is because at high volumes, momentum causes the vane to continue to move for a short time after flow has ceased. At low volumes, the proportion of energy used to start the vane rotating is a significant proportion of the total energy from the breath. This portion does not translate into movement of the needle and a reading of volume.

Electrical Volume Meter

The electrical volume meter (Figure 5.7) works in a very similar way to the Wright respirometer in that gas flows through the meter and is directed to spin a vane. The difference is that instead of the vane being attached directly to a dial, a beam of light is shone through the path of the vane tip. A detector allows the number of times the tip cuts the beam to be counted. This signal passes to a microprocessor and is displayed as a volume on a monitor. The advantages of such a system are that it leads to an electrical read-out, and that the system is bi-directional, allowing measurements of both inspiratory and expiratory volumes. As the vane is not attached to a dial, there is also less

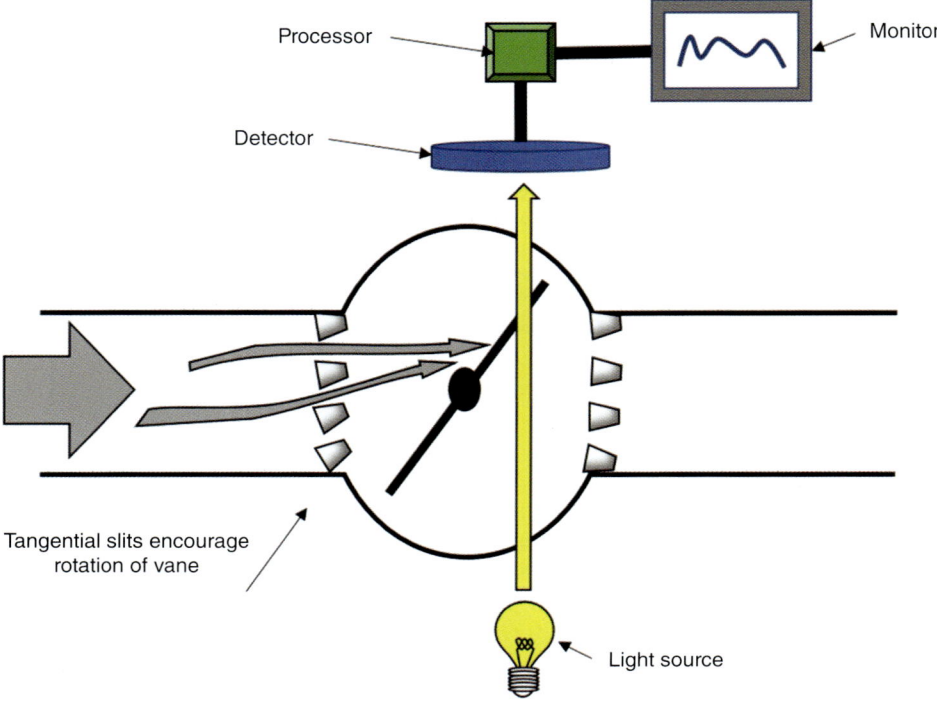

Figure 5.7 Electrical volume meter

resistance to movement so it is more accurate than the mechanical Wright respirometer, particularly for small volumes. The main disadvantages are that it requires an electrical supply and is relatively expensive compared to simpler technology.

Gas Flow Measurement

As discussed earlier, gas flow equates to volume of gas per unit time. Flow measurements are central to monitoring a patient's respiratory performance and in regulating the functions of equipment such as anaesthetic machines and ventilators. The most common gas flowmeter is the variable-orifice flowmeter. This is used on most wards for oxygen delivery and also within some anaesthetic machines (electronic systems are becoming more common in this setting, however). The flowmeter consists of a bobbin in a tapered gas tube (Figure 5.8). As gas flow increases, the force pushing the bobbin up increases. As the tubes are tapered, when the bobbin rises, the gap around the bobbin also increases allowing more of the gas flow to escape through this route; this means that the

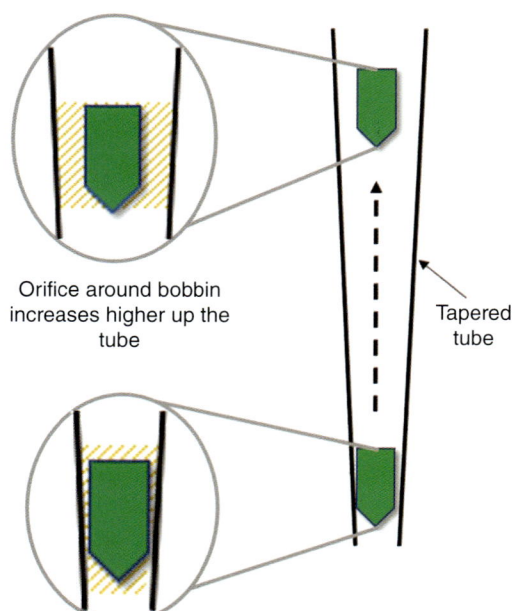

Figure 5.8 Anaesthetic machine flat-topped bobbin flowmeter within a tapered tube

pressure around the bobbin is constant. These types of flowmeter are therefore termed constant-pressure, variable-orifice flowmeters.

At low flows, the orifice around the bobbin is narrow and laminar flow predominates. At higher flows, the orifice opens up due to the taper of the tube. This predisposes to turbulent flow. Consequently, the pressure suspending the bobbin against gravity changes from being proportional to flow to being proportional to the square of flow. This means the scale on the tube will not be linear. Although, by designing the tube with a variable taper, the scale can be made linear.

In an anaesthetic machine, a flat-topped bobbin is generally used, with flow being measured from the top of the bobbin. This flat surface allows easier and more accurate readings to be made against the scale. Angled slits are cut into the bobbin to encourage it to spin when gas is flowing, as a visual clue that the bobbin has not got stuck. The spinning of the bobbin has the downside that it can induce an electrostatic charge if the bobbin does touch the wall; therefore, most anaesthetic machine flowmeters have a conducting strip down the side to dissipate this charge. On most wards, these problems are overcome by using a ball bobbin. For these, the readings should be made from the middle of the ball. This makes it less accurate as the middle of the ball is more difficult to define but less prone to sticking.

Flowmeters are specific to a particular gas. The height of the bobbin depends on the pressure of the gas generated by the flow into the bottom of the tube. As with a manometer, the balance of pressure and gravity determines the vertical displacement of the bobbin. The pressure exerted depends on density of the gas. Flowmeters for different gases can be designed to the same length to fit alongside one another in the anaesthetic machine simply by changing the weight of the bobbin. Additionally, at low flows, the gap around the bobbin is small, encouraging laminar flow to occur. The tendency to laminar flow is viscosity-dependent. At high flows, the gap is larger so turbulent flow occurs, at which point the density of the gas is important (see Chapter 4). Consequently, as different gases have different densities and viscosities, a single flowmeter cannot be accurate for all gases.

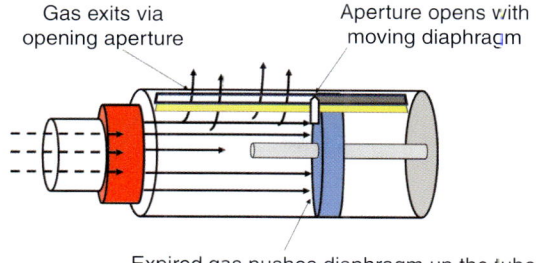

Figure 5.9 Peak-flowmeter

Peak-Flowmeter

Another variant of the constant-pressure, variable-orifice flowmeter is the peak-flowmeter (Figure 5.9). The incoming gas forces a diaphragm along the inside of a tube. As it moves, it progressively opens a lengthways slit in the tube, allowing the gas to escape. Eventually, the slit will have opened so much that the gas escapes this way rather than moving the diaphragm further; hence constant pressure, variable orifice. The final position of the diaphragm can be read off the calibrated scale for the peak flow reading. The classical precursor of this device is the Wright peak-flowmeter. This is slightly more compact and the linear movement of the diaphragm is replaced by rotational movement of a vane around a dial. The principle is the same, however.

Pneumotachograph

To measure gas flow in the breathing circuit of modern ventilators and anaesthetic machines, pneumotachographs, hot-wire anemometers or mechanical flow transducers tend to be used.

A pneumotachograph works by introducing a resistance to gas flow within the breathing circuit so that a pressure difference occurs across it. For practical purposes, this resistance has to be very small to allow spontaneous breathing. Designing the device to ensure laminar flow across it ensures accuracy. This is achieved by using a large number of small, parallel tubes (Figure 5.10). As the gas is moving in a laminar fashion, pressure drop is directly proportional to flow (as per the Hagen–Poiseuille equation) as long as the gas mixture, and consequently viscosity, remains constant.

A variant of the pneumotachograph is the pitot-tube pneumotachograph (Figure 5.11). Small tubes within, and parallel to, the breathing circuit are joined

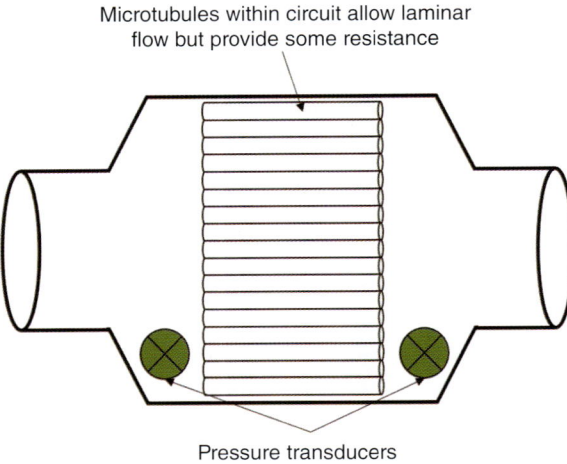

Figure 5.10 Pneumotachograph

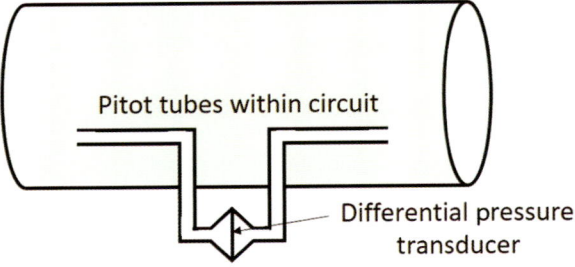

Figure 5.11 Pitot-tube pneumotachograph

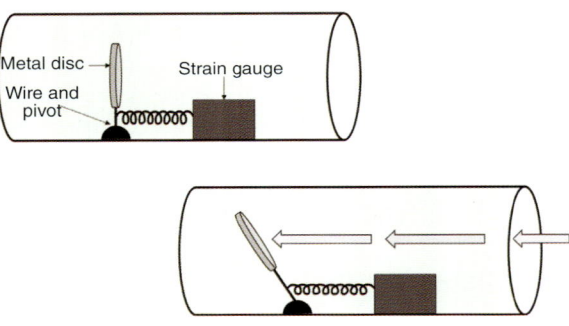

Figure 5.12 Mechanical strain gauge flowmeter

Pitot tubes are also found on aircraft and are used to determine air speed by comparing the pressure in the pitot tube to ambient pressure. Most such systems include a heating element and this is mandated on aircraft certified for instrument flying. The cold, wet air encountered in cloud predisposes to obstruction of the pitot tube by ice, leading to erroneous air-speed indications. An ice-obstructed pitot tube was the cause of the Air France Flight 447 disaster in 2009.

Mechanical Strain Gauge

The mechanical strain gauge flowmeter, as used in many intensive care ventilators, works by having a metal disc angled perpendicular to the flow of gas (Figure 5.12). This is attached to a flexible wire so that when gas is flowing, the wire is bent backwards. A strain gauge is positioned to measure the tension applied to the wire by this movement. This is transduced into an electrical signal. As this method causes significant obstruction to flow, the system is placed in a small side-channel, fed from the main circuit.

A different physical principle that can be utilized is that of cooling. A hot wire, positioned in the gas stream, will be cooled in proportion to the rate of flow: higher flow equates to a greater volume of gas moving past the wire and so a greater amount of energy can be absorbed from the wire. As the wire cools, the electrical resistance through it changes. When combined into a circuit, change in resistance with temperature will lead to a measurable change in current within the circuit (Figure 5.13). This change in current can be calibrated to gas flow. In most systems that utilize this principle, two variations are commonly employed. Firstly, the wire is incorporated

by a pressure transducer. As these tubes already contain gas, no fresh gas from the breathing circuit enters them. This ensures that the physical properties of the gas within the pitot tubes remain constant and water vapour build-up, which could cause inaccuracy, is limited. As the circuit gas flows past the opening of the tube facing the direction of flow, an increase in pressure occurs within the tube. It is the kinetic energy of the moving circuit gas that is responsible for generating this pressure effect. Since kinetic energy is proportional to the square of the flow velocity, very small changes in velocity cause relatively large pressure changes, making this system extremely sensitive.

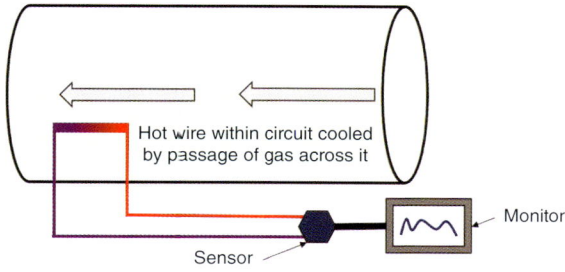

Figure 5.13 Hot-wire anemometer

Table 5.2 Gas cylinder identification

Gas	Shoulder colour	Pin position
Oxygen	White	2 & 5
Nitrous oxide	Blue	3 & 5
Entonox	Blue/white quarters	7 (single pin in the middle)
Air	White/black quarters	1 & 5
Carbon dioxide	Grey	1 & 6
Heliox	White/brown quarters	2 & 4

into a Wheatstone bridge to improve the sensitivity of the system. Secondly, a null-deflection philosophy is employed: the current required to maintain a constant wire temperature in the face of fluctuant cooling effects is used to deduce the gas flow.

A limitation to this simple system is that the direction of flow cannot be differentiated. To get around this, a shield can be used to ensure the wire is only cooled by flow from one direction and not the other. A pair of transducers then allows the direction and amount of flow to be measured.

Supply of Medical Gases

Within anaesthetic practice we use many different types of gas, most of which are stored in cylinders or, in the case of oxygen, in a large container outside the hospital called a vacuum-insulated evaporator (VIE). From these sources, the gas is piped to where we need it in the clinical areas. A working knowledge about the gases we use every day and the safety features that prevent harm to patients and the hospital itself is vital.

Cylinders

Medical gas cylinders are most commonly made of molybdenum steel. Lightweight aluminium alloy or carbon composite varieties are increasingly common though. Gases are contained within the cylinders at high pressures. A conventional molybdenum–steel oxygen cylinder contains the gas at 13,700 kPa when full. For safety, the cylinders are designed to withstand pressures 65–70% above their working range (approximately 23,000 kPa).

The gas contained within the cylinders can be identified in a number of ways (Table 5.2):

(1) The colour-coding system: this is an international standard to which the UK adheres; some countries, for example the USA, may still have non-standard colours in use
(2) Chemical symbol engraved onto the cylinder valve
(3) Name and chemical symbol on the cylinder label
(4) Pin index system (see below)

Cylinders have multiple safety features to ensure that they deliver the correct gas and minimize the risk of explosion. Between the body of the cylinder and the valve sits a plastic disc. This disc is colour-coded to indicate when the cylinder last underwent safety checks. The valve, which is engraved with the chemical symbol for the gas within, has a single exit port for the gas. Before a cylinder is attached, it should be briefly opened and closed to blow out any dust or oil that is sitting in the exit port, to prevent this entering the anaesthetic machine. The port sits close to the holes for the pin index system, an arrangement of pins and corresponding holes located in one of six possible positions to form a pattern unique to each gas. The valve stem features the holes and the attaching interface, e.g. the cylinder yoke on the anaesthetic machine carries the pins. This ensures that only the correct gas can be attached. The valve stem also includes a fusible plug, an alloy plug which melts at relatively low temperature to allow a controlled leak of the cylinder contents so as to prevent a potentially explosive increase in cylinder pressure if the cylinder is exposed to a fire. Between the exit port of the cylinder and the anaesthetic machine there is a Bodok seal. This is a neoprene washer, bonded within a brass ring, which ensures a gas-tight fit and prevents any leakage of the cylinder contents into the atmosphere.

Chapter 5: Gas Measurement and Supply

Once attached to the anaesthetic machine, cylinders should initially be opened slowly to prevent a rapid pressure rise within the machine pipework. A rapid increase in pressure within a fixed volume (that of the pipework) causes an increase in temperature. This is called an adiabatic temperature rise. An adiabatic process is any change in a system that does not involve transfer of energy between the system and its surroundings. In this example, the change in pressure is so rapid that the thermal energy doesn't have time to be conducted into the pipework of the machine. Consequently, as no energy has left the gas, its temperature increases and, in the presence of a small amount of grease or other contaminant, a fire or explosion may result.

Volume of Gas within a Cylinder

Cylinders have a standardized internal volume, independent of what they contain. This is quantified as the volume of water the cylinder could hold if full (Table 5.3). The volume of pressurized gas or vapour that the cylinder holds when full is dependent on the individual substance and also the region of the world in which it will be used.

For chemicals stored as a gas, such as oxygen, the volume of gas available can be worked out using Boyle's law (see Chapter 4). As long as the temperature stays constant, the product of the pressure in the cylinder and the volume of the cylinder will equal the product of the volume outside of the cylinder and the atmospheric pressure:

$$P_{cylinder} \times V_{cylinder} = P_{atmosphere} \times V_{atmosphere}$$

This can be rearranged to find the volume of gas available:

$$V_{atmosphere} = \frac{P_{cylinder} \times V_{cylinder}}{P_{atmosphere}}$$

A full oxygen cylinder is pressurized to 13,700 kPa. For a size E cylinder, as found attached to the back of an anaesthetic machine:

$$\text{Volume available} = \frac{13,700 \times 4.7}{101.325}$$

$$= 635.5 \text{ l of oxygen}$$

As oxygen is stored above its critical temperature of −118 °C, no matter how much pressure is applied it will never turn to liquid. As it always exists as a gas in the cylinder the pressure on the gauge will always be directly proportional to the volume of gas remaining.

Table 5.3 Cylinder volumes (data reproduced with permission from BOC Healthcare, Guildford, UK)

Cylinder size	Capacity (litres of water)
CD	2.0
D	2.3
E	4.7
F	9.4
G	23.6
J	47.2

This rule does not apply for nitrous oxide. As the critical temperature for nitrous oxide is 36.5 °C, at room temperature it exists in the cylinder as a liquid in equilibrium with a vapour above. A vapour, by definition, is any substance in the gaseous state but at a temperature below the critical temperature for that substance. What distinguishes a vapour from a true gas is that a vapour can be liquefied by application of pressure whereas a gas cannot. A full nitrous oxide cylinder is pressurized to 4,400 kPa but, due to the storage as a liquid and vapour, this can change significantly with changes in ambient temperature. Because of this, cylinders are only partially filled to allow some space for more liquid to vaporize if the temperature increases. The amount by which the cylinder is filled depends on the climate. In temperate climates, such as the UK, cylinders are filled with a mass of liquid 0.75 times the mass of water it would take to fill the cylinder. This ratio is called the filling ratio. In hotter climates, this is reduced to 0.67.

As the nitrous oxide vapour is used, the pressure within the cylinder falls, which results in more of the liquid turning to vapour to maintain the equilibrium. Consequently, the vapour pressure is maintained as a constant. This pressure is the only quantity a standard Bourdon gauge can measure. This means that the pressure in the cylinder does not drop until all of the liquid has been used and the cylinder is nearly empty. A small drop in pressure is sometimes seen during high-consumption use of the cylinder. In this circumstance, the constant vaporization of fresh liquid consumes latent heat of vaporization and thus causes the temperature to drop. As the volume in the cylinder is constant, Gay-Lussac's law states that if the temperature drops, the pressure will also drop.

To determine the volume of vapour within the nitrous oxide cylinder we must therefore use the mass of chemical within the cylinder. All cylinders have their tare weight (empty weight) printed on the label and engraved into the neck. By weighing the cylinder, we can then work out the mass of nitrous oxide within. This can be converted into the volume of gas using Avogadro's law (1 mol of gas will occupy 22.4 l at atmospheric pressure). For example, if a cylinder contained 2 kg (2,000 g) of nitrous oxide (which has a molecular mass of 44):

$$\frac{2{,}000}{44} = 45.45 \text{ mol}$$

$$45.45 \times 22.4 = 1{,}018 \text{ l of nitrous oxide vapour}$$

Further working examples of this principle can be found in Chapter 4. The behaviour of nitrous oxide is interesting because it can exist as a liquid, vapour and gas in anaesthetic practice. In the cylinders, vapour and liquid co-exist as described. In the anaesthetic machine, it is a vapour and, in the circle, which operates at around 38 °C to 40 °C on account of the heat from the reaction in soda lime, it can exist as a true gas. The interface between all these states can be described by the pressure–volume isotherm diagram (Figure 5.14). This can seem bewildering. To make sense of it, read the isotherms from right to left. By definition, the various lines describe the change in pressure of a fixed amount of gas at a constant temperature whose volume is gradually reduced. Compressing a gas usually leads to an adiabatic increase in temperature so, to construct these lines, the experiment must proceed very slowly so that the heat dissipates to the surroundings and the temperature of the substance remains constant at the desired value.

Convection within the atmosphere gives rise to a predictable drop in temperature with altitude known as the adiabatic lapse rate. Because warm air expands, it becomes less dense and rises. As a consequence, its temperature drops. This is an adiabatic process; energy in a parcel of air does work in expanding the volume of the parcel but no energy is added from the surroundings. In dry air, the temperature drops by 9.8 °C per 1,000 m. This persists to around 17 km at the tropopause where the troposphere gives way to the stratosphere. Above this point, the lapse rate becomes negative; temperature rises with altitude.

To start with, consider the 40 °C line. At this temperature, nitrous oxide is a gas and therefore obeys Boyle's law (pressure is inversely proportional

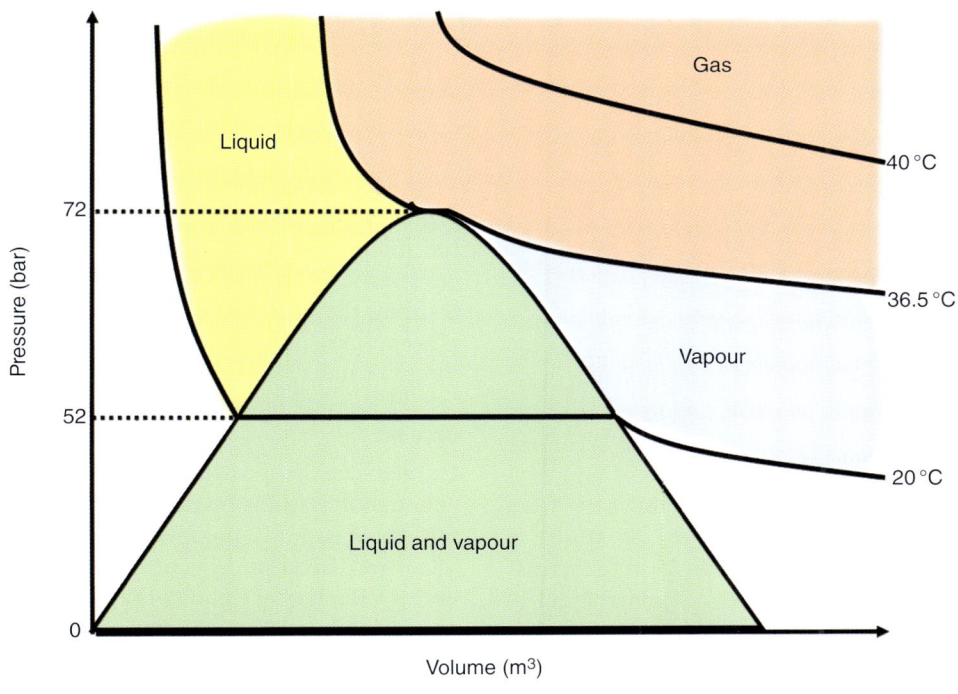

Figure 5.14 Isotherm diagram for nitrous oxide

to volume). The graphical representation of this is a parabola. At the critical temperature (36.5 °C), as the gas is compressed, it *just* liquefies at the critical pressure (the pressure required to liquefy a vapour at its critical temperature). This is why the line *just* kisses the shaded area where liquid and vapour co-exist: only at this perfect combination of temperature and pressure can liquefaction occur. At 20 °C, reduction in volume of the vapour causes an increase in pressure as per Boyle's law but, soon enough, liquefaction begins as the vapour is well below its critical temperature. In fact, if the volume is reduced sufficiently, all the vapour is liquefied. During this process, reduction in volume leads to liquefaction rather than an increase in pressure: this causes the flat-spot in the line. Eventually, however, when liquefaction is complete, the principles of hydraulics take over: liquids are very incompressible and further volume reduction causes a rapid increase in pressure. Similar lines could be drawn for experiments at multiple temperatures and the 'flat-spots' describing liquefaction at each temperature give rise to the shape of the 'liquid and vapour' area on the graph.

Entonox is a 50:50 mixture of oxygen and nitrous oxide, which is commonly used as an analgesic within emergency departments and maternity wards. This mixture is usually presented in cylinders although these may be as a part of a cylinder manifold (see later), connected by pipeline to the outlets in the hospital. A full cylinder is pressurized to 13,700 kPa. Entonox is created by bubbling oxygen through nitrous oxide. The production of a mixture of these two gases is an example of the Poynting effect: there is a change in vapour pressure and other physical properties observed when gaseous oxygen is combined with the nitrous oxide. In the case of Entonox, the mixture exhibits a pseudocritical temperature of −5.5 °C. If the mixture is cooled below this point, it liquefies in an uneven manner called lamination. When this occurs, more nitrous oxide liquefies, leaving an oxygen-rich mixture above. As this is used up, the composition of the mixture changes, becoming increasingly rich in nitrous oxide content and progressively more hypoxic. To prevent this from happening, Entonox cylinders should be stored at room temperature in a horizontal position to increase the surface area of the liquid for re-vaporization. In cold conditions, the cylinder should be up-ended to mix the contents before use.

The fusible plug in medical gas cylinders is made from a substance known as Wood's metal, after its discoverer, Barnabas Wood, a nineteenth-century, American dental surgeon. It is a eutectic mixture (one having a lower melting point than that of its constituents), consisting of bismuth, lead, tin and cadmium. It has a melting point of around 70 °C and has other applications including soldering, antiques repair and templating for radiotherapy.

Pipeline Gas Supplies

Most hospitals in the UK have pipeline gas supplies to the majority of clinical areas. These provide gases via uniform wall connectors called Schrader sockets. These sockets are colour-coded for the gases and have specific sizes of collars that are individual for each gas. This means there is both a colour identifier and a physical socket shape to ensure only the correct hose or flowmeter can be attached.

Nitrous Oxide

Piped supplies of nitrous oxide are usually provided from a cylinder manifold (Figure 5.15), situated outside the main building of the hospital. A cylinder manifold consists of two sets of cylinders, usually size J. The number of cylinders in each set depends on the amount of the gas used by the hospital. The cylinders within each set are connected in parallel so that they are all used at the same rate. Once one set is used, a shuttle valve automatically switches to the other side so that the secondary set is used. This allows the primary set to then be replaced without interrupting the supply. After leaving the cylinder manifold, the gas goes through a series of pressure-reducing valves to bring the cylinder pressure down to the 400 kPa pipeline pressure. A similar system is also used for Entonox and sometimes for oxygen.

Oxygen

Oxygen can be provided by a cylinder manifold, although due to the amount that most hospitals use this would require a huge number of cylinders in each set, or very frequent deliveries. Instead, most hospitals have a VIE on site (Figure 5.16). This allows for liquid oxygen to be stored on site, which is much more economical.

In a VIE, oxygen is stored as a liquid under a small amount of pressure at approximately −160 °C. The liquid oxygen is stored in a vacuum-insulated container as the absence of air between the layers of the container prevents convective and conductive heat loss. This is the same principle used to keep soup hot in a vacuum flask. Within the container, oxygen is present as both a liquid and as a vapour above the liquid. If oxygen is used, the oxygen vapour leaves the chamber where it is heated to ambient temperature by passing through a superheater (essentially a heat exchanger). This can be recognized, particularly in damp weather, as the ice-encrusted apparatus next to the VIE. As the gas is warmed, the pressure increases, as per Gay-Lussac's law, so it then passes through a pressure-reducing valve to reduce it to 400 kPa to enter the pipeline supply. As oxygen is used, some of the liquid oxygen then evaporates. This requires latent heat of vaporization, the energy for which comes from a drop in the temperature of the liquid oxygen and inner tank of the VIE. This maintains the VIE at approximately −160 °C without the need for a separate refrigeration system.

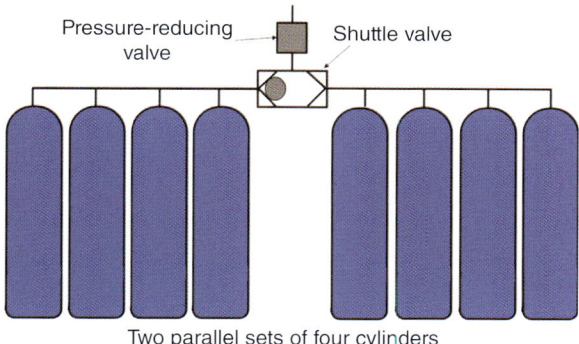

Figure 5.15 Cylinder manifold of nitrous oxide

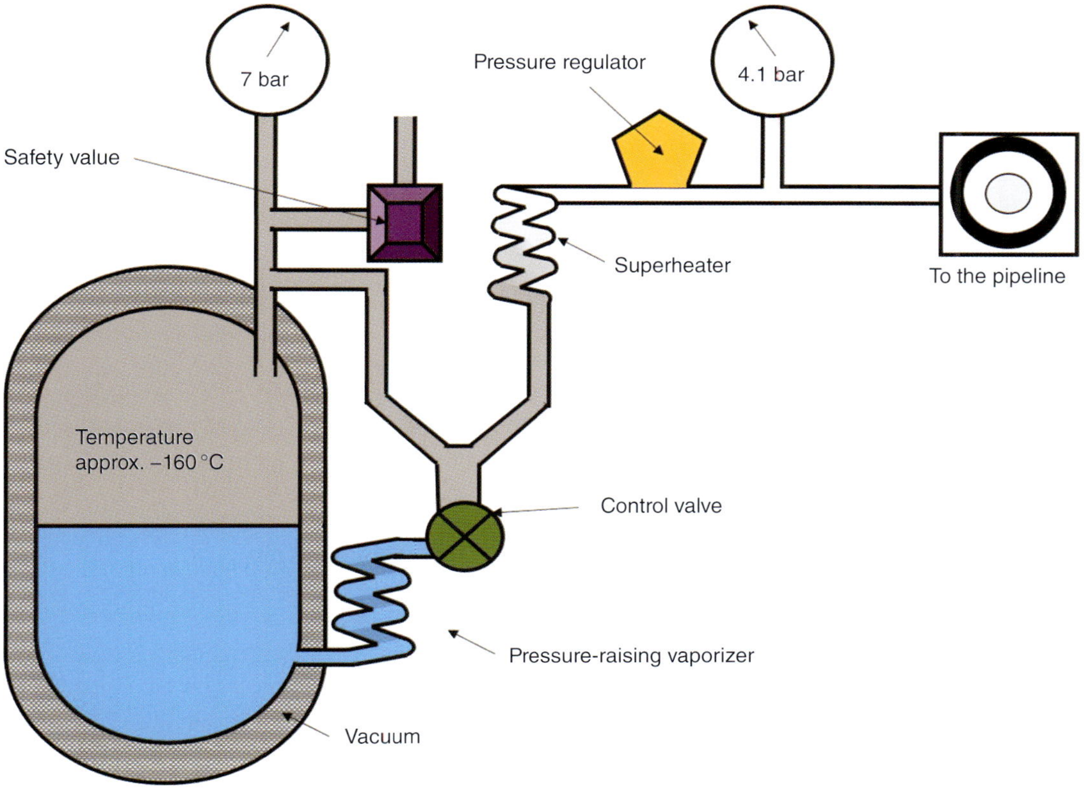

Figure 5.16 A vacuum-insulated evaporator (VIE)

If demand for oxygen is low, the pressure in the chamber can increase so a pressure-reducing valve is present to safely exhaust vapour at 700 kPa, to prevent explosion. If oxygen demand is high, constant vaporization of liquid cools the whole system to a point where no further vaporization is possible and pressure falls. In this situation, a control valve opens, allowing some of the liquid oxygen to leave the bottom of the tank and pass through a pressure-raising vaporizer (a similar apparatus to the super-heater) and be directly added to the pipeline supply. This gives the chance for ambient temperature to re-warm the whole VIE and re-establish a working pressure. One litre of liquid oxygen can provide 842 litres of gas at 15 °C, making this a very efficient method of storage.

The behaviour of oxygen under the conditions found in the VIE is identical to that exhibited by nitrous oxide in a cylinder in the anaesthetic room. A pressure gauge only serves to demonstrate if the safety-relief valve is stuck and says nothing about the remaining oxygen within. Consequently, the VIE stands on three legs; two are hinged and the third rests on a weighing-scale. This is how the remaining contents of the VIE are monitored.

An alternative method of supplying oxygen is the oxygen concentrator. This can be used for an individual patient, such as in a home system for long-term oxygen therapy, or larger systems can be used to supply pipeline oxygen. An oxygen concentrator works by compressing air to 137 kPa with an air compressor and then passing the air over a zeolite sieve. This selectively absorbs nitrogen, which is then released into the atmosphere. The remaining gas has an oxygen concentration that can be up to 95% but the flow rates are relatively low except in large systems.

Air

Air, like any of the gases, can be supplied via a cylinder manifold as described above for nitrous oxide. Most hospitals, however, utilize air compressors, which are more economical. An air compressor works by drawing air in and compressing it before storing it in cylinder reservoirs. This allows a constant-pressure supply to be maintained. Before the air is compressed, it must be dried by passing it over silica filters as the compression process would otherwise increase the relative humidity. The intake duct has to be carefully positioned so that it is not affected by weather conditions such as rain or snow. Once compressed, air can be released into a high-pressure supply (700 kPa) or the standard medical air supply system (400 kPa). The high-pressure system is reserved for powering tools and machinery. Importantly, the Schrader connectors for the different pressure pipelines are different to prevent patients and equipment being exposed to excessive pressure.

Summary

The ability to measure and manipulate gas flows, volumes and pressure is a key component of modern anaesthetic and intensive care treatment. It allows us to investigate and monitor patients' physiological status both preoperatively and during anaesthesia, allowing us to make informed decisions about treatment. It also allows us to ensure patient safety by protecting them from high-pressure storage systems and unsafe gas mixtures. A sound knowledge of gas pressure and volumes is essential to enable the high-risk activities such as the intra- and inter-hospital transfer of ventilated patients. Monitoring of safe ventilation volumes and pressures, as well as ensuring adequate supplies of gases, is vital in such circumstances.

Questions

MCQs – select true or false for each response

1. Regarding flowmeters:
   (a) They rely on viscosity of gas at low flows
   (b) They rely on density of gas at high flows
   (c) The nitrous oxide flowmeter can be used safely with oxygen attached
   (d) They are a type of variable-pressure, constant-orifice meter
   (e) Two flowmeters can be used in series for increased accuracy
2. Regarding pressure valves:
   (a) The Ritchie whistle relies on an electrical supply
   (b) The Entonox valve has a demand valve followed by a pressure-reducing valve
   (c) They are utilized as a safety feature on the vacuum-insulated evaporator (VIE)

(d) The valves in a circle breathing system are calibrated to approximately 50 Pa
(e) Medical gas supplies use pressure-increasing valves to provide gases at 400 kPa

3. Regarding measurement of gas flow and volume:
   (a) A Wright respirometer tends to under-read at high flows
   (b) A Wheatstone bridge can be used to increase the sensitivity of a hot-wire anemometer
   (c) Pitot tubes significantly increase the resistance during spontaneous ventilation
   (d) The Wright peak-flowmeter is an example of a constant-pressure, variable-orifice flowmeter
   (e) ICU ventilators incorporate pneumotachographs to measure flow

4. The VIE
   (a) Stores oxygen as a liquid between −160 °C and −180 °C
   (b) Utilizes latent heat of condensation to maintain its temperature
   (c) The amount of oxygen left is determined by the weight of the VIE
   (d) During periods of high demand, liquid oxygen is vaporized by the superheater coil
   (e) Allows oxygen to leave at 400 kPa

5. The contents of a gas cylinder can be identified by the
   (a) Colour of the cylinder shoulders
   (b) Engraving on the neck of the cylinder
   (c) The chemical formula on the label
   (d) The name of the gas on the label
   (e) The positions of the holes near to the gas outlet.

SBAs – select the single *best* answer

6. The nitrous oxide cylinder on the anaesthetic machine becomes cold during use because of:
   (a) The smaller amount of vapour inside the same cylinder volume exerting less pressure and consequently less temperature as per Gay-Lussac's law
   (b) Latent heat of vaporization using energy causing a temperature drop as vapour is used
   (c) The flow of vapour causing cooling by convective loss

(d) The low specific heat capacity of molybdenum steel
(e) The size E cylinder attached to the anaesthetic machine has a large surface area:volume ratio so is prone to temperature change

Answers

1. FFFFT
   At low flow, laminar flow predominates, the Hagen–Poiseuille equation applies and density is the key factor. As flow increases, so does the predominance of turbulent flow where viscosity is a more relevant phenomenon. Flowmeters are very much gas-specific. Flowmeters are constant-pressure, variable-orifice devices, not the other way around. Some anaesthetic machines used to feature two flowmeters for each gas, one reading up to 1 l min^{-1} and the other up to 15 l min^{-1}. This was to facilitate low-flow anaesthesia.

2. FFTTF
   The Ritchie whistle, unlike the Bosun's whistle, does not require anything but a gas supply to function. The sequence of valves in the Entonox delivery system is the other way around to that stated. Valves alone cannot increase pressure.

3. FTFTF
   The Wright respirometer under-reads at low flows due to the inertia of the vane. Pitot tubes are particularly good at avoiding extraneous additional resistance within the breathing system. Strain-gauge flow sensors are typical in modern ICU ventilators.

4. TFTFT
   The VIE utilizes the overall cooling effect of latent heat of vaporization to maintain the low temperature of the remaining contents of the system. Under normal conditions, oxygen vapour is passed through the superheater but in periods of high demand when the vapour supply will dwindle, liquid oxygen is utilized in addition. This passes through the pressure-raising vaporizer and the vapour output joins the vapour from the top of the VIE before entering the superheater.

5. TTTTT
   All are statements of fact.

6. (b)
   Unless there is no remaining liquid, the amount of vapour in the cylinder does not change (making (a) incorrect) because the vapour is replenished from the liquid. This transformation requires latent heat of vaporization, which cools the cylinder (so (b) is

correct). Answers (c), (d) and (e) are incorrect for the following reasons. The volume of the vapour and flow rates involved means that convective loss is trivial. The thermal conductivity is more relevant than the specific heat of the steel in perceiving the effects of a cooling process within the cylinder.

That said, both properties explain why the steel feels cold but the question specifically refers to the underlying cause of the temperature drop; vaporization in this case. The size of cylinder is irrelevant – any size of cylinder will become cold under the same conditions of use.

Chapter 6

Gas Concentration Measurement

Catriona Frankling

Learning Objectives

- To be able to state the place of gas concentration measuring in standards for anaesthesia monitoring
- To list and explain the basic principles behind the common gas analyzers: Raman effect, mass spectrometry, refractometry and chromatography
- To understand, compare and contrast and explain the various methods of oxygen analysis in common use today
- To explain the role of infrared and ultraviolet light in gas concentration analysis
- To understand the role of gas analysis in the measurement of dead space

Chapter Content

- Paramagnetic oxygen analyzer
- Infrared analyzer
- Raman effect
- Mass spectrometry
- Refractometry
- Piezoelectric absorption
- Ultraviolet absorption
- Chromatography
- Nitrogen meter

Scenario

A 57-year-old man requires general anaesthesia for an emergency laparotomy due to bowel perforation. To provide safe general anaesthesia, it is necessary to monitor the oxygen concentration in the gas mixture delivered to the patient. In addition, knowledge of the fraction of inspired and expired carbon dioxide concentration is needed to ensure adequate ventilation of the patient, and to alert the anaesthetist to any issues, such as disconnection of the anaesthetic circuit. Measurement of nitrous oxide and the volatile anaesthetics is also imperative to ensure adequate anaesthesia.

How would you measure respiratory oxygen and carbon dioxide concentrations? How do you measure the concentration of volatile anaesthetics and nitrous oxide within the anaesthetic circuit? Which techniques are suitable for clinical practice compared to those only suited to laboratory work?

Introduction

Respiratory gas analysis is part of the minimum monitoring requirements during general anaesthesia as recommended by the Association of Anaesthetists of Great Britain and Ireland (AAGBI) [1]. Measurements of environmental anaesthetic agent concentrations within the theatre suite are also required to ensure staff safety and adherence to Control of Substances Hazardous to Health (COSHH) regulations (see Chapter 10) [2]. It is important that measurement devices are cheap, small and light, long-lasting, quick and accurate. This chapter will explain the different devices and techniques available to measure gas concentrations.

Paramagnetic Oxygen Analyzer

Paramagnetism is the phenomenon of attraction of a substance into an external magnetic field. The external field induces a magnetic field within the substance, the alignment of which results in attraction to the inducing field. Gases will behave in this manner if they have unpaired electrons. Oxygen has two unpaired electrons in separate atomic orbitals, making it paramagnetic and so attracted by a magnetic field. Other gases, such as nitrogen, are weakly diamagnetic; the field induced in these substances is aligned in opposition to the original field and so they are repulsed by it. Paramagnetic gas analysis uses the paramagnetic quality of oxygen to measure the concentration of oxygen within a gas mixture. This is the

Chapter 6: Gas Concentration Measurement

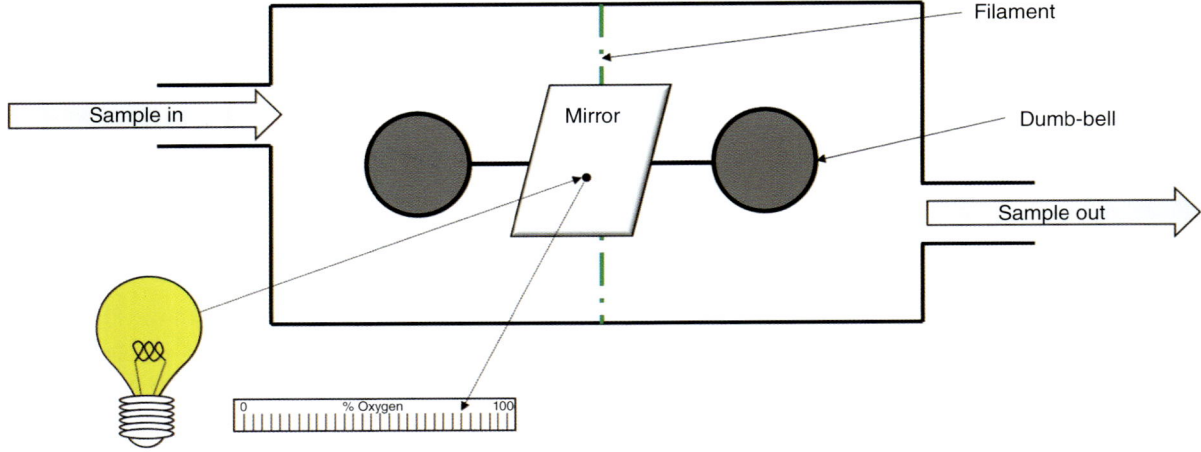

Figure 6.1 Paramagnetic oxygen analyzer

most commonly used technique for oxygen analysis in anaesthetic practice.

In the paramagnetic oxygen analyzer are two glass spheres filled with nitrogen that are attached to each other in the form of a dumb-bell. This is suspended on a filament within a chamber enveloped by a non-uniform magnetic field, allowing the dumb-bell to rotate. The gas sample enters the chamber, and the oxygen within the gas sample is attracted by the magnetic field, causing displacement of the glass spheres. This causes the dumb-bell to rotate. The extent of rotation corresponds to the concentration of oxygen in the sample. Classically, a mirror was attached to the dumb-bell, and a light source directed at the mirror to reflect onto a calibrated scale, depending on how much the dumb-bell has rotated (Figure 6.1).

A more accurate version of this simple paramagnetic oxygen analyzer uses null-deflection. The light beam is reflected onto two photocells rather than the calibrated scale. The output from the two photocells is compared and used to generate a current that flows through a coil that surrounds the dumb-bell. The current produces an opposing magnetic field to that within the analyzer and this keeps the dumb-bell in a resting position (the null-deflection). The magnitude of the current required to keep the dumb-bell in its resting position gives a measure of the concentration of oxygen present in the analyzer.

A further form of paramagnetic oxygen analyzer uses a differential pressure transducer and a pulsed magnetic field (Figure 6.2). It has no moving parts so is less prone to inaccuracy due to wear and tear. A sample gas and a reference gas enter the analyzer and are subjected to a pulsed magnetic field. When the magnetic field is on, oxygen within the sample gas is attracted into the field, which causes a reduction in pressure further upstream in the analyzer. This causes deflection of the pressure transducer diaphragm towards the gas stream with the higher oxygen concentration. When the magnetic field is off, there is no change in pressure and the pressure transducer diaphragm returns to its central position. This change in pressure corresponds to the amount of oxygen present in the gas sample.

Infrared Analyzer

To measure the concentrations of gases other than oxygen, including carbon dioxide, nitrous oxide and the volatile anaesthetic gases, paramagnetic analyzers are of no use. The infrared analyzer can measure all of these gases and works on the basis that any gas which contains two or more *different* atoms will absorb infrared radiation. Each gas absorbs radiation of a particular wavelength, such as 4.26 μm for carbon dioxide. In the infrared analyzer, infrared radiation is emitted by a hot wire, and the frequency of infrared required to measure concentration of a particular gas is obtained by passing the radiation through a filter (Figure 6.3). The infrared radiation then passes through a crystal window into the sample chamber

Chapter 6: Gas Concentration Measurement

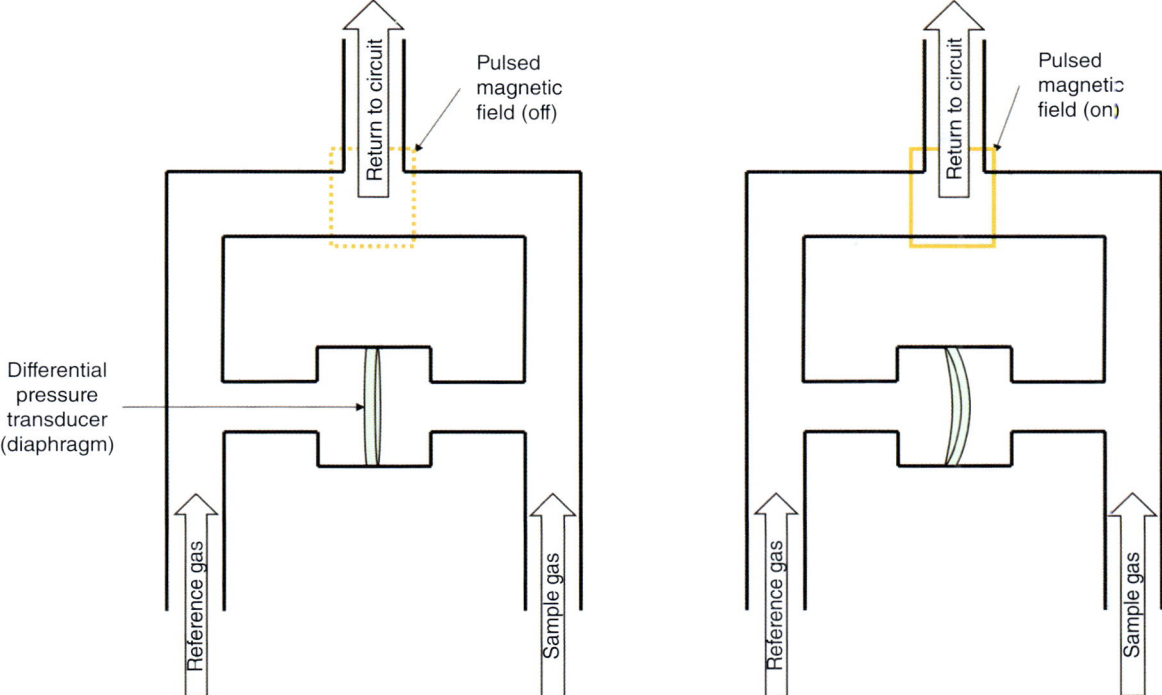

Figure 6.2 Differential pressure-measuring paramagnetic oxygen analyzer

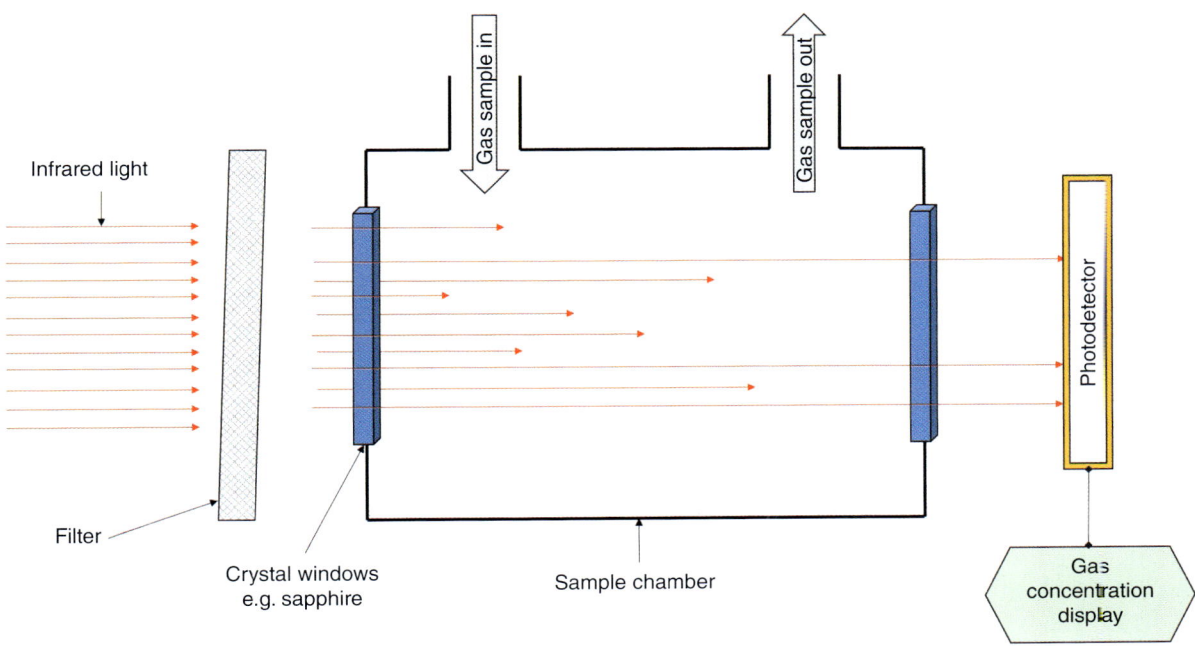

Figure 6.3 Infrared gas analyzer

that contains the gas to be analyzed. A glass window cannot be used as glass absorbs infrared radiation. Within the sample chamber, the gas present will absorb the infrared radiation. The amount of radiation absorbed depends upon the concentration of gas within the chamber. The higher the concentration of gas within the sample chamber, the more infrared radiation will be absorbed. The radiation passes through another crystal window and falls onto a photodetector. The detector output is processed electronically to give a reading of gas concentration. This follows the Beer–Lambert law which describes the relationship between the concentration of the measured substance and the path-length of the infrared beam travelled.

$$\text{Absorption} \propto \text{Path length} \times \text{Concentration}$$

In remembering the Beer–Lambert law, try the following: 'Beer' comes in different strengths and 'concentrations' and 'Lambert' is all to do with path 'length'. Of course, if you stand two pints of different types of beer side by side, the differing amount of light transmitted through the beers on account of their colour is given by Beer's law!

The infrared analyzer can be used to measure several different gases by mounting filters for different wavelengths of radiation onto a rotating disc. This also results in an alternating signal falling on the photodetector. An alternating signal is easier to amplify and is less prone to drift than constant signals, resulting in greater accuracy.

Raman Effect

In the infrared analyzer described above, radiation is absorbed completely by the molecule being measured. In contrast, Raman gas analyzers make use of the Raman effect, where there is partial transfer of energy between a molecule and the radiation. The Raman effect is the change in the wavelength of radiation which occurs when a beam of radiation is scattered by an atom or molecule. Most of the radiation that is scattered will be of the same wavelength (called Rayleigh scattering), but a small fraction will be of a different wavelength (usually a lower frequency), and this is called Raman scattering. The change in the wavelength will be typical of a specific molecule, so the partial pressure of different gases can be measured using the Raman effect. A helium–neon laser emits monochromatic light of wavelength 633 nm to enter the analysis chamber. When the light hits the intermolecular bonds of the gas to be analyzed, it is scattered and re-emitted at a different wavelength. There are photodetectors with filters that allow only radiation of a specified wavelength to pass through (Figure 6.4). The photodetectors can have filters fitted that are specific to Raman radiation, representative of oxygen, nitrogen, carbon dioxide, nitrous oxide and the volatile gases. Raman gas analyzers are more expensive than the infrared analyzers, but respond more quickly and with greater accuracy. Although used in industry, research and education, the Raman gas analyzer's need for a high sampling gas flow and its expense means that it is not used in modern clinical anaesthesia.

Mass Spectrometry

Even more accurate than Raman effect analyzers is the mass spectrometer. In this instrument, the gas sample is taken into the analysis chamber by a pump. A molecular leak allows a few molecules from the sample to enter an ionization chamber. Here they are ionized by a bombarding beam of electrons. The ions are then accelerated out of the chamber by accelerating and focusing plates. They then pass through a strong magnetic field, causing them to be deflected in an arc. The degree of deflection will depend upon the mass and charge of the ions, with those that have a low mass being deflected the most. Ions of a particular mass will be deflected to pass through a small slit to hit a detector (Figure 6.5). Changing the voltage on the acceleration and focusing plates will change the position and speed of the beam, so that ions of a particular mass will fall through the slit to be detected. In this way, the mass spectrometer can identify compounds by their mass numbers. However, some compounds have the same mass number, such as nitrous oxide and carbon dioxide (their mass number is 44). This can lead to inaccuracy in mixtures containing gases of identical mass. To compensate for this, the mass spectrometer can be used to measure an ionized fragment of the compound to be measured, such as nitric oxide fragments, which have a mass number of 30. In this way, nitrous oxide content can be measured without overestimation due to the presence of carbon dioxide.

Mass spectrometers have a rapid response time and can analyze very small samples. However, the

Chapter 6: Gas Concentration Measurement

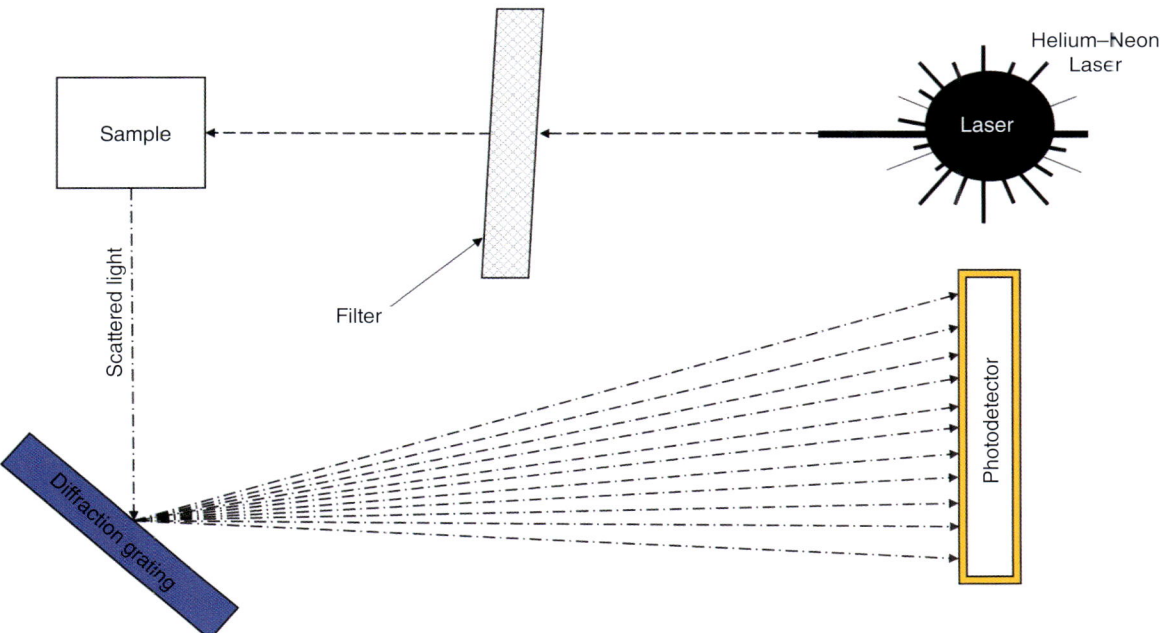

Figure 6.4 Raman effect gas analyzer

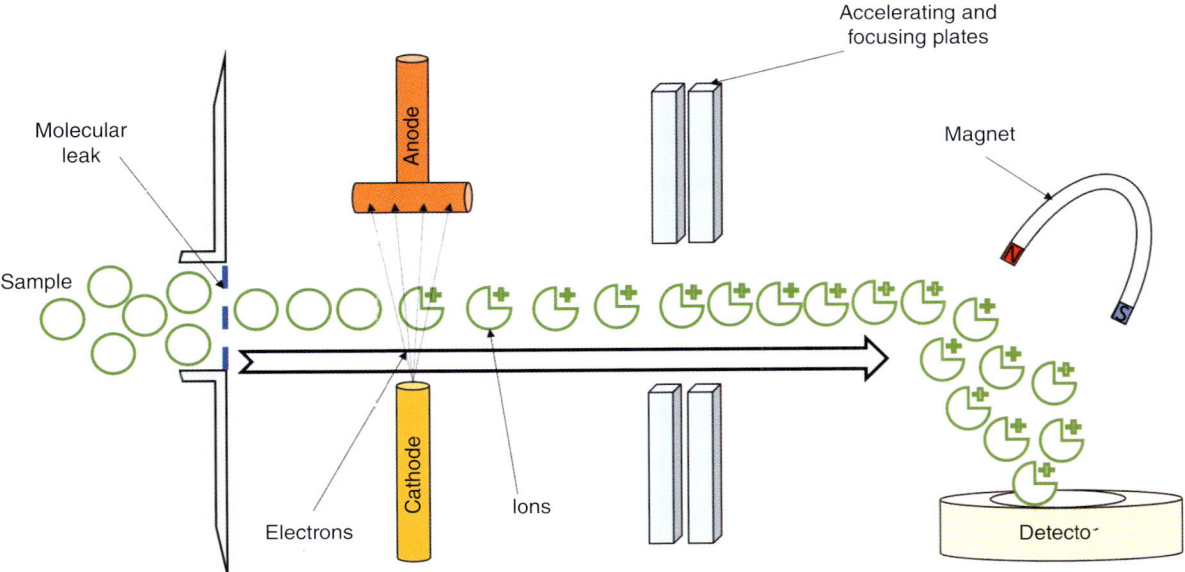

Figure 6.5 Mass spectrometer

Chapter 6: Gas Concentration Measurement

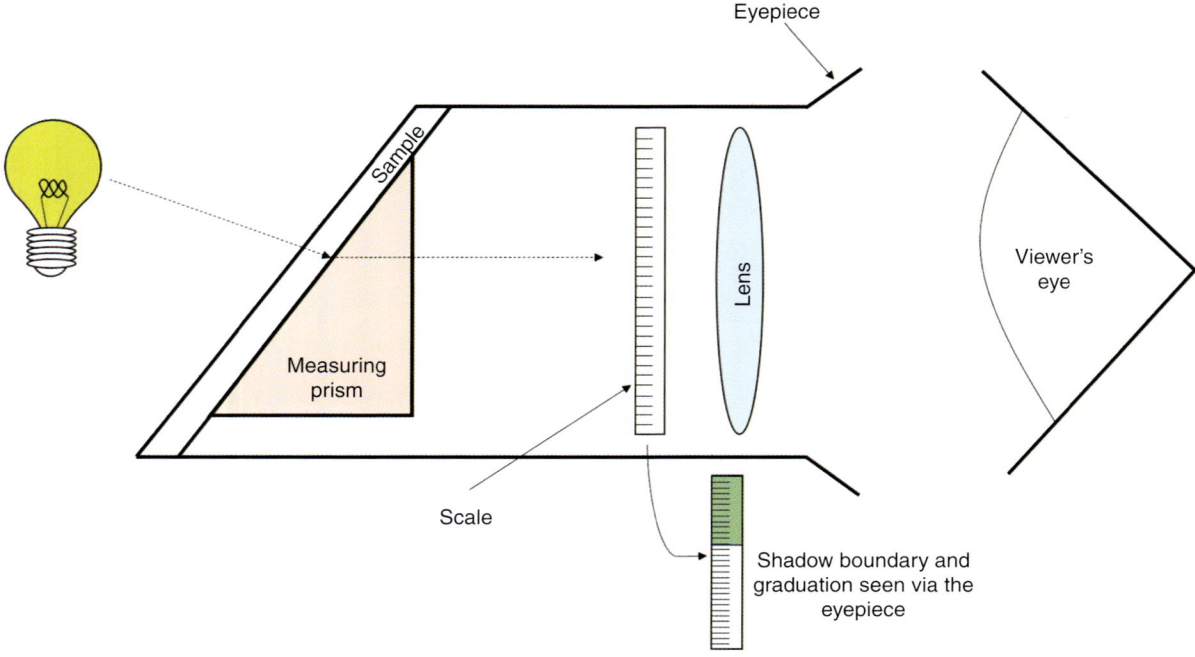

Figure 6.6 Refractometer

equipment is large and expensive and is therefore not used in routine clinical practice.

Routine continuous monitoring was still unheard of in the 1980s, but the introduction of the mass spectrometer into anaesthetic use in 1981 meant that intermittent monitoring of respiratory gases was possible. Side-stream sampling sent the gases from each theatre to a centrally located mass spectrometer for analysis.

Refractometry

Refractometry measures the refractive index of a substance. The refractive index is a dimensionless number that determines to what degree light is bent (refracted) when it enters a substance. This method of gas analysis is too slow to use for the breath-by-breath analysis of respiratory gases. However, it can be used for the calibration of vaporizers and to measure environmental anaesthetic agent concentrations within the theatre suite. In a refractometer, beams of monochromatic light are shone through the gaseous medium to be measured and focused onto a glass lens. Light and dark bands appear on the lens, the pattern of which will depend on the gaseous medium's refractive index and concentration (Figure 6.6). The Rayleigh refractometer uses a series of prisms to split the light source through sampling and control tubes. The refractometer will be calibrated for a particular gas. By aligning the patterns of light and dark bands created by each sample, a scale can be devised to correspond to gas concentration.

Why is the sky blue? It's because of Rayleigh scattering, named after the British physicist Lord Rayleigh, who also described the Rayleigh refractometer. Molecules in the air scatter blue light from the Sun. Rayleigh scattering is also responsible for the orange and red colour of sunsets. For a more complete answer, see Chapter 15.

Piezoelectric Absorption

The piezoelectric effect is the generation of an electrical potential when a crystal, such as quartz, is subject to a mechanical force. The inverse piezo effect is the deformation of the crystal in response to applying an electrical potential to the crystal. By using an alternating current, quartz crystals can be made to oscillate. The frequency of oscillation can be influenced by dissolving anaesthetic vapour from a sample into a silicone-based oil, which coats the crystal. The quantity of vapour dissolved in the oil is proportional to the partial pressure of the vapour present (Henry's law) and therefore the change in resonant frequency of the crystal will correspond to the anaesthetic vapour concentration. This type of analyzer has a slow response time, is not able to differentiate between different vapours and accuracy is affected by nitrous oxide and water vapour. In use in the 1980s, it has now been superseded by the infrared analyzer, which has a faster response time and greater accuracy, and can be used for the analysis of multiple gases.

The earliest gas monitor used a silicone rubber band. Anaesthetic gases would cause the silicone rubber band to relax and the change in tension could be measured mechanically by a lever attached to the band and a measuring scale. It was accurate to 3%.

The piezoelectric effect is not just used for the measurement of gas concentrations. It is used in the electric cigarette lighter, guitar pick-ups, loudspeakers and ultrasound probes. Smokers, rockers and pregnant women all benefit from the piezoelectric properties of quartz!

Ultraviolet Absorption

Historically, the absorption of ultraviolet light was used to measure halothane concentrations. This agent is no longer in clinical use in the UK due to its link with fulminant hepatic failure and so this type of gas measurement is no longer used. Halothane absorbs strongly in the ultraviolet region of the light spectrum. Gases composed of similar atoms absorb ultraviolet light. Halothane has a peak absorption of ultraviolet light at a wavelength of 206 nm. An ultraviolet spectrophotometer has a light source, such as a light-emitting diode (LED), a filter to ensure light of a single wavelength passes through to the sample chamber and a photodetector to measure how much ultraviolet light has been absorbed by the gas in the sample chamber. Like the infrared analyzer, the amount of

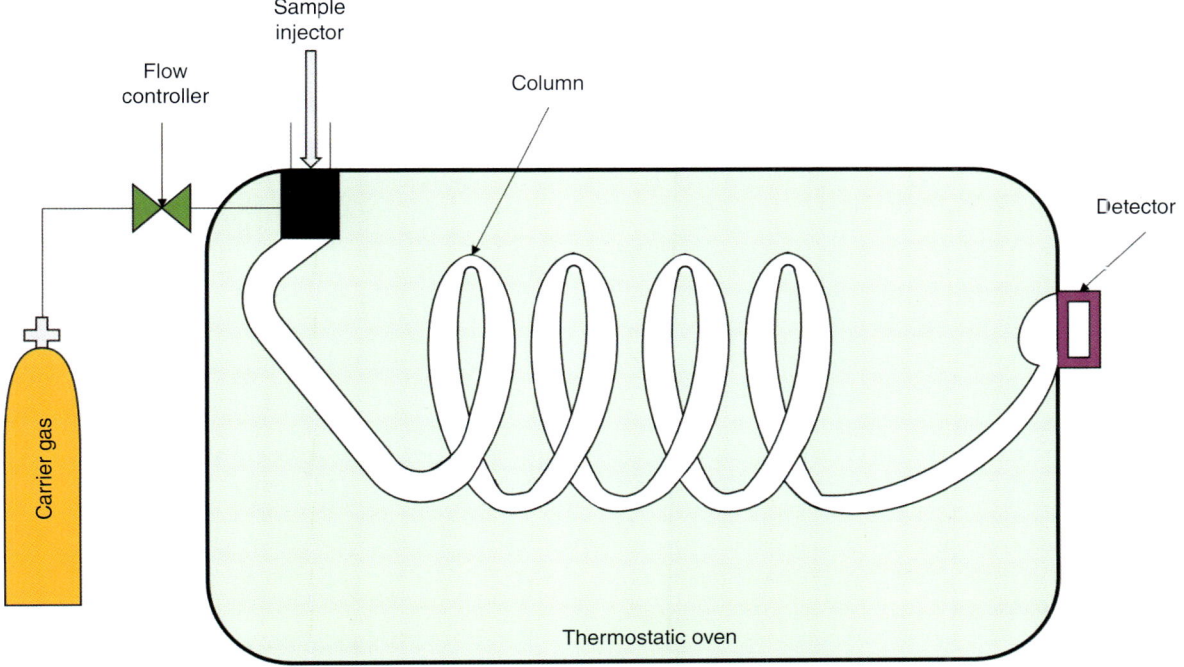

Figure 6.7 Gas chromatograph

ultraviolet light absorbed will depend upon the concentration of gas in the sample chamber, as explained by the Beer–Lambert law. The main disadvantage of this analyzer in clinical use was that it resulted in toxic breakdown products. These breakdown products needed to be passed through soda lime to be rendered safe before returning to the breathing circuit.

Chromatography

Gas chromatography can be used to identify very small concentrations of gases in a sample. This is useful for research purposes and for environmental and industrial use, but it cannot analyze gases continuously and therefore is not used to measure respiratory anaesthetic gases. Compounds separate depending on their affinity for the stationary or mobile phase of the system. A column is filled with small particles of silica–alumina that are coated with polyethylene glycol (the stationary phase) and an unreactive carrier gas such as helium (the mobile phase). The gas sample is injected into the column and the different gases in the sample will pass through the column at different speeds depending on their differential solubility between the two phases. A detector at the end of the column records the sample components (Figure 6.7).

Nitrogen Meter

This form of gas concentration measurement is not used in anaesthesia monitoring, but does have a role in the measurement of anatomical dead space. The nitrogen meter measures electromagnetic emission from nitrogen molecules. A voltage of 2,000 V is applied to the gas sample. This ionizes the sample and radiation is emitted that is measured by a photoelectric cell. It has a short response time of 20–40 ms and requires a logarithmic conversion of the non-linear output from the photodetector.

Summary

Gas concentration measurement has evolved greatly over time from simple, inaccurate devices to complicated machinery with greater accuracy but slow

Table 6.1 Summary table of gas analyzers and their properties

Technique	Gas detected					Can differentiate between gases	Uses
	Oxygen	Carbon dioxide	Nitrous oxide	Volatile anaesthetics	Nitrogen		
Paramagnetic oxygen analyzer	Yes	No	No	No	No	Not applicable	Anaesthetic machines
Infrared analyzer	No	Yes	Yes	Yes	No	Yes	Anaesthetic machines, capnography
Raman effect	Yes	Yes	Yes	Yes	Yes	Yes	Industry/research
Mass spectrometry	Yes	Yes	Yes	Yes	Yes	Yes	Industry/research
Refractometry	Yes	Yes	Yes	Yes	Yes	No	Industry/research
Piezoelectric absorption	No	No	No	Yes	No	No	Industry/research
Ultraviolet absorption	No	No	No	Halothane	No	Not applicable	Historical use
Chromatography	Yes	Yes	Yes	Yes	Yes	Yes	Industry/research
Nitrogen meter	No	No	No	No	Yes	Not applicable	Anatomical dead space

response times, through to the current continuous monitoring we now take for granted in the theatre suite.

Table 6.1 summarizes the different methods of gas analysis discussed.

Questions

MCQs – select true or false for each response

1. The paramagnetic oxygen analyzer:
   (a) Works on the principle that oxygen is weakly repelled from a magnetic field
   (b) Can be made more accurate by using null-deflection
   (c) Is the most commonly used method of respiratory oxygen measurement in anaesthesia
   (d) Which uses a differential pressure transducer is more prone to inaccuracy than the paramagnetic oxygen analyzer that uses a dumb-bell
   (e) Can be used to measure nitrogen as well as oxygen

2. With regard to the infrared analyzer:
   (a) It can be used for any gases that contain two or more different atoms
   (b) Carbon dioxide absorbs radiation with a wavelength of 4.26 cm
   (c) Glass windows cannot be used in the analyzer
   (d) It can be used to measure several different gases using one analyzer
   (e) It can be used to measure oxygen

3. Nitrous oxide can be measured using the following methods:
   (a) Mass spectrometry
   (b) Piezoelectric absorption
   (c) Ultraviolet absorption
   (d) Raman spectrometry
   (e) Infrared analyzer

SBAs – select the single *best* answer

4. During a left-knee arthroscopy on a 65-year-old lady, you maintain anaesthesia using isoflurane and nitrous oxide in oxygen. What is the most likely method of gas analysis used in this case?
   (a) Mass spectrometry and a paramagnetic oxygen analyzer
   (b) Mass spectrometry using a central mass spectrometer for intermittent gas analysis
   (c) Infrared analyzer and a paramagnetic oxygen analyzer
   (d) Raman spectrometry and a paramagnetic oxygen analyzer
   (e) Piezoelectric absorption, infrared analyzer and a paramagnetic oxygen analyzer

5. You are undertaking research into environmental pollution with anaesthetic gases and you need to measure very small quantities of unknown anaesthetic gases from the air. What would be the best method to do this?
   (a) Piezoelectric absorption
   (b) Silicone rubber band
   (c) Ultraviolet absorption
   (d) Chromatography
   (e) Paramagnetic oxygen analyzer

6. A company is designing new equipment for gas analysis. Which piece of equipment would you pick for gas analysis in a new anaesthetic machine?
   (a) Cost: £300. Shelf-life: 6 months. Weight: 500 g. Accuracy: 0.1%. Response time: 10–20 ms
   (b) Cost: £5,000. Shelf-life: 10 years. Weight: 800 g. Accuracy: 0.1%. Response time: 10–20 ms
   (c) Cost: £20. Shelf-life: 10 years. Weight: 1 kg. Accuracy: 3%. Response time: 10s
   (d) Cost: £100. Shelf-life: 6 months. Weight: 35 kg. Accuracy: 0.1%. Response time: 10–20 ms
   (e) Cost: £2,000. Shelf-life: 3 years. Weight: 500 g. Accuracy: 1%. Response time: 10–20 ms

Answers

1. FTTFF

   Oxygen is weakly paramagnetic. The differential pressure transducer increases accuracy compared to the dumb-bell paramagnetic oxygen analyzer. Nitrogen is weakly diamagnetic so cannot be measured using paramagnetism.

2. TFTTF

   Carbon dioxide absorbs radiation at wavelength 4.26 µm not 4.26 cm. Glass absorbs infrared radiation so cannot be used in the analyzer. It cannot measure oxygen because oxygen doesn't contain two different atoms and therefore does not absorb infrared radiation.

3. TFFTT

Piezoelectric absorption is used for volatile anaesthetics. Ultraviolet absorption was used for measurement of halothane.

4. (c)

The paramagnetic oxygen analyzer is the most common method of oxygen measurement in modern anaesthesia. The infrared analyzer can measure carbon dioxide, nitrous oxide and the volatile anaesthetic gases and is the most common method of analysis of these gases in modern anaesthetic machines.

5. (d)

Piezoelectric absorption will not be able to measure quantities of nitrous oxide and can only be calibrated for one volatile gas at a time. The silicone rubber band will not be able to detect such small quantities of anaesthetic gases. Ultraviolet absorption is used for halothane and the paramagnetic oxygen analyzer is used for oxygen. Chromatography will be able to analyze several different gases in small quantities.

6. (b)

Gas analyzers need to be cheap, long-lasting, lightweight, accurate and have a fast response time. (a) is fairly cheap, but needs to be replaced more often than (b), making it less economical overall. (c) is very cheap, but is too inaccurate and too slow. (d) is cheap, but has a short life span and is too heavy to be of any practical use. (e) appears to be almost equal to (b), but again over the years it will need to be replaced more often and ends up being less economical than option (b).

References

1. Association of Anaesthetists of Great Britain and Ireland. Recommendations for standards of monitoring during anaesthesia and recovery 2015. *Anaesthesia* 71, 2016; 85–93.
2. Health and Safety Executive. *EH40/2005 Workplace Exposure Limits* (The Stationery Office, 2018).

Chapter 7

Blood Gas Analysis

David Connor

Learning Objectives

- To understand the principles and limitations of pulse oximetry, including the relevance of the presence of various haemoglobin species
- To understand the difference between the terms SpO_2, SaO_2 and FO_2Hb
- To understand the principles underlying the measurement of blood gas variables, including co-oximetry
- To appreciate the importance of avoiding pre-analytical errors during blood gas analysis
- To understand which arterial blood gas parameters can be reliably estimated by venous or capillary samples

Chapter Content

- Pulse oximetry
- Errors in pulse oximetry
- PO_2 electrodes
- pH electrode
- PCO_2 electrode (Severinghaus electrode)
- Blood gas machine and derived variables
- Errors in blood gas measurement
- Comparing arterial, venous and capillary samples
- Transcutaneous methods

Scenario

A 32-year-old female is admitted to the emergency department following rescue from a house fire. She is unconscious and her face is covered in soot. There is no evidence of traumatic injury and her blood pressure is normal. Her oxygen saturation on pulse oximetry (SpO_2) reads 98% and she is receiving supplementary oxygen via a non-rebreathe oxygen mask. On blood gas analysis, she has a pH of 7.1 with a lactate of 10 mmol l^{-1}, her PO_2 is 70 kPa and her PCO_2 is 3.5 kPa. Her arterial oxygen saturation (SaO_2) is 100%, whilst her fractional oxyhaemoglobin content (FO_2Hb) is 90%.

Which of these parameters is the best measure of the patient's oxygenation? What is the likely explanation of the discrepancy between the FO_2Hb and the SpO_2? What is the most likely explanation for her raised lactate and what are the treatment options?

Introduction

Over the past few decades, technological innovation has revolutionized patient monitoring systems, leading to a significant improvement in patient safety. Although pulse oximetry was first used experimentally in 1941, it was not employed clinically until 1972, and commercial pulse oximeters only became available in 1981. Now the device is a ubiquitous part of modern-day medical practice and is even readily available for purchase by the general public.

The first commercially available blood gas analyzer was developed in 1954 by a Danish scientist called Poul Astrup, following a devastating polio epidemic. Polio patients were originally treated with negative pressure ventilation, via either a cuirass or a cabinet respirator, and had a mortality of 87%. Astrup began to provide regular blood gas analysis for polio patients, which facilitated the introduction of manual intermittent positive pressure ventilation by an anaesthetist called Bjørn Ibsen. These measures, among others, reduced patient mortality to 26% and laid the foundations for the specialty of critical care medicine. Manufacturers today are focused on reducing sample processing time on ever-smaller blood samples with some machines capable of producing results for 19 variables in less than 35 seconds. Despite rapid development, these devices are still based on the same physical principles as their predecessors.

Chapter 7: Blood Gas Analysis

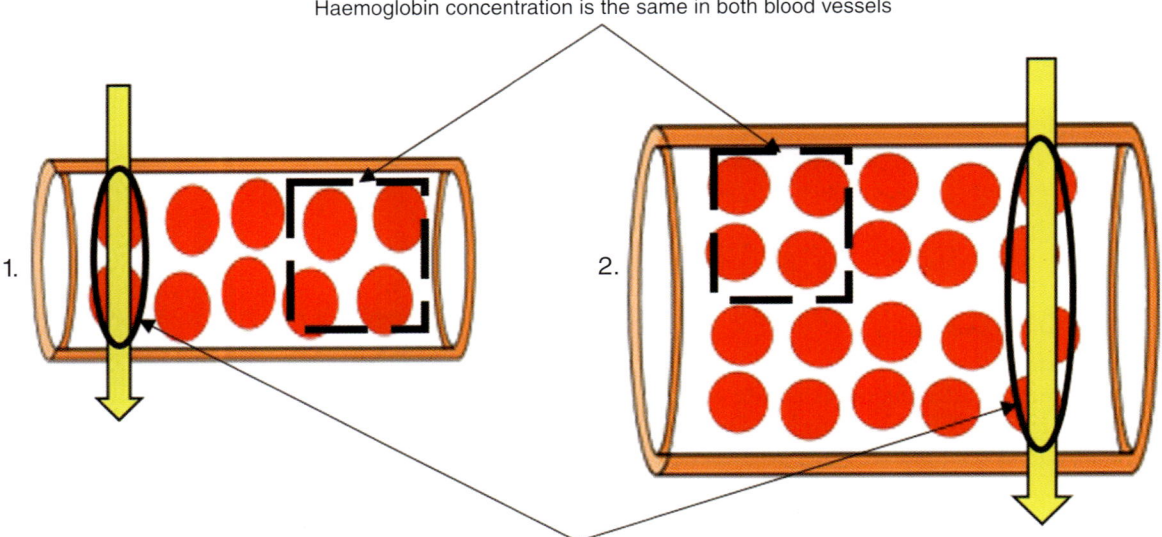

Figure 7.1 Illustration of Lambert's law

Pulse Oximetry

Arterial oxygen saturation (SaO_2) is defined as the percentage of total haemoglobin in the blood that is oxygenated. Traditionally, this was measured with a co-oximeter using an arterial blood sample. The pulse oximeter provides an indirect measure of this parameter (SpO_2). It achieves this by using a combination of red (wavelength 660 nm) and infrared (wavelength 940 nm) light to determine the oxygen saturation of blood as it passes through a peripheral vascular bed such as a finger.

A photoemitter is positioned on one side of the finger and a photodetector on the other. As the light passes through the finger, a proportion of it is absorbed and the remaining light is picked up by the detector. The amount of incident light which is absorbed by a substance is known as its absorbance. This is inversely related to the transmittance, which measures the quantity of light which passes through a substance. There are several variables which affect the proportion of light which is absorbed by a finger:

1. The concentration of light-absorbing molecules in the path of the beam (Beer's law): the greater the concentration of haemoglobin in the finger, the greater the proportion of light absorbed.

2. The distance travelled by the light between the photoemitter and -detector (Lambert's law): even if the concentration of haemoglobin in the finger remains the same, if the arteries in the finger are wider, light will have to cross more haemoglobin before it reaches the detector (Figure 7.1). Therefore, the greater the distance travelled by the light, the more light will be absorbed.

3. Differences in the absorption properties of oxygenated haemoglobin (oxy-Hb) and de-oxygenated haemoglobin (deoxy-Hb): Figure 7.2 illustrates that deoxy-Hb absorbs more light than oxy-Hb when red (660-nm wavelength) light is used. The opposite is the case when infrared (940 nm) light is used. Comparing readings at these two light wavelengths allows the pulse oximeter to ascertain the relative quantities of deoxy-Hb and oxy-Hb. If light with a wavelength of 805 nm was used, it would be impossible to differentiate deoxy-Hb and oxy-Hb; this wavelength is the isosbestic point for these haemoglobin forms, in other words the wavelength at which they both absorb light equally.

Light is clearly absorbed by other tissues in the finger apart from just the oxy-Hb and deoxy-Hb present in the arteries and this must be taken into account (Figure 7.3).

The pulse oximeter assumes that any pulsatile flow must be arterial and measures the fluctuating light absorption as AC current from the photodetector. A DC current component is also measured and this represents non-pulsatile absorption by the remaining tissues. These measurements are performed with both red and infrared light and entered into the equation below to calculate the modulation ratio (R).

$$R = \frac{AC_{red}/DC_{red}}{AC_{Infrared}/DC_{Infrared}}$$

In a situation where the patient has an SaO_2 of 100%, only oxy-Hb will be present and the deoxy-Hb curve can be ignored. Therefore, when measured with red light, absorption will be low but, when using infrared light, absorption will be high. This corresponds to an R value of 0.43 (see Table 7.1).

At any given saturation, the relative quantities of deoxy-Hb and oxy-Hb contribute to an overall absorption curve for the blood known as a composite

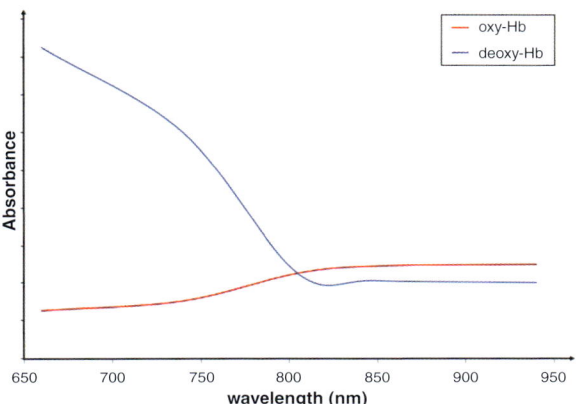

Figure 7.2 Graph of absorbance for both oxy-Hb and deoxy-Hb at different wavelengths

Table 7.1 Modulation ratios (R) for the pulse oximeter and their corresponding SpO_2 readings

SpO_2 (%)	Light absorption at 660 nm (red)	Light absorption at 940 nm (infrared)	R
0	High	Low	3.4
85	Medium	Medium	1.0
100	Low	High	0.43

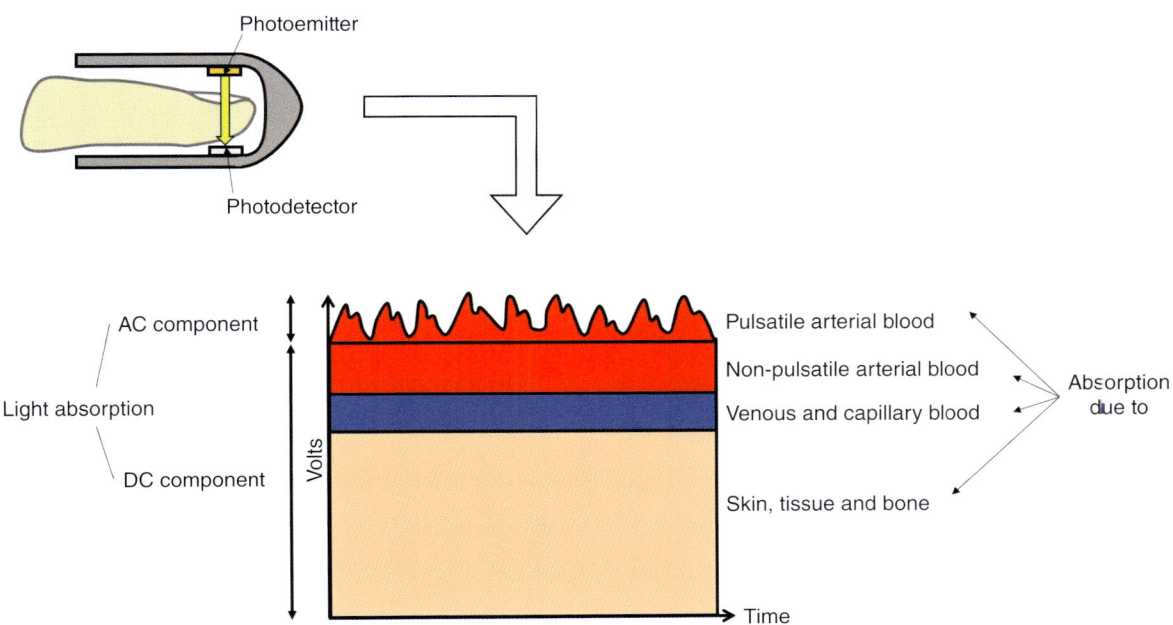

Figure 7.3 Light absorption by various tissues in the finger

Chapter 7: Blood Gas Analysis

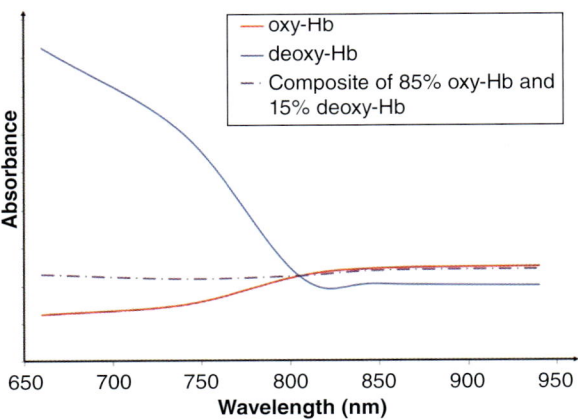

Figure 7.4 Composite absorbance curve for oxy-Hb and deoxy-Hb at different wavelengths

Table 7.2 LED sequence for a pulse oximeter

LED		Purpose
660 nm	940 nm	
On	Off	Quantifies absorption of light in 660-nm spectrum
Off	On	Quantifies absorption of light in 940-nm spectrum
Off	Off	Quantifies amount of ambient light

Table 7.3 Causes of incorrect pulse-oximeter readings

Low or high SpO_2	Low SpO_2	Normal or high SpO_2
Methaemoglobinaemia	Venous pulsations	Carbon monoxide poisoning
Sulph-haemoglobinaemia	Movement artefact	
	Fingernail polish	
	Intravenous pigmented dyes	
	Poor perfusion	
	Haemoglobinopathy	
	Anaemia with co-existing hypoxia	

curve (it is an average of the deoxy-Hb and oxy-Hb curves, weighted by proportion of each species present).

In the scenario where the patient has an SpO_2 of 85%, there is a predominance of oxy-Hb present, although there will also be some deoxy-Hb. The absorption curve is now a composite of the curves for both oxy- and deoxy-Hb (purple line, Figure 7.4). For this particular oxygen saturation, the absorption is the same when measured with either red light or infrared light; this corresponds to an R value of 1.

The R value is converted to an SpO_2 reading by cross-referencing to a calibration table, stored in the machine. Construction of this table involves the exposure of healthy volunteers to hypoxic mixtures, followed by arterial blood sampling. These samples are analyzed in controlled conditions in a laboratory and SaO_2 is determined using a co-oximeter. The laboratory-determined SaO_2 is compared to the equivalent R value obtained by pulse oximetry. This is repeated for different levels of hypoxia and used to populate the calibration table. For volunteer safety, the pulse oximeter is not calibrated below 70% and thus it is presumed to be less accurate below this level. One popular myth is that it was US service personnel who underwent such hypoxia experiments to calibrate the pulse oximeter during its invention. In reality, the FDA requires in vivo testing down to 70% for every new design of pulse oximeter prior to granting a product licence.

The photoemitter contains two LEDs that activate 30 times per second (30 Hz) according to the sequence detailed in Table 7.2. This allows the pulse oximeter to quantify and subtract the effect of any ambient light.

Errors in Pulse Oximetry

Like any monitoring device, however, pulse oximetry has its limitations, which are summarized in Table 7.3.

Before we discuss these limitations in more depth, there are some important terms and principles which must first be understood. The pulse oximeter assumes that only oxy-Hb and deoxy-Hb are present in the blood. It cannot differentiate other species of haemoglobin such as carboxyhaemoglobin (carboxy-Hb) or methaemoglobin (met-Hb) because it only uses two wavelengths of light (660 nm and 940 nm). This is important because different species of haemoglobin are also capable of absorbing the light and their

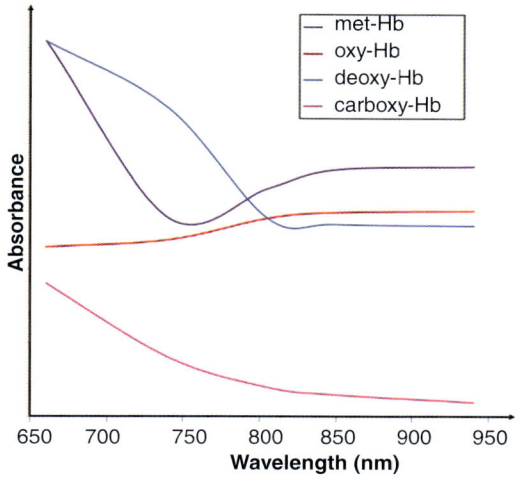

Figure 7.5 Absorbance spectra of several different species of haemoglobin

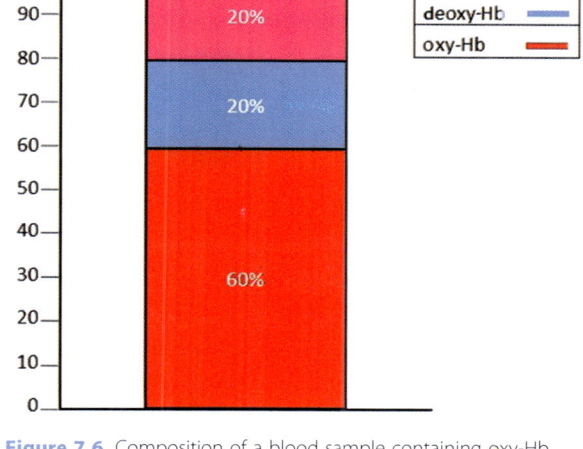

Figure 7.6 Composition of a blood sample containing oxy-Hb, deoxy-Hb and carboxy-Hb

presence may lead to inaccurate pulse-oximeter readings. The absorption spectra of different haemoglobin species are illustrated in Figure 7.5.

Terminology used in oximetry can be confusing and it is important to understand the difference between the terms SpO_2, SaO_2 and FO_2Hb. Consider a blood sample that has 60% oxy-Hb, 20% deoxy-Hb and 20% carboxy-Hb, as depicted in Figure 7.6.

The arterial oxygen saturation (SaO_2) is measured directly by a co-oximeter and is defined as:

$$SaO_2 = \frac{\text{oxy-Hb}}{\text{oxy-Hb} + \text{deoxy-Hb}}$$
$$= \frac{60}{80}$$
$$= 75\%$$

This does not take into account the presence of carboxy-Hb or met-Hb and consequently, in this case, overestimates oxygen availability to the tissues. Pulse oximeters provide an indirect measurement of the SaO_2 (the SpO_2). In normal conditions, the SpO_2 correlates well with the SaO_2. In the conditions described above, the SpO_2 will overestimate the SaO_2 because carboxy-Hb mimics oxy-Hb (see the more detailed explanation later in the chapter).

Blood gas machines actually employ a co-oximeter with multiple light wavelengths, which allows them to quantify the presence of other species of haemoglobin, such as carboxy-Hb and met-Hb. This is reported as the fractional oxyhaemoglobin content (FO_2Hb), which is defined as:

$$FO_2Hb = \frac{\text{oxy-Hb}}{\text{oxy-Hb} + \text{deoxy-Hb} + \text{carboxy-Hb} - \text{met-Hb}}$$
$$= \frac{60}{60 + 20 + 20 + 0}$$
$$= 60\%$$

The FO_2Hb measure provides a more accurate picture of the availability of oxygen to the tissues in the presence of haemoglobin variants. If the original blood sample contained no carboxy-Hb or met-Hb, then the values for FO_2Hb and SaO_2 would be identical.

The blood of almost all invertebrates contains haemoglobin. As discussed, haemoglobin is the main carrier of oxygen to the tissues. One of nature's oddities is the crocodile icefish. Living mainly around Antarctica, it does not have functional haemoglobin. Indeed, its blood is almost colourless! Due to its extremely low metabolic rate, a crocodile icefish can survive simply by the oxygen dissolved in its plasma. It lives in water that is constantly around 0 °C; the colder the water, the greater the dissolved oxygen. It is believed to be the only living invertebrate with clear blood!

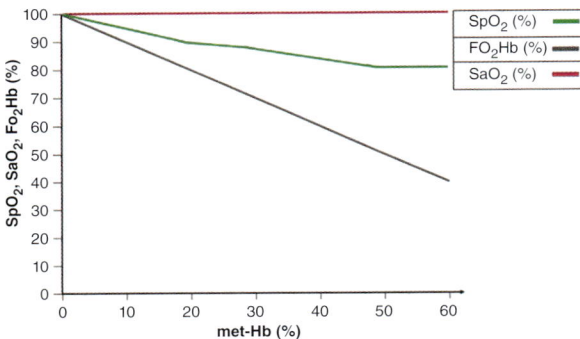

Figure 7.7 Values of SpO_2, SaO_2 and FO_2Hb at different levels of methaemoglobinaemia

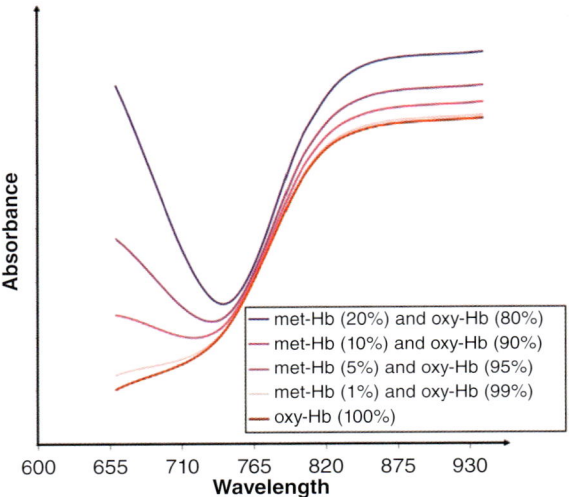

Figure 7.8 Composite absorbance spectra of blood as the level of methaemoglobin increases

Methaemoglobin

Methaemoglobinaemia occurs when some of the ferrous iron (Fe^{2+}) within haemoglobin exists in the oxidized ferric (Fe^{3+}) state. This prevents the affected haem groups from carrying oxygen. In addition, a conformational change is induced in the unaffected haem groups that increases their affinity for oxygen, shifting the oxygen–haemoglobin dissociation curve to the left and resulting in less oxygen being released to the tissues.

Methaemoglobinaemia is either congenital or may be acquired as a side-effect of several drugs (such as prilocaine, aniline dyes or nitrates). It is clinically significant because it reduces the ability of haemoglobin to carry oxygen, causing tissue hypoxia. Met-Hb levels of between 20% and 45% cause headaches, lethargy, breathlessness and low conscious level. Levels as high as 50–60% are usually fatal and present with cardiovascular instability, seizures and coma.

The effect of met-Hb on the pulse oximeter reading is proportional to the quantity present. Figure 7.7 illustrates the effect of increasing levels of met-Hb when the patient is breathing 100% oxygen.

This can be explained by observing the effect of met-Hb on the composite absorbance spectrum of the blood. For relative simplicity, let us consider a patient who, on blood gas analysis, has an SaO_2 of 100% and varying concentrations of met-Hb. This example allows us to ignore the effects of deoxy-Hb on the scenario because there is none present in the sample. The composite absorbance curve is now simply derived from the varying contributions of the oxy-Hb and met-Hb absorbance curves (Figure 7.8).

The pulse oximeter lacks the correct wavelengths of light to determine the concentration of met-Hb. It essentially assumes that any absorption of light must be due to the presence of the two conventional forms (oxy-Hb and deoxy-Hb). This allows met-Hb to mimic the effect of deoxy-Hb in the red spectrum and oxy-Hb in the infrared spectrum. In Figure 7.8, as the concentration of met-Hb increases (each different line on the graph), the absorbance values at 660 nm and 940 nm begin to become similar to each other. When they are identical (as they are, almost, for the met-Hb 20% line), this will equate to an R value of 1 and the pulse oximeter will present a reading of 85%.

High met-Hb levels therefore cause the SpO_2 to trend towards 85% irrespective of the true patient saturation (as revealed by FO_2Hb). Depending on the patient's true oxygen saturation, this means that the SpO_2 may be either an over- or underestimate: an SpO_2 of 85% would be an overestimate if the true oxygen saturation was 70% or an underestimate if the true oxygen saturation was actually 92%. Treatment of methaemoglobinaemia involves stopping the precipitant and administration of a reducing agent such as methylene blue.

In severe methaemoglobinaemia, the blood develops a blueish colouration. The disease may be acquired or congenital. There have been documented families throughout the world who have suffered greatly with the condition. One such family were the 'Blue Fugates' of Hazard, Kentucky, in the early 1800s. Due to inter-marriages within the close community, the otherwise recessive genes became phenotypically dominant. Many Fugate descendants had a blue complexion. However, the author can find no evidence of suspected methaemoglobinaemia within the Smurf family!

Sulph-haemoglobin

Sulph-haemoglobin (sulph-Hb) also occurs when some of the ferrous iron (Fe^{2+}) within haemoglobin is irreversibly oxidized to the ferric (Fe^{3+}) state. It has a similar effect to met-Hb but with the addition of a sulphur atom in the porphyrin ring of the haemoglobin molecule. Like met-Hb, sulph-Hb cannot carry oxygen. However, unlike met-Hb, sulph-Hb shifts the oxygen–haemoglobin dissociation curve to the right which facilitates oxygen unloading to the tissues. Consequently, sulph-haemoglobinaemia generally has a milder clinical course than methaemoglobinaemia at equivalent blood levels.

Sulph-Hb is also caused as a side-effect of drugs (such as aniline dyes, nitrates, sulphonamides and metoclopramide). It behaves in a similar fashion to met-Hb by mimicking oxy-Hb and deoxy-Hb, which causes the SpO_2 to trend towards 85%.

Interestingly, most co-oximeters cannot differentiate between met-Hb and sulph-Hb. The diagnosis is usually considered when presumed methaemoglobinaemia does not improve with methylene blue treatment. The addition of cyanide to a blood sample can help to differentiate between the two as sulph-Hb will remain intact, whilst met-Hb will disappear. There is no specific antidote for sulph-haemoglobinaemia and treatment is supportive. Sulph-Hb will spontaneously resolve as new erythrocytes are created and an exchange transfusion may be performed to expedite this process in severe cases.

Venous Pulsations

The mathematical algorithm for the pulse oximeter assumes that any pulsatile flow in the vascular bed is arterial. Venous blood flow can sometimes become pulsatile, for example if the patient has tricuspid regurgitation or a finger probe is applied too tightly. This causes a low SpO_2 reading because venous oxygen saturation is now averaged with the arterial.

Movement Artefact

High-frequency movement such as seizure activity, shivering or tremor can mimic the frequency of the cardiac cycle and lead to venous blood being measured as pulsatile by the pulse oximeter. In addition, patient movement can alter the path length of the light travelling from the LED to the photodiode. Manufacturers have developed improved algorithms to detect and minimize the effect of movement artefact.

Fingernail Polish

Traditionally, fingernail polish was noted to lower the recorded SpO_2 by around 10%. Modern pulse oximeter design has reduced this effect to less than 2%.

Intravenous Pigmented Dyes

Pigmented dyes, such as methylene blue and indocyanine green, are not uncommonly used in medical practice. Methylene blue mimics deoxy-Hb and can spuriously reduce the measured SpO_2 by up to 30%. Intravenous indocyanine green causes a minor reduction in SpO_2 of around 3–4%.

Poor Perfusion

Pulse oximeters rely on pulsatile flow to distinguish between arterial blood and that in the veins or tissue. In low perfusion states, this pulsatile flow may be diminished to the degree that the pulse oximeter produces a spuriously low reading.

Haemoglobinopathy

A few rare haemoglobin variants (such as Hb-Bonn, Hb-Hammersmith, Hb-M and Hb-Köln) have been noted to artificially lower recorded SpO_2. Fetal haemoglobin (Hb-F) has no effect on the measured SpO_2.

Anaemia with Co-existing Hypoxia

Anaemia itself does not cause an inaccurately low SpO_2. However, in patients who are both anaemic and hypoxaemic, the pulse oximeter can overestimate the severity of hypoxaemia. This effect is not observed in normoxic patients with anaemia. The underlying

Table 7.4 Values of FO$_2$Hb and SpO$_2$ with increasing levels of carboxyhaemoglobin

Carboxyhaemoglobin (%)	FO$_2$Hb (%)	SpO$_2$ (%)
0	90	90
1	90	90
5	90	92
10	90	94
20	90	98

mechanism is thought to involve limitations in the application of the Beer–Lambert law, which assumes that light travels in a straight, defined path through the finger. The reality is that light is scattered by red blood cells so the Lambert law is not strictly followed because the true path length is longer than the physical breadth of the finger-tip. This error is automatically corrected for by calibrating the sensor algorithms in real subjects. This scatter effect is, however, observed to a lesser extent when there are fewer red blood cells (anaemia); the device is therefore not accurately calibrated in this clinical setting.

Carboxyhaemoglobin

Carbon monoxide binds to haemoglobin, forming carboxyhaemoglobin (carboxy-Hb), with 250 times the affinity of oxygen. This reduces the availability of haemoglobin for oxygen transport and causes the oxygen–haemoglobin dissociation curve to be shifted to the left, which results in less oxygen being released to the tissues. The arterial PO$_2$ (PaO$_2$) is unaffected. The effect of carboxy-Hb on the pulse oximeter reading is proportional to the quantity present. Table 7.4 illustrates that when the patient is actually 90% saturated, the pulse oximeter increasingly over-reads as the levels of carboxy-Hb rise.

Carboxy-Hb has similar light-absorption properties to oxy-Hb in that it has a low absorbance of light in the red spectrum (660 nm). Its presence effectively dilutes the quantity of deoxy-Hb (which absorbs red light significantly) and allows more red light to pass through. This causes the R value to be lower than it would be otherwise and this corresponds to a higher SpO$_2$ reading from the pulse oximeter.

In essence, mimics of oxy-Hb (for example, carboxy-Hb) will cause the SpO$_2$ to tend towards the value of pure oxy-Hb. Mimics of both oxy-Hb and deoxy-Hb (for example, met-Hb and sulph-Hb) will cause the SpO$_2$ to tend towards the value of 85%. The uniting feature of all these haemoglobin states is that they make the SpO$_2$ unreliable.

Pulse oximetry is a very convenient, portable, non-invasive method of monitoring the oxygenation of a patient. However, the limitations that have been described above highlight the importance of arterial blood gas analysis in the care of a critically unwell patient.

PO$_2$ Electrodes

Two systems are commonly used to measure the partial pressure of oxygen (PO$_2$) of a sample (sometimes referred to as the oxygen tension): the Clark (polarographic) electrode and the fuel cell.

Clark (Polarographic) Electrode

Oxygen molecules diffuse through the membrane from the blood sample at a rate proportional to their partial pressure (Figure 7.9). They reach the cathode where they are reduced (**R**eduction **I**s **G**ain of electrons; remember 'OIL <u>RIG</u>') and OH$^-$ ions are formed. The OH$^-$ ions react with the electrolyte to form chloride ions in solution. These chloride ions are oxidized (**O**xidation **I**s **L**oss of electrons; '<u>OIL</u>') to silver chloride at the anode. The current through the circuit is measured by an ammeter and is proportional to the PO$_2$.

The Clark electrode is battery-powered (0.6 V) and is relatively robust and portable. Disadvantages of the device include a limited lifespan of around 3 years due to the consumption of its silver anode and degradation of the Teflon™ membrane. It also requires a high level of maintenance, regular electrolyte replacement and a power supply, and must be maintained at a constant temperature of 37 °C. It has a slow response time of around 30 seconds which means that it is unable to perform breath-to-breath gas analysis.

The Clark electrode is most commonly used in modern-day blood gas analyzers, although it can measure PO$_2$ in both liquid and gas samples. The electrode will over-read the PO$_2$ in the presence of strong oxidizing substances (such as halothane or nitrous oxide) as they are also reduced at the cathode. It will also over-read in conditions of high ambient pressure (such as in mechanical ventilation). Humidity in a gas sample will cause the electrode to under-read due to impairment in the diffusion of oxygen across the membrane.

Fuel Cell (Hersch or Galvanic Cell)

Oxygen molecules diffuse through the membrane at a rate proportional to their partial pressure where they

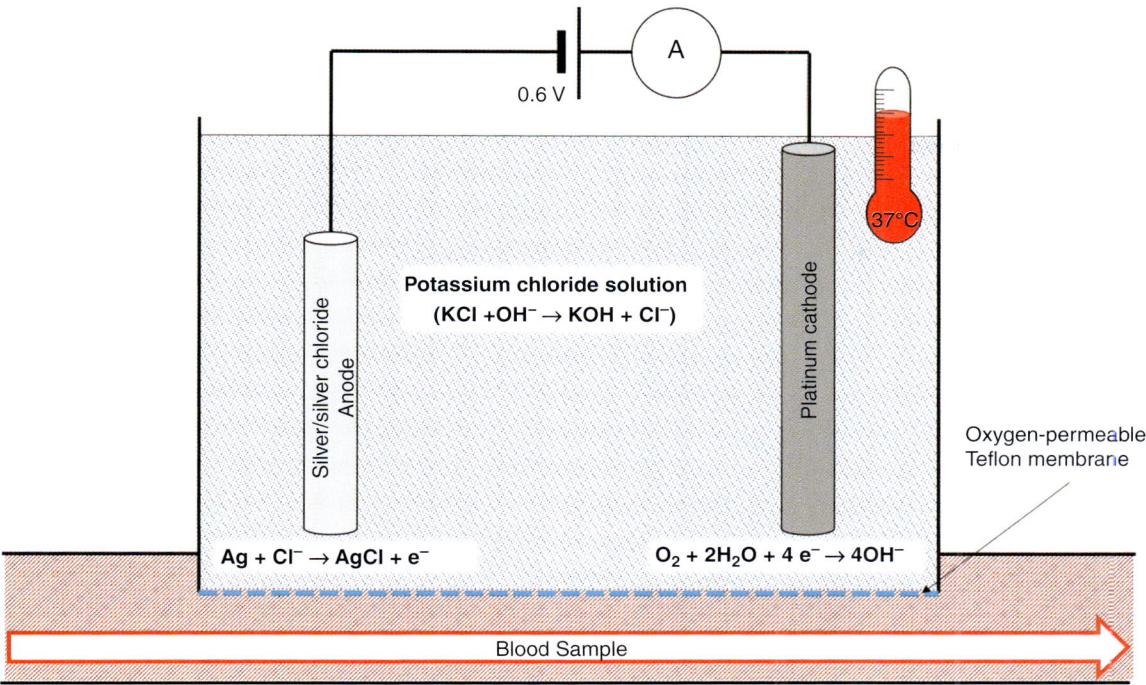

Figure 7.9 Clark (polarographic) electrode

are, as in the Clark electrode, reduced at the cathode to form OH⁻ ions. These serve to replace those OH⁻ ions being oxidized to form lead oxide at the anode (Figure 7.10).

The fuel cell has several advantages over the Clark electrode. First, it requires significantly less maintenance and is more compact. In addition, it functions as a battery and therefore does not require an external power source. These advantages have led to its use in 'rebreather' scuba-diving equipment.

The fuel cell has a limited lifespan of around 1 year due to exhaustion of the cell; this is shorter still if exposed to high concentrations of oxygen. It over-reads and under-reads in the same conditions described for the Clark electrode and has a similarly slow response time. Like the Clark electrode, the fuel cell requires conditions of constant temperature and pressure to maintain its accuracy. The addition of a thermistor in parallel to the circuit allows temperature compensation of the cell. The fuel cell was traditionally used for monitoring PO_2 in anaesthetic breathing circuits, although it has now largely been superseded by paramagnetic analysis.

pH Electrode

The pH is defined as the negative logarithm to the base 10 of the H^+ ion concentration. In blood samples, it can be measured using the pH electrode which is essentially two half-cells that are in electrical continuity via the sample. One half-cell is pH-dependent (glass electrode) and the other is not (the reference electrode), which means that when they are connected, a potential difference can be measured that is reflective of the sample pH. The reference electrode is commonly made from silver/silver chloride or mercury/mercurous chloride (calomel) (Figure 7.11). Unlike the Clark electrode and fuel cell, there are no reduction or oxidation reactions occurring and therefore the cell does not have an anode or cathode.

The principle of the pH electrode is instead based on ion interactions within the pH-sensitive glass. The glass is a complex framework of silicon oxides in which calcium and sodium ions are embedded. Hydrogen ions from the blood sample displace sodium ions from within the glass but do not cross it. This draws chloride ions from the buffer solution to

Chapter 7: Blood Gas Analysis

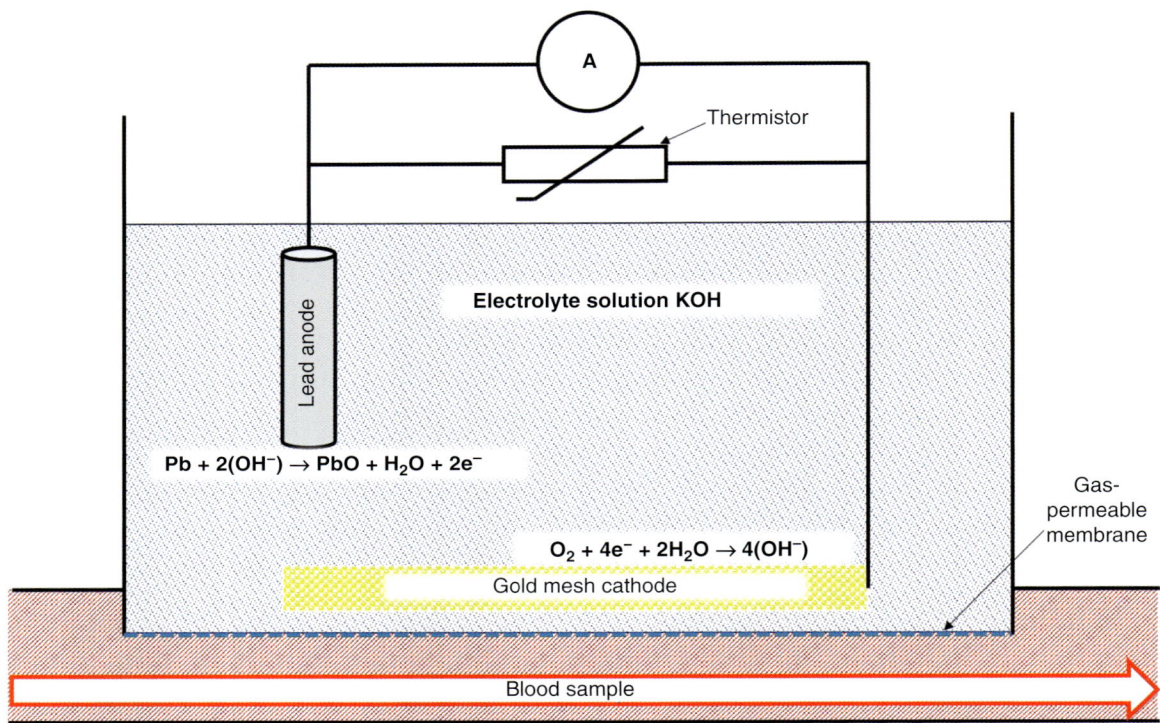

Figure 7.10 Fuel cell

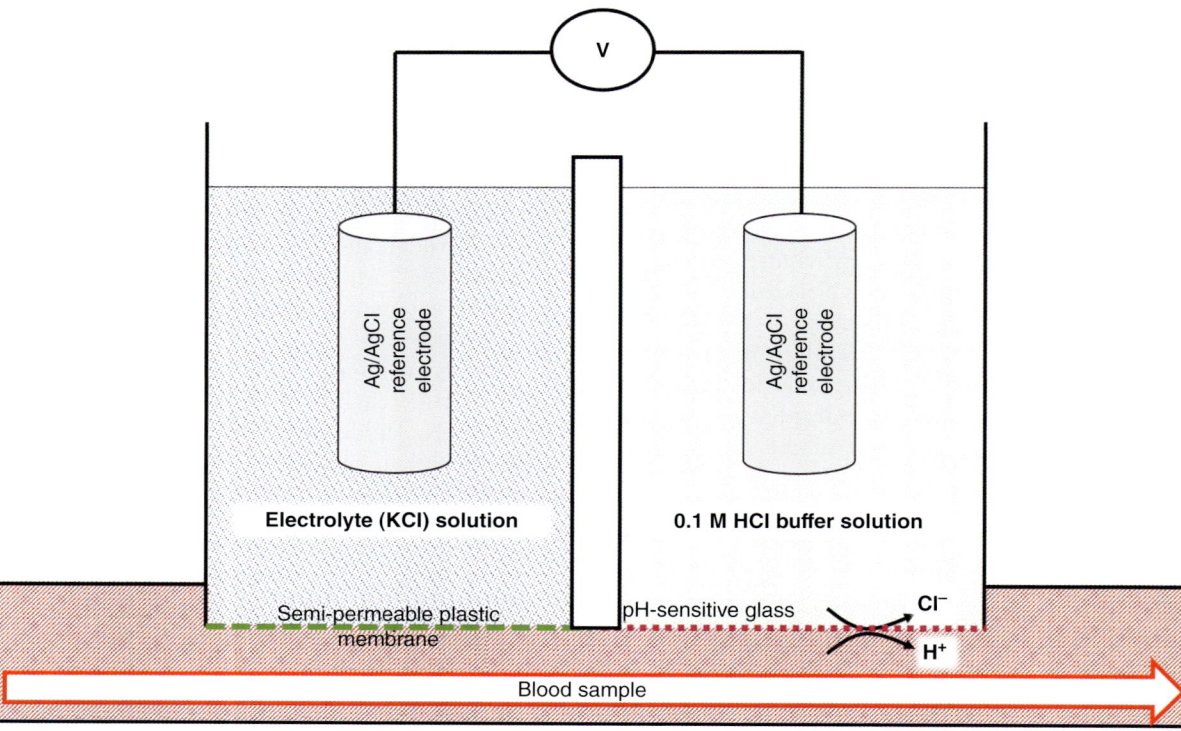

Figure 7.11 pH electrode

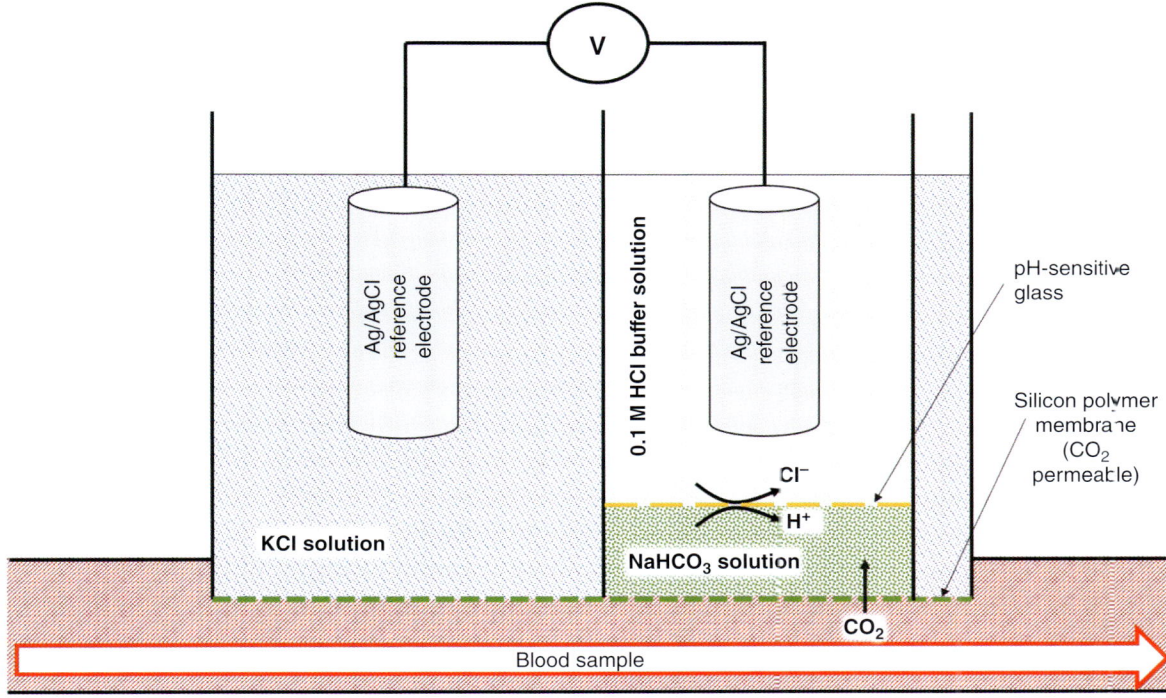

Figure 7.12 Severinghaus electrode

the internal surface of the glass. A potential difference is therefore generated across the glass (equivalent to 60 mV per unit of pH) which can be measured and calibrated to determine the pH of the sample. Two different samples of known pH are used for calibration. The electrodes must be kept at a constant temperature of 37 °C. Hydrogen chloride (0.1 M) is one example of a buffer solution but potassium chloride can also be used.

PCO_2 Electrode (Severinghaus Electrode)

The Severinghaus electrode is essentially a modified version of the pH electrode (Figure 7.12). Carbon dioxide (CO_2) from the blood sample crosses a permeable membrane, entering a solution of bicarbonate.

$$CO_2 + H_2O \rightarrow H_2CO_3 \rightarrow H^+ + HCO_3^-$$

Hydrogen ions are generated, which leads to a potential difference across the pH-sensitive glass which is measured and calibrated to determine the PCO_2. The relationship between PCO_2 and H^+ is described in the Henderson–Hasselbach equation:

$$pH = pK_a + \log_{10} \frac{[HCO_3^-]}{[H_2CO_3]}$$

$$= pK_a + \log_{10} \frac{[HCO_3^-]}{0.003 \times PCO_2}$$

where 0.003 mmol l^{-1} mmHg^{-1} represents the Ostwald solubility coefficient.

The electrodes should be kept at a constant temperature of 37 °C. Diffusion of CO_2 across the silicon polymer membrane causes a slow response time of 2–3 minutes. Perforation of the membrane will cause inaccurate results.

Blood Gas Machine and Derived Variables

The blood gas machine combines the pH, Severinghaus and Clark electrodes, using a single common silver/silver chloride reference electrode. Modern blood gas analyzers also have an array of electrolyte modules, which allows point-of-care testing for a wide number of variables.

Some blood gas variables are calculated from other measured parameters and these are summarized in Table 7.5.

Chapter 7: Blood Gas Analysis

Table 7.5 Methods by which the blood gas machine determines its variables

Variables measured directly	Variables calculated using the Siggaard-Anderson nomogram	Variables determined differently in different machines
pH PCO_2 PO_2 carboxy-Hb met-Hb deoxy-Hb fetal-Hb Haemoglobin Na^+ K^+ Cl^- Ca^{2+} Glucose Lactate Bilirubin	HCO_3^- (actual) HCO_3^- (standard) BE	SaO_2 is measured with a co-oximeter in some machines. In others, it is calculated using the pH and PO_2 using the standard oxygen-dissociation curve. This method assumes a normal P_{50} with no abnormal haemoglobin species (which doesn't necessarily apply to hospitalized patients). FO_2Hb is usually measured

Errors in Blood Gas Measurement

Protein

Protein deposits from the sample commonly build up on the membranes of electrodes, hindering the diffusion of gas to the electrode and therefore reducing its accuracy. Regular maintenance is required to remove these.

Air Bubbles

A common source of error in blood gas analysis is the presence of air bubbles within the sample and the impact of these on the results increases with the length of time prior to analysis. Bubbles cause an increase in PO_2, a fall in PCO_2 but a negligible change in pH.

Excess Heparin

Blood gas samples are anticoagulated with either liquid heparin or lyophilized (dry) heparin. An excess of liquid heparin impairs the accuracy of the result, predominantly by diluting the blood sample (although this is only clinically significant if the heparin volume exceeds 10% of the total blood sample volume). The observed effects include an increased PO_2 with a decreased PCO_2 and HCO_3^- and a slight reduction in pH. Interestingly, similar results can be obtained if the sample is diluted with normal saline, illustrating the predominance of the dilution effect. Chemically, heparin is acidic in both dry and liquid forms and would be predicted to reduce pH. In reality, pH changes are buffered by serum proteins and therefore pH changes are negligible.

Patients with Haematological Malignancy

Cellular metabolism and oxygen consumption continue in arterial blood samples prior to analysis. Spurious hypoxaemia may result from significant leucocytosis (leucocyte larceny) or thrombocytosis, as may occur in patients with haematological malignancy. Anomalously elevated serum potassium (pseudo-hyperkalaemia) may also be observed in this cohort of patients and occurs due to cell lysis prior to laboratory analysis. The impact of both of these processes can be mitigated by transporting the sample on ice and minimizing the time between blood sampling and analysis.

Reverse Pseudo-hyperkalaemia

This describes the phenomenon where the potassium result derived from a heparinized plasma sample is anomalously high compared to that from an unheparinized serum sample. It is usually observed in patients who have leukaemia or lymphoma and is thought to be due to a heparin effect on the fragile white blood cell walls.

Hypothermia

Blood gas analyzers adjust the temperature of the blood sample to 37 °C prior to performing their analysis. If the patient is normothermic, this merely recreates the *in vivo* environment and has no impact on interpretation of the results. If the patient is actually hypo- or hyperthermic, however, the values obtained from the machine will not accurately reflect those in the patient unless the values are mathematically corrected to allow for the effects of temperature on gas solubility. As blood temperature decreases in the hypothermic patient, the solubility of oxygen and carbon dioxide increases and they exhibit lower partial pressures. When a blood sample is taken from a hypothermic patient and warmed by the blood gas analyzer, PO_2 and PCO_2 increase with a corresponding reduction in pH. There are two schools of thought about how this should be interpreted clinically (see below). As a general rule, for every degree temperature drop below 37 °C, the PO_2 is reduced by 0.66 kPa and the PCO_2 is reduced by 0.26 kPa. pH can be temperature-corrected using the Rosenthal correction factor which adds 0.015 to the measured pH for every degree drop in patient temperature.

Let's consider those two different approaches a little further: using the values straight from the machine without any alterations made for temperature (alpha-stat), versus mathematically correcting the values to account for the patient's temperature at the time of sampling (pH-stat). Imagine that an arterial blood gas is taken from a patient undergoing deep hypothermic circulatory arrest (DHCA) at 20 °C on cardiopulmonary bypass. The temperature-corrected sample (pH-stat) might show pH 7.6 and PCO_2 2.3 kPa. If this same sample was analyzed at 37 °C and not temperature-corrected (alpha-stat), the values might read pH 7.4 and PCO_2 5.2 kPa. Applying a pH-stat approach ('**p**H is **p**ushed back (corrected) in a **p**erishingly-cold **p**atient'), the anaesthetist uses the temperature-corrected values, interprets them as a respiratory alkalosis and manipulates the pH to 7.4 and PCO_2 to 5.2 kPa by adding CO_2 to the inspired gas. Adopting the alpha-stat approach ('**a**lpha **a**ssumes a normal temperature and leaves the values **a**s-is'), the anaesthetist interprets the values as within the normal range and takes no action.

Traditional proponents of pH-stat management argue that the addition of carbon dioxide causes cerebral vasodilation, facilitating more reliable cerebral cooling and improves cerebral oxygen delivery by adjusting the oxygen dissociation curve. However, its detractors highlight the risks of increased cerebral blood flow, including microembolism and intracranial hypertension. There is no good quality evidence to support either strategy but there is a suggestion of improved outcome using a pH-stat approach in paediatric DHCA cases and an alpha-stat approach for adults (**p**H for **p**aediatrics, **a**lpha for **a**dults). The basis for this is that the paediatric brain is still developing and the more even cooling offered by pH-stat may be particularly advantageous for neuroprotection. In addition, as children don't tend to have vessel calcification, the risk of embolic phenomenon associated with pH-stat management can largely be discounted.

Comparing Arterial, Venous and Capillary Samples

Obtaining an arterial blood gas sample can be a potentially challenging procedure with associated morbidity for the patient. Consequently, venous blood (sampled from a central venous catheter, pulmonary artery catheter or peripheral venous catheter) or capillary blood is sometimes used as a substitute although there are some important limitations.

Capillary blood should be obtained from the earlobe in adults and is usually obtained from a heel prick in neonates. In theory, capillary blood contains a mixture of venous and arterial blood from damaged venules and arterioles, with a higher proportion of arterial blood due to its higher pressure. Traditionally, 'arterialization' of the sample (achieved by pre-warming the puncture site or using vasodilator cream) was used to encourage free blood flow and reduce the arteriovenous difference. This practice is generally recognized as ineffective and is now less commonly used.

Table 7.6 illustrates how these alternative samples compare to the gold standard of an arterial blood gas.

The alternatives to arterial blood gases cannot reliably measure oxygenation although this deficit can be ameliorated by the concomitant use of pulse oximetry. Generally, there is good concordance between arterial and capillary or venous blood gases for pH, PCO_2 and HCO_3^-. However, this concordance does not apply in a haemodynamically unstable patient or at higher levels of PCO_2 (PCO_2 >6 kPa). Arterial samples must therefore be taken in these patient cohorts.

When using capillary or venous blood samples to monitor acid–base status, it is good practice to intermittently calibrate them with an arterial sample to ensure that they remain representative.

Lactate is comparable between arterial and central or mixed venous samples. However, caution must be exercised if a peripheral venous sample is used since this concordance is not maintained for lactate levels above 2 mmol l^{-1}.

Transcutaneous Methods

Modern transcutaneous monitors measure both transcutaneous carbon dioxide (PtcCO$_2$) and oxygen (PtcO$_2$) using Severinghaus and Clark electrodes, respectively (Figure 7.13). They avoid invasive arterial blood sampling and, unlike venous or capillary blood gases, provide information about oxygenation. They were traditionally used in neonates and were thought to be unreliable in adults. Technological advances have improved the accuracy of transcutaneous monitors, allowing them to maintain accuracy, even in adult critical care patients with hypercarbic respiratory failure on vasopressors. Manufacturers nevertheless recommend that arterial blood gases are used to intermittently calibrate the results.

A heating element is used to increase the skin temperature to 42–45 °C in order to optimize local skin perfusion and, consequently, the device site should be changed regularly to avoid thermal injury. Sensor placement should avoid areas of excessive oedema or subcutaneous tissue, and the earlobe is commonly selected.

Table 7.6 Comparison of blood gas values from capillary, mixed venous and peripheral venous samples with the gold standard arterial sample

Arterial variable	Capillary sample	Central/mixed venous sample	Peripheral venous sample
pH	~0.01 lower	~0.04 lower	~0.03 lower
PCO$_2$ (kPa)	~0.1 higher	~0.6 higher	~0.8 higher
PO$_2$ (kPa)	Unreliable		
HCO$_3^-$ (mmol l^{-1})	No data found	~1 lower	~1.5 higher
BE	No data found	~0.18 lower	~0.4 higher
Lactate (mmol l^{-1})	~0.08 higher	~0.08 higher	0.18–1 higher

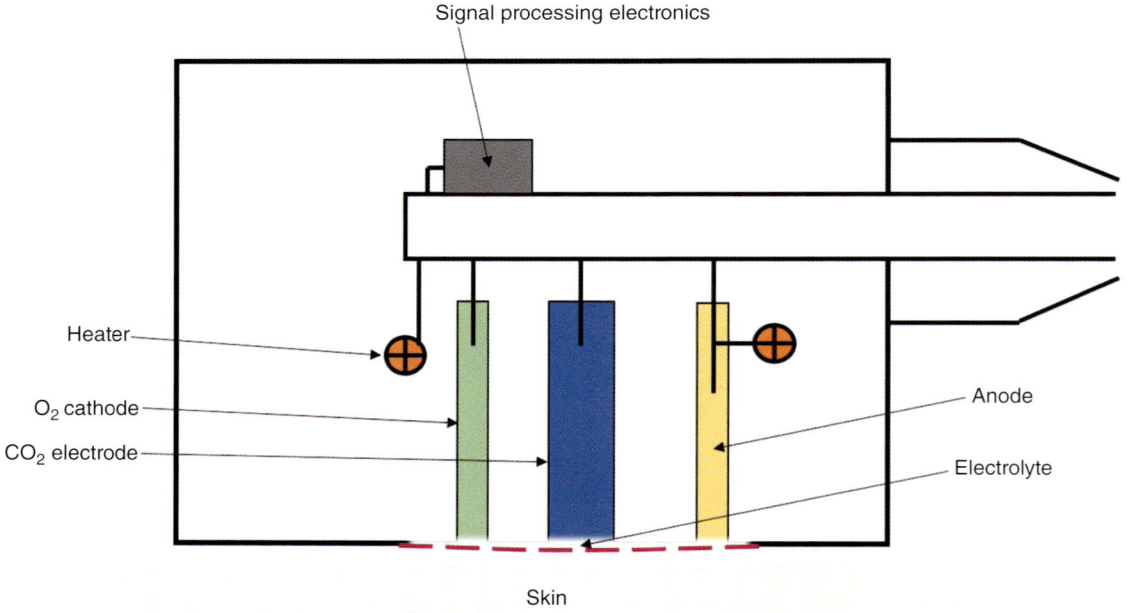

Figure 7.13 Transcutaneous oxygen and carbon dioxide monitor

Summary

Technological development of near-patient monitoring continues at an astounding pace and provides a wealth of information about each patient we treat. However, it is important to appreciate the limitations of each device and interpret the results accordingly, always taking into account the clinical context.

To go back to our house-fire survivor, we now know that, where available, the FO_2Hb is superior to the SaO_2 as there is a high likelihood of non-oxy/deoxy-Hb species in this clinical scenario for which the SaO_2 will not account. The discrepancy between the SaO_2 and FO_2Hb in her case should prompt the clinician to measure her carboxy-Hb level. The detrimental effect of carbon monoxide on oxygen carriage is one possible explanation for her elevated lactate but cyanide toxicity should also be considered. Understanding the principles of co-oximetry allows the clinician to have a better appreciation of the limitations of the pulse oximeter and to interpret its values with caution in certain situations.

Questions

MCQs – select true or false for each response

1. With regard to pulse oximetry:
   (a) Carboxyhaemoglobin absorbs more light in the red spectrum (660 nm) than oxyhaemoglobin
   (b) Lambert's law states that the absorbance of a substance is proportional to its concentration
   (c) The isosbestic point is defined when light absorption is independent of the degree of saturation and occurs at 815 nm
   (d) Methaemoglobinaemia causes the pulse oximeter to under-read
   (e) Methaemoglobinaemia occurs when haemoglobin exists in the oxidized Fe^{3+} state
2. With regard to the fuel cell used in partial pressure analysis:
   (a) It requires a power source supplying 0.6 V of electricity to function
   (b) Lead forms the anode
   (c) Potassium chloride is the most commonly used electrolyte solution
   (d) Unlike the Clark electrode, it over-reads in the presence of nitrous oxide
   (e) A thermistor is used to adjust the temperature of the electrolyte solution
3. With regard to the Severinghaus electrode:
   (a) Silver/silver chloride is used for the anode
   (b) H^+ ions diffuse across the pH-sensitive glass creating a potential difference of 60 mV per unit of pH
   (c) Sodium bicarbonate solution is a commonly used buffer
   (d) It has a fast response time and can be used to analyze gas samples
   (e) Potassium chloride is used as an electrolyte

SBAs – select the single *best* answer to each stem

4. A 70-year-old male is on the cardiac ICU following an uneventful two-vessel coronary artery bypass. During his first post-operative night, he develops hypertension and an infusion of sodium nitroprusside is commenced to treat it. Within a few hours, he develops cyanosis and his pulse oximeter reads 87%. His FiO_2 is turned up to 0.6 but there is no improvement in his SpO_2 and his blood gases following this are shown:

pH	7.37
PCO_2	5.2 kPa
PO_2	50 kPa
HCO_3^-	23 mmol l^{-1}
Base excess	0
Lactate	0.1 mmol l^{-1}
SaO_2	100%

What is the most likely cause of the cyanosis?
   (a) Cyanide toxicity
   (b) Shunt
   (c) Methaemoglobinaemia
   (d) Thiocyanate toxicity
   (e) Pulmonary embolus
5. Which of the following patients has the highest blood oxygen content?
   (a) Haemoglobin 100 g l^{-1}, SpO_2 85%, SaO_2 100%, FO_2Hb 90%, PO_2 40 kPa
   (b) Haemoglobin 100 g l^{-1}, SpO_2 100%, SaO_2 85%, FO_2Hb 75%, PO_2 40 kPa

(c) Haemoglobin 80 g l^{-1}, SpO$_2$ 100%, SaO$_2$ 100%, FO$_2$Hb 100%, PO$_2$ 20 kPa

(d) Haemoglobin 80 g l^{-1}, SpO$_2$ 100%, SaO$_2$ 100%, FO$_2$Hb 100%, PO$_2$ 40 kPa

(e) Haemoglobin 110 g l^{-1}, SpO$_2$ 85%, SaO$_2$ 100%, FO$_2$Hb 90%, PO$_2$ 20 kPa

Answers

1. FFFFT

    Deoxyhaemoglobin (deoxy-Hb) absorbs more light in the red spectrum than oxyhaemoglobin (oxy-Hb). Beer's law states that the absorbance of a substance is proportional to its concentration. Lambert's law states that the greater the distance travelled by the light, the more light will be absorbed. The isosbestic point for oxy-Hb and deoxy-Hb is 805 nm. Methaemoglobinaemia causes the pulse oximetry reading to trend towards 85% and therefore usually under-reads. However, if the patient is severely hypoxic, the pulse-oximeter reading may well be an overestimate.

2. FTFFF

    The fuel cell is itself a battery and does not require an external power source. Potassium hydroxide is the most common electrolyte solution. Both the Clark electrode and the fuel cell over-read in the presence of nitrous oxide. A thermistor provides temperature compensation by changing the electrical resistance (and thus the electrical output) of the fuel-cell circuit. It does not change the temperature of the electrolyte solution.

3. FFTFT

    The Severinghaus electrode is a modified version of the pH electrode and, as such, does not have an anode or a cathode. Silver/silver chloride is, however, used for both the electrodes. H$^+$ ions do generate a potential difference of 60 mV per unit of pH but are not thought to cross the pH-sensitive glass. Due to slow diffusion across the silicon polymer membrane, the Severinghaus electrode has a slow response time.

4. (c)

    Cyanide toxicity would usually be observed after a prolonged infusion of sodium nitroprusside and would cause a lactic acidosis, which is not present in this case. Shunt would cause an elevated arterial–alveolar gradient but in this case the gradient is normal. Thiocyanate toxicity can occur with sodium nitroprusside but causes psychosis, tinnitus and seizures rather than cyanosis. Pulmonary embolus causes an increase in both physiological shunt and dead space. The majority of patients with a pulmonary embolus exhibit an increased arterial–alveolar gradient (although a normal gradient does not exclude a pulmonary embolus) and an improvement in SpO$_2$ with oxygen therapy would be expected.

5. (e)

    Pulse oximetry is an indirect measurement of the SaO$_2$. Therefore, if the SaO$_2$ is available, this value should be used in preference to the SpO$_2$. In normal individuals, the SaO$_2$ is the same as the FO$_2$Hb. Where there is a discrepancy, the FO$_2$Hb should be used since it accounts for the presence of abnormal haemoglobin species. With this in mind, before doing any calculations, it should be clear that (c) is lower than (d) because (d) has a higher PO$_2$; this means the plasma-dissolved oxygen content of (d) will be higher even though the oxygen content bound to haemoglobin will be identical in both (c) and (d). It should also be clear that (a) is greater than (b) because the only difference between the two is the higher FO$_2$Hb. This means that (b) and (c) can be excluded.

    Since haemoglobin has a much larger impact on oxygen content than PO$_2$, it can be concluded that (e) is greater than (a). This means that (a) can be excluded.

    The remaining choice is between (d) and (e) and, for this, a calculation is needed: the calculation of the oxygen-carrying capacity of blood:

    Oxygen content (ml) in 100 ml blood
    $$= \left(1.34 \times Hb \times \frac{SaO_2}{100}\right) + (0.023 \times PO_2)$$

    where Hb is expressed in g dl^{-1}, SaO$_2$ as a percentage and PO$_2$ in kPa. 1.34 ml g^{-1} Hb is known as Hüfner's constant.

    For part (d):

    Oxygen content = (1.34 × 8 × 1) + (0.023 × 40)
    = 11.63 ml per 100 ml blood

    For part (e):

    Oxygen content = (1.34 × 11 × 1) + (0.023 × 20)
    = 15.2 ml per 100 ml blood

Chapter 8

Vapours and Vaporizers

Ed Copley

Learning Objectives

- To understand the behaviour of substances as they change phase
- To understand the working of vaporizers in common use
- To gain a knowledge of the safety mechanisms employed in vaporizer design
- To have an appreciation of the dangers inherent in the use of vapour anaesthesia
- To understand how vapours and gases behave in unusual environments

Chapter Content

- Physics of phase changes
- Anaesthetic vapours
- Vaporizers
- Hyperbaric systems
- High altitudes

Scenario

During an anaesthetic, it is uncommon for the pipeline gases to fail. It is, however, vital to be able to maintain safety should this occur.

You are delivering anaesthesia for a surgical procedure of approximately 2 hours' duration. The patient is stable and the anaesthesia has reached equilibrium, with end-tidal oxygen, nitrous oxide and sevoflurane concentrations of 40%, 58% and 2%, respectively. Unexpectedly, the oxygen supply alarm sounds and you are forced to switch from pipeline gases to bottled gases. This is accomplished without incident and, to preserve your supply for as long as possible, you opt for low-flow anaesthesia.

How do the pressure changes within a cylinder of oxygen versus a cylinder of nitrous oxide compare during consumption of the substance? Why do the physical properties of the individual vapour agent used for anaesthesia have so much relevance to vaporizer design? Does this design need to be modified for emergency anaesthesia at high altitude?

Introduction

Delivering safe mixtures of gases to patients is central to the practice of anaesthesia. This can only be achieved if you have a good understanding of the physical principles of how substances change their state (particularly, in this case, from liquid to vapour) and how that affects the designs and limitations of the equipment we use to achieve this phase change. Similarly, once the proper concentration of anaesthetic vapour is produced, we need to safely convey it to the patient in a carrier gas at a suitable pressure. These and other topics will be covered in this chapter. Chapter 9 will cover the physical concepts of the delivery system itself, i.e. anaesthesia breathing systems and associated equipment.

Physics of Phase Changes

In this chapter, the focus will be on the three principal phases of matter: the gas, liquid and solid phases (Figure 8.1). Plasma, the fourth phase, is not commonly encountered and so will not be discussed to a significant degree. It is helpful to have a very clear understanding, before we go further, as to what defines and differentiates these three phases:

Solid: A substance in its non-fluid state; it is characterized by structural rigidity, and resists changes to shape and volume

Liquid: A substance in a state of constant volume, which flows freely

Gas: A fluid substance that expands to fill the container in which it is placed, irrespective of its quantity; the atoms are so far apart as to have negligible inter-particulate interaction

Chapter 8: Vapours and Vaporizers

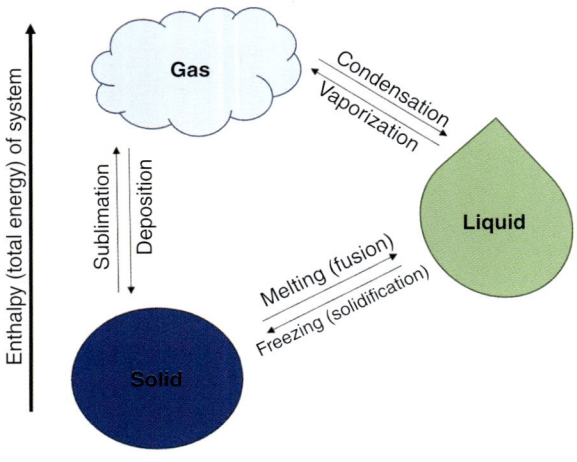

Figure 8.1 Phases and transitions

In addition, you will notice these definitions introduce another, that of a fluid:

Fluid: A substance that conforms to the shape of its container; liquids, gases and vapours are fluids

The distinction between gas and vapour will be dealt with in detail later in the chapter.

Phase changes for a given substance can be conveniently represented in a phase diagram (Figure 8.2). Conventionally, these diagrams are two-dimensional, with temperature increasing along the *x*-axis and pressure increasing along the *y*-axis. They generally show a region above and below both the critical temperature and critical pressure.

The phase diagram in Figure 8.2 shows how a typical substance responds to alterations in pressure and temperature. Nitrous oxide is an example of a

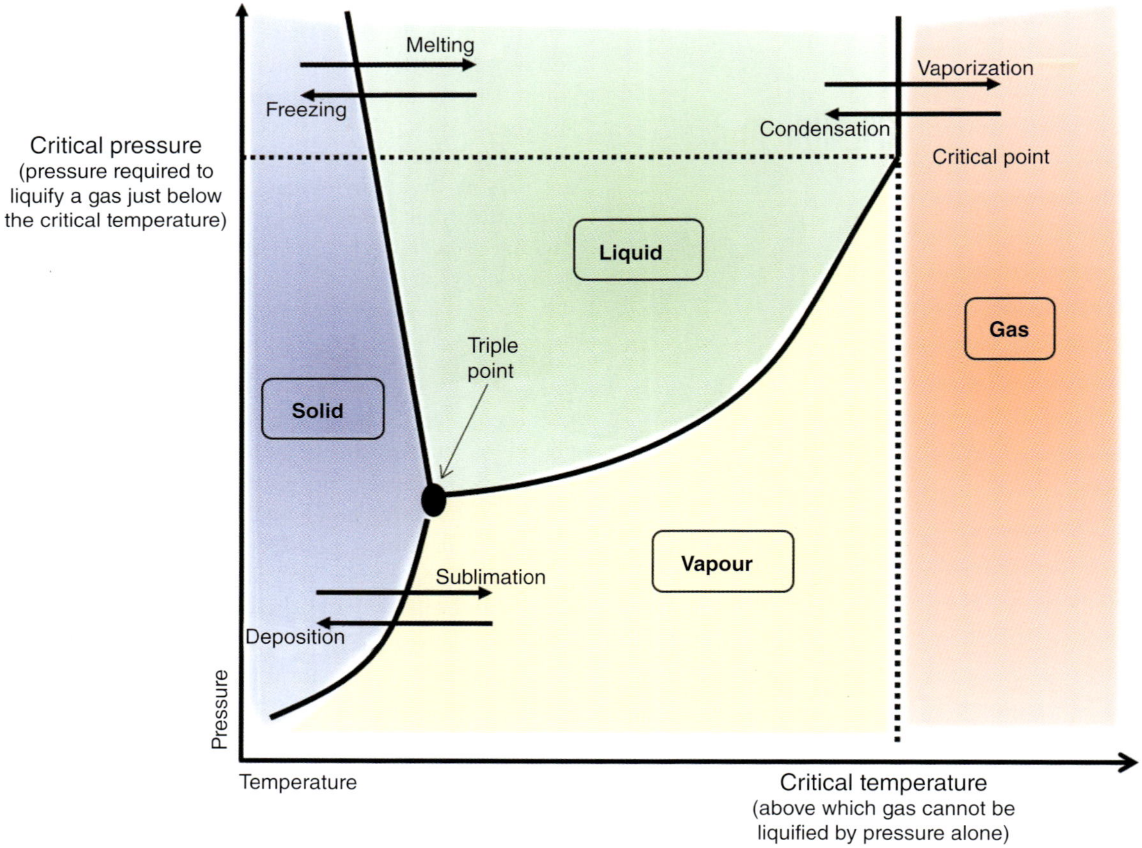

Figure 8.2 A typical phase diagram

substance with a characteristic phase diagram, which is a common topic in examinations (see Chapter 5).

To the left of the diagram is the solid phase (blue). This is the state of matter which does not flow. For example, ice is the solid state of water and quartz is solid at room temperature. The transition from solid to liquid is referred to as melting and requires energy input, the latent heat of fusion (see later). This energy does not necessarily result in an increase in temperature. Similarly, evaporation requires energy to overcome the liquid bonds and results in a vapour or gas, which may or may not be hotter than the liquid. As the diagram shows, the liquid may, in fact, depending on the accompanying pressure changes, be colder than the solid and the vapour may be colder than the liquid.

Liquids are of a relatively fixed volume but assume the shape of their container. As one further heats a liquid, it will evaporate into the vapour phase (yellow) or the gas phase (red), depending on the prevailing temperature and pressure. Vapours are often confused with gases (red) but they differ in that, unlike a vapour, it is impossible to condense a gas by applying pressure alone. A reduction in temperature in conjunction with an increase in pressure can, however, compress a gaseous substance to its liquid, or, in some cases, solid phase. The transitions are condensation and deposition respectively (see Figure 8.1).

Above the critical temperature, the vapour becomes a gas and can no longer be liquefied (or solidified) by pressure alone. The definition of the **critical temperature** of a substance is 'the temperature above which it is not possible to compress the matter from the gaseous phase to the condensed (liquid or solid) phase'. When a substance is held at its critical temperature and steadily compressed, liquid will begin to condense when the critical pressure is reached. Above the critical temperature there is no pressure which will result in transition from the gaseous to liquid phase.

The critical point is defined as 'the point on the phase diagram where both liquid and vapour phases have the same density'. The triple point is the point where the substance exists in equilibrium between its solid, liquid and vapour phases.

The words 'gas' and 'vapour' are often incorrectly used interchangeably in a similar way to the words 'fluid' and 'liquid'. Although readily understood in most situations, this is not strictly correct. A gas is the gaseous phase of a substance above its critical temperature. It cannot undergo any phase change by the application of pressure alone. A fluid is any substance in a phase that is capable of changing its shape. Liquids, gases and vapours are all fluids.

Vapour Pressure

The phase diagram also shows that there is a range of temperatures and pressures in which the substance can exist in both the liquid and gaseous phase. If the substance is in a closed container, the system is said to be in equilibrium with a gaseous region above the liquid. Under these conditions, the gas will exert a pressure on the surface of the liquid. This pressure is proportional to the temperature and is known as the vapour pressure. When the vapour pressure is equal to the ambient pressure, bubbles of the substance will form in the liquid and it is said to be boiling. At this point, the vapour pressure above the liquid will be the *saturated vapour pressure*. For ease of comparison of volatile anaesthetic agents, this property is typically quoted at a standard temperature of 293 K.

It is important to understand a further point here. Vapours and gases are not separate phases – vapours are simply a subset of gases. Vapours are gases – but gases are not necessarily vapours. A vapour is a gas below its critical temperature.

For a vaporizer which goes unused for some time, the vapour within the chamber will have had time to reach equilibrium. By definition, therefore, the pressure exerted by the vapour will equate to the saturated vapour pressure for the agent at that temperature. If vapour is released from the chamber then the vapour pressure will be restored through evaporation of more liquid. Le Chatelier's principle states that, in a dynamic equilibrium, any change to the conditions will be counteracted by movement of the equilibrium. In this case the change (removal of vapour and therefore a fall in the vapour pressure in the vessel) will be counteracted by evaporation of molecules from the liquid. In turn, this causes the temperature to drop as heat from the liquid is used in the phase change from liquid to vapour. The lower temperature results in a new equilibrium with a lower vapour pressure within the container.

Energy, Temperature and Latent Heat

In order to change from one phase to another, energy must be either given to or taken from the system. It is very important to understand that this does not

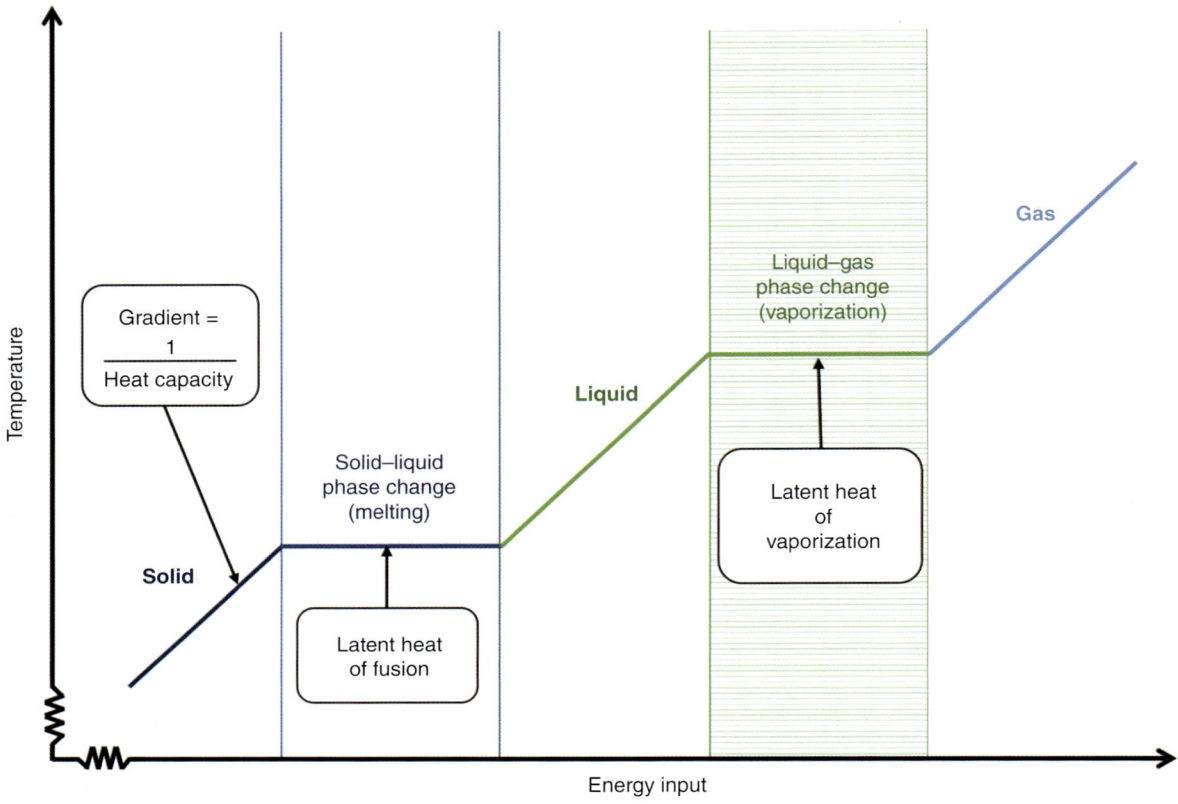

Figure 8.3 Latent heat and temperature changes in a substance as energy is added and the phases transitioned

necessarily mean the temperature will change (Figure 8.3). Temperature is a measure of the average kinetic energy of the molecules in a system. The total energy of all the molecules in that system, meanwhile, quantifies its capacity to do work. The difference is subtle but important. If one takes a quantity of a solid substance, such as candle wax, and applies heat, the temperature will steadily rise until the substance begins to melt. At this point, the heat added to the system does not raise the temperature but, instead, changes the phase of the material. Only once all the wax is liquid will the addition of energy cause a further temperature rise. The energy deposited in the system which does not change its temperature is known as the latent heat of fusion. Instead of increasing the temperature of the wax it contributes to the phase change by overcoming the intermolecular forces (e.g. hydrogen bonding, dipole–dipole interactions and van der Waals forces). A similar increase in energy without an accompanying rise in temperature occurs during the change from liquid to vapour.

A visible example of this phenomenon is the 'superheater' of a vacuum-insulated oxygen evaporator. As the liquid oxygen passes through the superheater, it gains energy from the atmosphere and is changed from liquid to gaseous oxygen. The atmosphere, on the other hand, is rapidly cooled and the water vapour contained in the air loses so much energy that it first condenses, then freezes onto the outer surface of the superheater tubes.

In gas cylinders containing liquid with vapour in equilibrium above (such as Entonox or pure nitrous oxide), the temperature falls as the vapour is consumed and further liquid evaporates to maintain the vapour pressure and restore the equilibrium. This is a result of the energy used in supplying latent heat of evaporation when the substance changes from a liquid to gaseous state within the cylinder. This can result in dew or even ice formation on the outside of the cylinder.

Mixtures of gases behave differently to single gases and have a pseudo-critical temperature: that at which one or other of the component gases can be liquefied under pressure. Cylinders of mixed nitrous oxide and oxygen in a 50:50 ratio (known as Entonox) are susceptible to separation because drawing off the gaseous mixture from the cylinder causes a drop in temperature, which can result in the remaining mixture falling below the pseudo-critical temperature (around –6 °C). This, in turn, can result in liquefaction of the nitrous oxide while the oxygen remains gaseous. If this occurs, depending on the cylinder design and its orientation, either an oxygen-rich or a nitrous oxide-rich mixture could be delivered. An oxygen-rich mixture would be deficient in analgesic effect whilst a nitrous oxide-rich mixture may be dangerously hypoxic.

Entropy and Enthalpy

In considering phase changes, it is also important to consider entropy and enthalpy. Enthalpy refers to the total energy content of a system and includes not just the heat, which we generally represent as the temperature of a material in a given phase, but also the pressure exerted by the substance on its container.

Entropy refers to the disorder present in a system. In general, entropy increases as a system changes in the solid-to-liquid-to-gas direction. This is because a crystal has a regular structure and is therefore a more ordered system than an equivalent mass of the same substance in liquid form. The molecules of the liquid form, e.g. water, can take a wider range of positions than the solid form, e.g. ice. Similarly, molecules in the gas form can take a wider range of positions than the molecules in either the liquid or solid forms. The larger number of possible positions of the molecules is roughly analogous to the increase in entropy.

The second law of thermodynamics (see Chapter 3) states that the entropy of an isolated system always increases and that this progression is irreversible. It is possible to locally reverse the entropy increase by 'shunting' entropy from one place to another. This is the mechanism by which refrigerators work. They use a cycle of evaporation, which occurs in tubes in the cold section of the unit, and condensation, which occurs outside the device. There are radiator coils on the back of the fridge that transfer the heat to the room air. By this means, it is possible to reverse the increase in entropy inside the fridge at the cost of increasing entropy outside. It is important also to note that the entropy increase outside the fridge is greater than the entropy decrease inside the fridge.

This is due to the expenditure of electrical energy by the fridge itself, which contributes to the entropy increase. It is this overall increase in entropy which allows the system to work without violating the second law of thermodynamics.

One area of relevance of the second law of thermodynamics in anaesthesia is that the increase in entropy of a system means that liquids, which have relatively low entropy, tend to evaporate to a gaseous phase, which has a higher entropy. This is how vaporizers work.

Anaesthetic Vapours

Most of the physical characteristics listed in Table 8.1 are self-explanatory but some merit further discussion. The global warming potential (GWP) is a relatively new concept. This is a measure of the effectiveness of heat capture of the gaseous form of the agent once it is released into the atmosphere. The numbers represent the equivalent mass of carbon dioxide in kilograms that would be needed to exert the same degree of 'greenhouse' effect as 1 kg of the agent in gaseous form. Other measures are also used – for example, the GWP_{20} which represents the effect of 1 kg of vapour over 20 years. This may be important because the different vapours have different atmospheric lifetimes. Although clinical considerations are extremely important, it can be seen from the table that some of the chemicals used in anaesthesia have the potential to cause great ecological damage. This should have at least some weight in the consideration of their use.

The minimum alveolar concentration (MAC) is a measure of anaesthetic potency. Numerically, it is the concentration of the gaseous form of the agent in exhaled gas (assumed to be the alveolar concentration at equilibrium) which achieves a depth of anaesthesia sufficient to prevent 50% of subjects from moving in response to a standard supra-maximal stimulus. For comparative purposes between agents, this is quoted for a pressure of 1 atm at a temperature of 20 °C.

Biotransformation describes the percentage of absorbed vapour which is metabolized to other forms. Usually, this is under the influence of liver microsomal enzymes. Biotransformation can result in the formation of compounds which cause renal and hepatic toxicity.

The oil:gas (O/G) and blood:gas (B/G) partition coefficients (PCs) are pharmacokinetic properties of

Table 8.1 Key properties of various volatile anaesthetic agents

Agent name	Desflurane	Sevoflurane	Isoflurane	Enflurane	Halothane	Ether	Chloroform	Nitrous oxide
Boiling point °C (1 atm)	23.5	58.6	48.5	56.5	50.2	34.6	61.2	−89
SVP (kPa) (20 °C)	88.5	20.9	31.7	22.9	32	55	21.2	5115
Density (g cm^{-3}) at 20 °C	1.465	1.52	1.496	1.496	1.868	0.713	1.49	1.98
Molecular weight (g)	168	200	184.5	184.5	197.4	74.1	119.4	44.003
MAC	6%	2.1%	1.15	1.68	0.75	1.92	0.77	105
Biotransformation	0.02%	3%	0.2%	2.5%	10–20%	10%	~95%	0%
O/G	19	47	98	98	224	65	400	1.4
B/G	0.42	0.68	1.4	1.9	2.3	12	8	0.47
Molecular structure								
GWP	3714	349	1401	—	—	—	—	289

the agent. They represent the relative solubility of the vapour in oil (representing cell membranes, most importantly of brain tissue) and blood respectively. The standard measurements are taken with olive oil or octanol (for oil) and blood or water (for blood). An equal volume of gas and liquid is allowed to equilibrate and the change in gas volume is then measured. For example, a B/G PC of 0.33 means that, at equilibrium, the vapour will be present in blood at one-third of the concentration present in the alveoli. The potency of agents tends to be related to their O/G PC but the speed of onset tends to be inversely related to the B/G PC; a low B/G PC tends to result in a high concentration gradient across the alveolar membrane, which facilitates rapid loading of the bloodstream. In practical terms, this means that the more fat-soluble an agent, the more potent it tends to be and the less water-soluble an agent, the more rapid tends to be its onset of action. Less water-soluble agents also tend to be excreted more quickly and so the patient will tend to emerge from anaesthesia more rapidly.

The ideal anaesthetic vapour would have the following properties:

- Non-irritant
- Non-toxic
- Non-flammable
- Non-explosive
- Rapid onset/offset (low blood solubility)
- High potency (high oil solubility)
- Analgesic
- Stable in storage
- Non-reactive with carbon dioxide absorber
- Low pungency
- Non-depressant (cardiovascular, respiratory)
- Economical
- Does not cause damage to equipment

No agent fulfils all these criteria but there are agents which are a more acceptable compromise than others.

Vaporizers

Vaporizers are precision devices for accurate mixing of fresh gas flow with a volatile agent to deliver a controlled concentration of anaesthetic to the patient. There have been numerous designs over the years but, in modern practice, these can be divided into those used in the circuit (the draw-over types) and those used outside the circuit. Those used outside the circuit generally fall into either the plenum or direct-vapour-injection design where common practice is concerned. Other types exist and these will be discussed briefly below.

The majority of modern vaporizers are designed to work only with one agent, being incompatible with any other. Each agent has its own thermal characteristics (saturated vapour pressure, latent heat of evaporation) which means the dial is calibrated to accurately reflect the vapour output of the vaporizer over a range of temperatures and gas flows, but only for that agent. Some, such as halothane, contain preservatives (in this case, thymol) which could damage the vaporizer for another agent. Consequently, vaporizers have a number of safety features to ensure the correct agent is used (see below). Modern anaesthesia in developed countries almost invariably includes agent concentration monitoring but the dials are useful and the vaporizers should be regularly serviced to ensure and maintain accuracy. The differing clinical characteristics of the agent dictate particular ranges of output concentrations for each agent. For agents that are more soluble in fat, the potency is higher so less of the agent is required to achieve surgical anaesthesia. For this reason, more fat-soluble anaesthetic vapours are delivered at lower concentrations and their vaporizer dials are marked accordingly.

Plenum Vaporizers

Plenum vaporizers are simple in concept but often include a number of safety mechanisms. They require no external power for their basic function, though some may have powered servo mechanisms to allow for varying degrees of automated anaesthesia maintenance. The basic mechanism is a chamber full of liquid anaesthetic through which a fraction of the total fresh gas flow (FGF) from the anaesthetic machine is directed (Figure 8.4). The ratio of gas passing through the plenum chamber compared to the total gas flow is called the splitting ratio.

The FGF entering the chamber containing the liquid displaces the gas already present in the chamber. This gas will be saturated with anaesthetic vapour. The new fresh gas also quickly becomes saturated with vapour and, as more fresh gas enters, this saturated gas is pushed from the chamber.

This anaesthetic mixture is then delivered to the breathing system where it mixes with the existing gas mixture. It is important to note that only at very high

Chapter 8: Vapours and Vaporizers

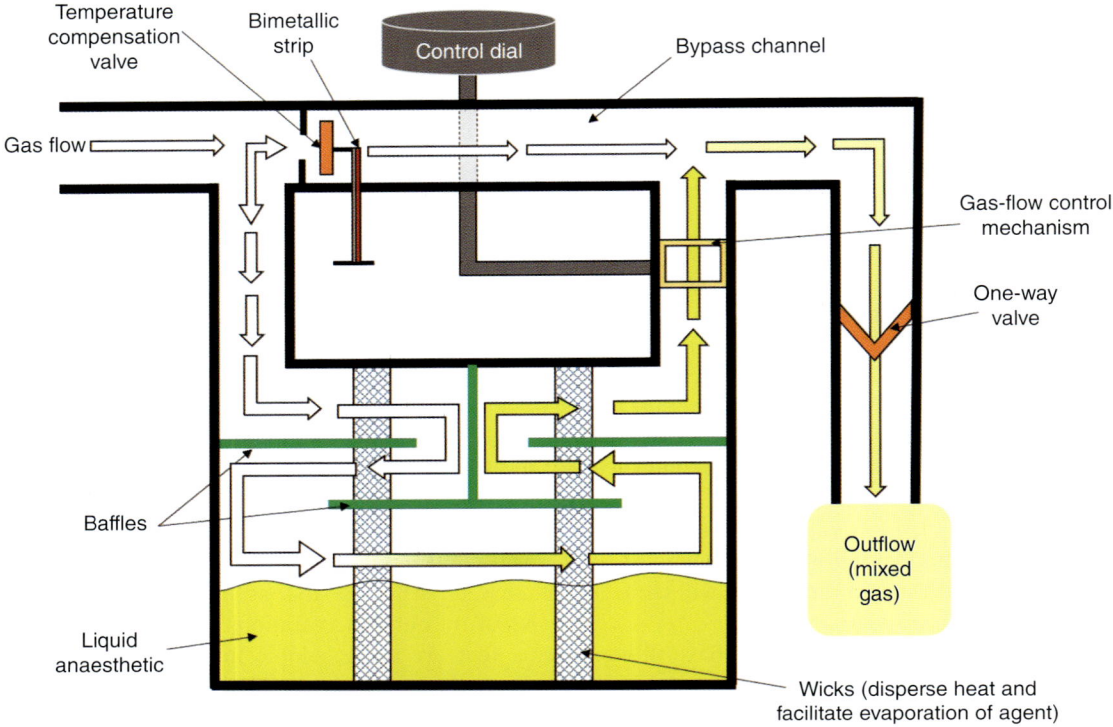

Figure 8.4 A schematic of a plenum vaporizer

gas flows does the composition of the mixture leaving the machine resemble that in the breathing system. Generally, the composition leaving the machine will be close to that set on the vaporizer but the composition in the breathing system will be quite different. This is particularly true of the circle system when being used in low-flow anaesthesia because the FGF replaces a relatively small proportion of total system volume. An analogy for the mixing process would be the addition of 1 l min^{-1} of water at a temperature of 50 °C to a bucket containing 5 l of water at 20 °C. Assuming thorough mixing of the water, the bucket contents will begin to overflow at some point but the water in the bucket will never reach 50 °C. There will always be some cooler water for the 50 °C water to mix with (even if we could abolish all heat losses from the contents of the bucket during the experiment). In the same way, if we were to add 2 l min^{-1} of FGF containing 2% sevoflurane to a circle breathing system, circle gas will be displaced via the adjustable pressure-limiting (APL) valve but the concentration of sevoflurane in the remaining gas in the circle will approach, but never actually reach, 2%. The 2% mixture is always diluted by the contents of the circuit and some sevoflurane is always taken up by the patient.

In plenum vaporizers, the energy required to evaporate the liquid anaesthetic into vapour is provided by a large heat sink inside and around the plenum chamber. This is the principal reason for the impressive weight of the devices; the heat sink is usually copper, with a density nearly nine-times that of water. While the specific heat capacity (energy to increase 1 kg of substance by 1 °C) is only one-third of water, the difference in their densities means copper is far more practical than a water jacket to ensure an effective heat sink. The thermal conductivity of copper is also significantly higher than that of water. This is important as the heat sink not only provides energy during use but also assists in transferring heat from the ambient air to the liquid to maintain the internal vapour pressure. A complex arrangement of wicks and baffles provide a large surface area from which liquid can evaporate efficiently, ensuring that the gas in the plenum chamber remains saturated with vapour.

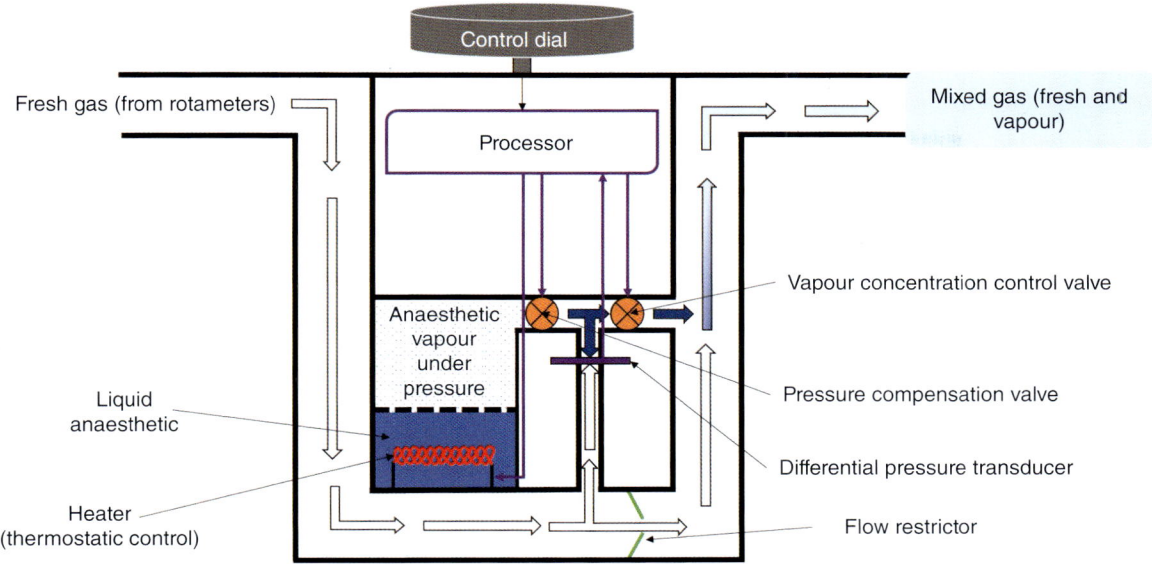

Figure 8.5 A vapour-injection vaporizer

If the ambient temperature rises then the temperature in the plenum chamber will also rise once the entire unit reaches thermal equilibrium with the environment. This will, in turn, cause the saturated vapour pressure to increase. To ensure that the composition of the anaesthetic gas remains constant, a mechanism, such as a bimetallic strip or aneroid bellows, restricts flow through the chamber. This changes the splitting ratio without any change in the dial setting on the vaporizer. At the higher temperature, the saturated vapour pressure in the plenum chamber is higher so a lower flow of gas through the chamber is sufficient to maintain a given vapour concentration at the output. The opposite occurs if the ambient temperature falls; vapour pressure falls so the temperature-compensation devices must allow the FGF through the chamber to increase in order to maintain the set concentration.

Vapour-Injection Vaporizers

Figure 8.5 shows a schematic of a vapour-injection vaporizer. This is also known as a measured flow vaporizer or dual-circuit gas-vapour blender. It uses a different mechanism from the plenum system. This vaporizer is used for some agents because of their physical characteristics, in particular, the relationship of their boiling point to typical room temperatures.

As the temperature within the vaporizer rises, the saturated vapour pressure also rises. For some agents, the change in saturated vapour pressure is so rapid across the typical range of storage and room temperatures that the agent will tend to boil off, forming vapour very quickly. This, at first glance, would seem a good thing but rapid phase changes require large amounts of energy. If a large amount of energy is removed from a system then its temperature will fall. If the temperature falls then the saturated vapour pressure will fall with it. This could, under some circumstances, result in a saturated vapour pressure so low that the plenum mechanism described above is unable to deliver the required anaesthetic vapour concentration.

The vapour-injection vaporizer provides a solution to this problem. Unlike the plenum vaporizer this is a powered device. It consists of a heated reservoir which contains the liquid anaesthetic and maintains it at a constant temperature, above its boiling point. This ensures a constant vapour pressure. The FGF is never introduced to the vessel containing the vapour/liquid mixture but, instead, the dial controls the introduction of saturated vapour directly from the vapour reservoir into the FGF in the required proportions.

The most common application of this system is for desflurane, which has a very low solubility and, consequently, is used at relatively high concentrations. The delivery of stable and clinically usable concentrations of desflurane would be impractical and expensive with a plenum design. Instead, the liquid is heated to 39 °C, producing a reliable saturated vapour pressure of 194 kPa (it boils at 23.5 °C and has a saturated vapour pressure of 88.5 kPa at 20 °C). The importance of the boiling point of desflurane should be noted. At normal theatre temperatures, desflurane would be a liquid, with vapour above. In a warm theatre, as encountered in a burns centre for example, desflurane may be above its boiling point, purely as a vapour. By actively heating the vapour chamber to 39 °C, the vapour pressure can be more reliably maintained, whatever the environment and whatever the rate of vapour consumption.

In vapour-injector vaporizers, there is no need to compensate for temperature changes because the temperature of the anaesthetic vapour is kept constant by a thermostatic controller.

Both plenum and vapour-injector vaporizers require high-pressure gas systems to ensure proper function and accuracy; this limits their use in resource-poor or remote locations.

Direct-Injection Systems

These vaporizers work by introducing the anaesthetic agent, in its liquid form, into a heated evaporation chamber adjoined to the breathing circuit. In this way, the concentration of vapour can be controlled by injecting liquid at the correct rate, as dictated by the temperature and pressure of gas within the circuit. This differs from a direct-vapour injector: for direct injection, liquid is metered out and vaporized; for vapour injection, the liquid is warmed and the resulting vapour is metered out.

As the FGF increases it will be necessary to increase the rate of anaesthetic liquid injection. All this is accomplished by the use of proprietary computer algorithms. Such vaporizers are available for use with various agents, including desflurane.

Draw-Over Vaporizers

The draw-over vaporizer is typically used in remote locations or where pressurized gases are unavailable. It is similar to a plenum vaporizer except that, rather than having fresh gas forced through it, the gas flow changes within the circuit and vaporizer are the result of the respiratory effort of the patient. These vaporizers behave very differently to plenum vaporizers.

As the patient inhales, gas is drawn towards the patient in the inspiratory limb of the system (which includes the vaporizer). As the gas moves through the vaporizer, some of the liquid contained in the device is evaporated into the gas stream. It is this process which provides the anaesthetic vapour. At a nominal minute volume there is a corresponding time during which the incoming gas is exposed to the liquid and can pick up vapour. If the minute volume of the patient changes, gas flow through the system changes and then so too will the time available for the liquid to evaporate. This means that the amount of vapour delivered by a draw-over vaporizer is inversely related to the minute volume of the patient; the higher their inspiratory flow, the lower the agent concentration will be. This is the opposite of the familiar effect seen with a plenum vaporizer whereby the spontaneously breathing patient will become more deeply anaesthetized, should their minute-volume increase.

Systems of Historical Interest

The Schimmelbusch mask was a wire-framed mask with a cloth insert. The patient breathed through the cloth as ether (diethyl ether) was dripped onto it. The ether evaporated as the patient breathed and the vapour was delivered. Depth of anaesthesia was crudely controlled by varying the rate of dripping of the ether.

The ether inhaler was a vessel which contained liquid ether soaked into a sponge. There was a mouthpiece on one side and an opening through which air could freely enter the vessel. The sponge both increased the surface area from which ether could evaporate and helped to prevent the ether from being spilt or inhaled in liquid form. As the patient inhaled, fresh air was drawn through the device and some of the ether evaporated into it.

Both these systems delivered unpredictable concentrations of vapour and are not suitable for use in modern anaesthesia. However, a modern presentation of methoxyflurane exists for pre-hospital care. This is based on an improved design of the ether inhaler.

Vaporizer Safety Features

Most of the safety features inherent in modern vaporizers focus on two key aims:

- To ensure the correct agent is used with the correct vaporizer
- To ensure only one agent can reach the patient at a time and in the correct concentration

Each agent has, by international convention, an associated colour; for example, purple for isoflurane. The colours are bright and prominently shown on all items associated with the particular agent, from the bottles the agent is supplied in to the vaporizers themselves. On many anaesthetic monitoring systems, the agent concentrations are also shown in the colour associated with the agent.

Filling is achieved by one of two systems. For some vaporizers, a system of non-interchangeable keyed filler tubes is used. These are attached to the bottle in which the agent is delivered by means of a colour-coded and specially shaped screw-top which will fit only bottles of the correct agent. On the other end of the filler tube is a connector, the same colour as the collar and of a shape that fits only into the appropriate vaporizer for the agent. In some systems, there is simply a specially shaped nozzle on the storage bottle that fits into a receptacle on the front of the corresponding vaporizer.

The dial on the vaporizer will not turn away from the zero position unless the vaporizer is securely locked into its correct position on the anaesthetic machine back-bar. It is important to note that this interlock does not prevent the leaks which can occur if the seals between the machine and the vaporizer are damaged or missing. It merely prevents the use of an improperly fixed unit.

At the rear of modern vaporizers there are, on both sides, protruding pins. As the dial is turned from the zero position, the pins extend from their resting position. As they do, they push against the pins of any adjacent vaporizer, preventing the second vaporizer from being switched on. This mechanism will disable both unused vaporizers on a back-bar of three. However, it does not allow a vaporizer at position 1 to lock a vaporizer at position 3 if position 2 is empty. This would allow two vaporizers to be used together, which is potentially dangerous. This is one reason for the relative scarcity of machines with three vaporizer positions.

Hazards Associated with Vaporizers

In spite of the many safety mechanisms, it is possible to misuse vaporizers in a number of potentially dangerous ways.

There are various modes of 'flow failure' which can occur during the delivery of vapour anaesthesia. In modern machines these are ameliorated to some extent but knowledge of the failure modes is important.

During positive pressure ventilation with some ventilators (particularly 'bag in bottle ventilators') the entire breathing system is pressurized during the inspiratory phase. With some vaporizer designs this can cause either or both of two issues, which are collectively known as 'backflow'.

In some instances, mixed gas can be forced back into the vaporization chamber where it will become fully saturated with anaesthetic vapour. When the pressure is released the fully saturated gas is released into the circuit, causing a higher than expected concentration of vapour in the outflow gas. This effect can be reduced by the use of a one-way valve at the exit of the vaporization chamber to prevent the outgoing mixed gas from being re-introduced into the chamber.

It is also possible for fully saturated gas to be forced back out of the vaporization chamber into the inlet port of the vaporizer. When the pressure is released this gas can, rather than re-entering the vaporization chamber, become part of the bypass stream. If this occurs, the delivered concentration will increase because, in addition to the chamber gas, the bypass gas now contains some vapour. This effect is also prevented by a one-way valve at the vaporizer exit but, in addition, it can be reduced by adding an extra length of tubing to the inlet port. This extra length means that, under most scenarios, any backflow pressure will be insufficient to cause the vapour-laden gas to get as far back as the bypass channel.

Vaporizers can be over- or under-filled. This would result in unpredictable agent delivery. It is easily avoidable by keeping the level of liquid between the minimum and maximum markers on the fill-level indicator. In some situations, if these indicators are not used correctly, it might be possible to mistake a completely empty vaporizer for a completely full one. This should be detected quickly because, whatever agent level is selected on the dial, the agent concentration monitor will always read zero. Newer vaporizers have the filling port in a position which makes it difficult to over-fill them without determined effort.

Vaporizers must be used in the correct orientation. They are generally designed to function correctly within a range of tipping angles but they can behave unpredictably if these limits are exceeded.

It is important to ensure that all the seals, caps and fittings are secure and that the vaporizer is locked into position. If any of the seals are damaged or missing, the filler system is open or the vaporizer is improperly locked in position, it may be possible for gas to leak either around or through the vaporizer. Should this occur, it may result in unpredictable vapour concentrations. Gas leaks will also make it difficult to maintain pressure within the breathing system, particularly during low-flow anaesthesia. A complete machine check reduces these hazards significantly but proper use and full monitoring with a competent and vigilant anaesthetist are required to ensure maximum patient safety.

Hyperbaric Systems

Hyperbaric systems are those in which the gas is above atmospheric pressure. This can refer to a range of situations but the most common are hyperbaric chambers and diving.

In self-contained underwater breathing apparatus ('scuba') diving, breathing is made possible by the use of high-pressure air tanks which, through the use of valves and pressure reducers, allow the user to breathe gas at the correct pressure to expand their lungs against the pressure of the water around them.

Hyperbaric chambers are used for a limited range of medical treatments, some of which are also related to diving. Details of hyperbaric systems will be divided into the difficulties and dangers associated with them and the treatment options they offer.

Dangers of Hyperbaric Systems
Barotrauma

Barotrauma is the most obvious danger of any high-pressure system. In fact, barotrauma can be a problem at the relatively low pressures supplied by modern anaesthesia machines. The maximum recommended inspiratory pressure varies according to the patient and their particular characteristics but caution should be used with pressures above 35–40 cmH$_2$O of peak pressure and slightly lower plateau pressures. Work is ongoing to determine optimal ventilation strategies in a range of both physiological and pathophysiological situations but it is generally recognized that attempting to ventilate patients with pulmonary damage to blood gas values within normal healthy ranges risks worsening the damage.

More extreme barotrauma results from the use of higher pressures. In scuba diving with properly maintained and correctly used equipment, it is difficult to breathe very high-pressure gas because there is a system of valves and pressure reducers to prevent this.

It is, however, relatively easy to suffer barotrauma by, for example, taking a breath at depth and then failing to exhale on ascent. For every 10-m reduction in depth the pressure to which the diver is subjected reduces by about 1 atm. This means that the transthoracic and transpleural pressures are increased by the same amount. A pressure of 1 atm (approximately 100 kPa) is more than enough to cause barotrauma. This scenario is explained by Boyle's law; volume increases with reducing pressure.

Narcosis and Toxicity

All non-toxic gases, with the exception of helium and possibly neon, cause narcosis if they are breathed at sufficient partial pressure. For some, such as xenon, the narcotic partial pressure is attainable within an atmospheric system (hence its role as an anaesthetic agent) but, for most others, partial pressures above 1 atm are required before narcosis sets in. In some people, nitrogen narcosis begins to be noticeable when breathing compressed air at about 30 m (about 4 atm of pressure and a nitrogen partial pressure of around 3 atm).

The mechanism of narcosis is thought to be similar to the mechanism of action of anaesthetic agents. This is, at least in part, due to the relationship between the fat solubility of the gas in question and the physical conditions required for it to cause narcosis. In the majority of cases, narcosis is rapidly reversible by reducing the partial pressure of the gas which is causing it. In the case of scuba diving with compressed air, this is accomplished by ascending to a lesser depth. If ascent does not resolve the symptoms, an alternative diagnosis should be sought.

Oxygen toxicity is caused by the production of reactive oxygen species (for example the superoxide anion (O_2^{2-}) and the hydroxyl radical (OH·)). These are naturally produced in cells as signalling molecules and as a by-product of oxygen metabolism. Levels of these species are controlled by the body's antioxidant systems, such as superoxide dismutase and glutathione. Increased oxygen delivery can cause these substances to be formed at a rate greater than that with which these mechanisms are able to cope. When oxygen is breathed at high partial pressures, the tissues with the highest blood flow receive the most oxygen and are therefore the most susceptible to oxygen toxicity. Perhaps the most dangerous element of oxygen toxicity while diving is the possibility of central nervous system toxicity, resulting in a seizure.

This is almost invariably a fatal event when underwater, due to loss of the mouthpiece and involuntary inhalation of water.

Decompression

The pressure of gas breathed by a diver must increase as they descend through the water to enable them to breathe against the increasing hydrostatic pressure of the water (management of this pressure is the task of their scuba regulator). Henry's law states that a greater amount of gas will be dissolved in blood as gas pressure increases. As the diver re-ascends to a lesser depth, the converse happens: dissolved gas will begin to come out of solution, forming gas bubbles in the blood. The bubbles result in a range of intravascular and extravascular effects, which include both embolic and inflammatory phenomena. The signs and symptoms caused by the formation of gas bubbles are collectively known as decompression sickness. Decompression sickness is the umbrella term for decompression illness, arterial gas embolism and pulmonary barotrauma.

The mass of a given gas that will dissolve in a diver's blood varies in proportion to the percentage of that gas in the breathing mixture, the depth of the dive and the time spent at that depth. A greater gas load requires a more gradual ascent to allow time for off-gassing of nitrogen in order to avoid decompression-related symptoms (unless, as commercial divers do, you are breathing a nitrogen-free mixture such as Heliox). Dive tables and computers give some guidance as to suitable ascent regimens. The most common symptoms of decompression illness are joint and muscle pain, particularly in the joints of the upper body. Cutaneous manifestations also occur. Neurological symptoms are rare but can be particularly serious and may include coma and death.

Decompression Chambers

Decompression chambers can be used to reduce the occurrence of decompression illness or to treat it if it does occur. A decompression chamber is a sealed unit, which can be pressurized to simulate a deep dive. Divers suffering or at risk of decompression illness can enter the chamber on completion of a deep dive and, when pressure is applied, the gas bubbles that are causing the symptoms redissolve. Once this is done, the pressure in the vessel is decreased at a rate that allows safe off-gassing.

Hyperbaric oxygen therapy is another use for decompression chambers. There is widespread interest in the use of hyperbaric oxygen therapy for treatment of a range of disease processes. There have been evidence reviews for a number of conditions, ranging from myocardial infarction to necrotizing fasciitis. There is no conclusive evidence to support hyperbaric therapy (other than for the treatment of decompression illness) and some evidence to suggest it may be harmful. The risks of hyperbaric oxygen therapy must be fully understood and balanced against the likelihood of successful treatment before its use can be justified.

High Altitudes

Atmospheric pressure is a result of the weight of the atmosphere above the surface of the Earth. As one ascends through the atmosphere there is less of it above and so the ambient pressure drops. At about 6,000 m, the atmospheric pressure will drop to approximately half of the surface pressure. At around 12,000 m it will be approximately one-third. The drop in pressure slows with increasing altitude because, for example, the atmosphere between 6,000 m and 12,000 m is less compressed by the atmosphere above than the atmosphere between the surface and 6,000 m. Tables are available to assist in calculating air pressure. They typically relate altitude, temperature and humidity to air pressure. It is also possible to use air pressure, temperature and humidity values to determine the altitude. This is the mechanism of action of barometric altimeters.

In the same way that ascent from a deep dive can cause decompression sickness, climbing from the surface to high altitudes can do the same. Long-duration flights above 6,000 m (around 18,000 ft) carry a risk of decompression sickness. Long-haul commercial flights cruise at 10,000–12,000 m but the cabin is maintained at a pressure equating to an altitude of about 2,500 m. It is important to take this into account when advising patients in respect of flying. At an altitude of 2,500 m, air pressure is about 75–80 kPa. Subsequently, the partial pressure of oxygen will be 20–25% lower than usual. In most people this will make very little difference but, in those with closely matched oxygen supply and demand, the reduction of oxygen partial pressure may have serious consequences. In addition, the pressure change itself may cause undesirable effects, for example 'popping' of the ears.

The effects of flying are particularly dangerous after diving to what would otherwise be safe depths, because the combination of ascent from a dive and the reduction in pressure associated with flying might cause bubbles of gas to form in the same way as ascent from a deeper dive. It is worth noting that to double the pressure, a diver only has to dive to 10 m whereas to halve the pressure, a pilot has to climb to 6,000 m. This also means that, in terms of pressure change, a dive to 10 m followed by a flight at 6,000 m is roughly equivalent to either a dive to 20 m or a flight to over 12,000 m in an unpressurized cabin.

> The humidity and pressure effects of travelling at 2,500-m pressure-altitude affect our sense of taste. That is the reason why airline food can taste particularly bland and recipes are specifically modified to try to account for these effects.

Anaesthesia at Altitude

Consider delivering an anaesthetic in a hospital in La Rinconada, Peru, the highest settlement in the world. It has an altitude of 5,170 m, so the atmospheric pressure will be a little over half of what it would be at sea level, with a corresponding reduction in the oxygen partial pressure in the air. In spite of the difficulties posed by pressure changes, you choose to use a vapour-based anaesthetic technique.

The drop in the partial pressure of oxygen on ascent into the atmosphere can be partially compensated for by increasing the oxygen content of the delivered gas. Before commencing the anaesthetic, you should consider the patient's oxygen requirement and how this might change over the course of the anaesthetic, deciding whether it is safe to proceed or whether the risks outweigh the potential benefit.

The monitoring systems of gas-based anaesthetic systems usually measure the partial pressure of the component gases. These partial pressures might be converted to percentages for convenience. In most situations, partial pressure and percentage are almost interchangeable (as 1 atm is 101 kPa so 20% oxygen would give a partial pressure of just under 20 kPa). At altitude, though, the difference between percentage and partial pressure becomes more pronounced, and it becomes more important to know which is being measured and what, exactly, is being displayed.

The minimum alveolar concentration (MAC) of a volatile agent is defined as the concentration of vapour measured at 1 atm that prevents movement in response to a supramaximal stimulus in 50% of subjects. A question about how the MAC changes with altitude is therefore a trick question – the definition dictates the altitude as being sea level (1 atm). It is, however, important to understand the effects of altitude on the delivery of an agent by a vaporizer and the difference between the partial pressure and the percentage of a given gas in a mixture. In addition, some questions are phrased specifically in terms of the partial pressure of an agent or the vaporizer setting required at altitude.

In plenum vaporizers, the delivery of vapour is determined by the difference between the saturated vapour pressure of the agent and the barometric pressure. In simple terms, as the air pressure decreases it becomes easier for the anaesthetic liquid to evaporate and form vapour. This increase in vapour production is approximately in proportion to the decrease in pressure, and thus partial pressure of the atmosphere. This, in turn, means that if the atmospheric pressure halves then the vapour output of the vaporizer approximately doubles. If we take the situation of a patient being anaesthetized at about 6,000 m, for example, there will be a doubling of vapour output from the vaporizer. This, however, is compensated for by the approximate halving of the atmospheric pressure; the partial pressure of the agent will be approximately the same as it would have been at sea level. Since it is the partial pressure of the anaesthetic vapour that causes the anaesthetic effect, it is not necessary to make any alterations to the splitting ratio of the vaporizer in order to use it at altitude and therefore the dial can be set as normal (provided it has not been specifically recalibrated for use at altitude).

It is important to note that some types of vaporizer, for example the desflurane vaporizer, work by a different method. Since this vaporizer is already heated and pressurized it will, within all but the most extreme environments, deliver vapour as per its calibration. Systems using these vaporizers may behave unpredictably as the ambient atmospheric pressure changes; for example, with altitude. The unpredictability is, in part, due to the delivery of the expected quantity of vapour into a gas stream at lower-than-expected pressure.

In all cases of vapour use at altitude, careful monitoring must be maintained and it is vital to understand the monitors so that the data they display can be correctly interpreted to deliver the safest treatment for the patient.

Summary

Anaesthesia is commonly maintained using vapour-based techniques. To safely manipulate vapour-based anaesthetics and the gases used to deliver them it is important to understand the mechanisms of phase changes. We have looked at this from a perspective of energy, temperature, entropy and enthalpy. In turn, these factors dictate the properties of the individual anaesthetic agent, such as latent heat of vaporization and saturated vapour pressure. Vaporizers must be designed to account for these and ensure that the device can provide suitable concentrations of agent which, in turn, account for the pharmacological properties such as MAC.

We have discussed the working mechanisms of vaporizers in common use as well as the associated potential dangers. Backflow problems through a vaporizer would be particularly dangerous but any such flaws are generally addressed at the design stage. Leaks, however, present a much more common, day-to-day risk to safe delivery of vapour anaesthesia. Although less common in developed-world anaesthesia, it is useful to have a working understanding of the key differences between vaporizer-in-circuit and vaporizer-out-of-circuit configurations.

There are also some important points of anaesthesia related to extremes of depth or altitude. These are not everyday clinical scenarios but they do neatly illustrate the physical principles of everyday practice. This makes them a popular examination topic. To answer the initial question, however, for those who may find themselves delivering an emergency anaesthetic in the Himalayas, a standard sevoflurane vaporizer would work well without any modifications or alterations in use as long as it could be kept warm enough to maintain the evaporation of the liquid sevoflurane and as long as the monitoring was well understood and properly used.

Questions

MCQs – select true or false for each response

1. Oxygen:
   (a) Is always beneficial
   (b) Causes narcosis at high pressures
   (c) Is supplied at pipeline pressure of 7 bar
   (d) Is present at a lower percentage at higher altitudes
   (e) Is impossible to compress to a liquid form

2. Entropy:
   (a) Cannot be decreased
   (b) Is a measure of the level of disorder in a system
   (c) Is directly related to temperature
   (d) Is higher in a vapour than a liquid
   (e) Represents unusable energy

3. Plenum vaporizers:
   (a) Require high-pressure gas inputs
   (b) Are heavy in order to prevent tipping
   (c) Contain large heat sinks
   (d) Can only be turned on when locked in position
   (e) Cannot leak when locked in position

SBAs – select the single *best* answer

4. There is a range of vaporizer technologies in current use. Each has its advantages and disadvantages. Which of the following features is most important in maintaining safety when using a vaporizer?
   (a) The vaporizer should have a standard pin index fitment to attach to the anaesthetic machine
   (b) The vaporizer should have a chamber capacity of at least 400 ml
   (c) The vaporizer should be electrically heated to maintain the correct temperature
   (d) Vaporizers should be clearly colour-coded to ensure they are filled with the correct agent
   (e) The agent details should be included in Braille on the front of the vaporizer

5. Phase diagrams can be used to help understand and predict the behaviour of a substance with changes in temperature and pressure. Which of the following statements best fits with phase diagrams in use in anaesthesia?
   (a) They should show extremes of temperature and pressure
   (b) They can be used to deduce the triple point of a substance
   (c) Pressure is shown as a logarithmic scale

(d) They are most useful when the melting, boiling and critical pressure and temperature are clearly shown
(e) Behaviour of the gaseous phase is the most accurately represented

Answers

1. FFFFF

Oxygen is well-recognized to have potentially harmful effects, even in therapeutic applications. Oxygen causes harm through toxicity, rather than narcosis (the latter is a different biological mechanism). The likelihood of toxicity is directly related to the partial pressure of oxygen and this can be particularly relevant at deep diving depths, even breathing compressed air. The atmosphere is relatively homogeneous with respect to gas concentration but, as the pressure reduces at altitude, the partial pressure of oxygen represented by the 20.5% also reduces. Gaseous substances, including oxygen, can be compressed to a liquid state if they are cooled below the critical temperature for that substance.

2. TFFTF

The total entropy in the universe can never decrease although it is possible to locally decrease entropy in one part of a system at the expense of an increase elsewhere in the system. This mechanism is exploited in, for example, the refrigerator (see earlier). In this system, heat can be moved from one place to another and a localized decrease in entropy can be demonstrated. Entropy is defined as a thermodynamic quality which represents the degree to which the thermal energy of a system is unavailable for work. Put very simply the more ordered the energy, the easier it is to use. This unavailability of energy for work, then, can also in some cases be represented by disorder but this is not a strict definition of the term.

Entropy tends to increase with temperature but the increase is not directly related. This can be shown by watching what happens to the temperature of water ice as it is heated through melting and then past its boiling point. The temperature will increase until the ice begins to melt. At this point, the temperature will stop increasing until the ice is fully melted. Once the ice has all turned to liquid water the temperature will rise again until the water starts to boil off to vapour, when the temperature will again remain constant until the water is all boiled. The two points where the temperature stops increasing are the melting of the ice and the boiling of the water. These are two points of large entropy change but no temperature change. This process also neatly illustrates the difference between heat and temperature. A great deal of heat energy is required to change the phase of water from solid to liquid but there is no temperature change at all. The entropy of a vapour system is higher than the entropy of an equivalent mass of the same substance in liquid form. The molecules in the liquid are held in a relatively rigid structure compared to the same molecules in a vapour, which are free to move throughout their container. Entropy is often described as a measure of the disorder or randomness in a system. A more formal thermodynamic definition is that entropy represents the unavailability of thermal energy for doing mechanical work.

3. TFTFF

Most vaporizers in use in modern anaesthetics require high-pressure gas systems. They have high internal resistance to flow and cannot be powered by patient respiratory effort alone. Vaporizers for use with low-pressure gas have different designs and include the draw-over vaporizer. Modern plenum vaporizers are generally heavy because they contain a large mass of metal. This is to provide a source of heat energy to ensure that the liquid is vaporized in the vaporization chamber. The heat is absorbed from the ambient air and no electrical power is required. Modern vaporizers include interlocks to prevent their activation unless they are fully locked into position. This mechanism can be defeated and does not ensure that there are no leaks. If, for example, the rubber seals between the machine and the vaporizer are damaged or missing, the interlock will still allow the use of the vaporizer even in the presence of a large leak.

4. (d)

Vaporizer safety has been covered in detail in this chapter. The only one of these statements which is absolutely mandatory is that each vaporizer should be clearly identified for use with a specific agent. This is invariably accomplished by colour-coding the vaporizers, accessories and the bottles in which the agents are supplied. There are many attachment safety measures but the pin index system is not for vaporizers – it is used to reduce the possibility of attaching gas cylinders to the wrong connections on the machine. While Braille markings might be useful under some circumstances, it would be very difficult to deliver anaesthesia safely without being able to see. Braille is not commonly included on the vaporizers but it is sometimes embossed on the agent bottles to allow those with poor vision to identify substances in similar-shaped and -sized bottles. This is similar to drug containers which are increasingly commonly embossed with Braille.

5. (d)

Phase diagrams should show the region of interest as clearly as possible. In anaesthesia, this generally means that temperatures and pressures close to the atmospheric conditions should be included but sometimes more extreme ranges are required (but not always, so (a) is incorrect). For example, high pressures may be needed to describe how a gas behaves within a cylinder, or low temperatures may be required to show how oxygen behaves within the VIE. The diagram can illustrate the triple point but only if the relevant temperature and pressures are included on the diagram. Logarithmic scales can be used but they are not necessarily any more useful than linear. The accuracy of the diagram depends on the experimental data available with which to construct it but, also, if the temperature and pressure scales allow other phases to be included, there is no reason why these will be any less well represented than the gaseous phase.

Chapter 9

Ventilators and Breathing Systems

Dan Shuttleworth and Nick Dodds

Learning Objectives

- To describe the history and development of breathing systems used in anaesthetic practice, with a focus on the relative advantages and disadvantages of different systems
- To compare the important principles underlying the function of the different breathing systems
- To apply the engineering and physical principles of breathing systems to pulmonary mechanics and physiology
- To demonstrate the impact of invasive ventilation on the lungs
- To describe the different modes of ventilation, with an emphasis on the differing clinical situations in which they may prove vital

Chapter Content

- Bernoulli principle and Venturi effect
- Non-invasive respiratory support
- Breathing systems overview
- Mapleson classification of breathing systems
- Circle breathing system
- Mechanical ventilation
- Portable ventilators
- Alternative modes of ventilation
- ECMO and $ECCO_2R$

Scenario 1

A previously well 53-year-old male is in the recovery room after a laparotomy for large bowel obstruction. His BMI is 43. His oxygen saturation is 91% on room air and he is feeling drowsy. He has a thoracic epidural. Anaesthesia consisted of propofol and remifentanil TIVA with a single 40-mg dose of rocuronium at induction. Sugammadex was given at the end of the case. What are the possible explanations for hypoxia in this scenario? What are the treatment options in such a circumstance and why do they work?

Introduction

In this chapter, we will describe the physical principles underlying the delivery of gases from the anaesthetic machine to the patient. Through a sound understanding of these principles you will gain greater insight into the utility of these systems in different circumstances, in addition to their limitations and potential problems. The physical principles relating to the mechanical ventilation of the patient are also considered and the utility of different modes of ventilation in different clinical circumstances is examined. Despite an exhaustive understanding of the breathing systems and ventilators, occasionally difficult circumstances will occur, and alternative means to ventilate and oxygenate patients may be called for. Although we use these techniques less frequently, it is still important to consider the principles underlying their operation as they relate to the disturbances in physiology we deal with on a daily basis, both in anaesthetic and intensive care environments.

Bernoulli Principle and Venturi Effect

The Bernoulli principle and Venturi effect underpin the operation of many breathing systems used in anaesthetic practice. These two terms refer to the behaviour of fluids as they encounter different conditions. The Bernoulli principle describes the change in pressure of a fluid as it flows through a constriction; its kinetic energy increases as the fluid accelerates through the narrowing. This increase in kinetic energy derives from the potential energy. As the fluid emerges from the constriction and begins to decelerate, the pressure exerted by the fluid falls. This fall in pressure can be utilized; a second fluid placed as a side-stream within the constriction will be drawn into the original fluid as a result of the fall in pressure. This process of entrainment is the basis of the Venturi effect (see Chapter 4).

The degree of pressure drop is dependent on the flow of the original or driving fluid – the faster the flow, the greater the pressure fall, the greater the degree of entrainment of the second or 'entrained' fluid. Other factors that are usually fixed, but also affect the degree of entrainment, include the dimensions of the tubing and the density and viscosity of the two fluids. As these variables are constant, flow is, in practical terms, the principal determinant of the degree of entrainment.

Venturi masks use the same effect to deliver oxygen (the driving gas), diluted to a predictable inspired fraction by entrainment of atmospheric air. These devices are cheap, robust and disposable. Due to the degree of entrainment, flow rates are usually high enough to meet or exceed peak inspiratory flow demands and to flush any alveolar gas from the mask to prevent rebreathing (the re-inspiration of carbon dioxide-containing gas from the last exhalation). In general, they therefore guarantee the FiO_2, regardless of the minute volume, and are referred to as 'fixed-performance devices'. Nasal cannulae and standard face masks comprise the variable-performance devices: the FiO_2 delivered is highly variable as patient effort determines the degree of air entrainment. That said, in the high-FiO_2 Venturi mask, a patient's peak inspiratory flow may exceed the rate of gas delivery, resulting in a greater degree of entrainment around the mask, and delivery of a lower than expected FiO_2. This can result in a 5–10% under-performance of these masks.

In Venturi devices, total entrained gas flow is defined by:

$$\text{Entrained flow} = \left(\frac{\text{Driving gas flow} \times (1 - FiO_2)}{FiO_2 - 0.2} \right)$$

For example, if a 60% Venturi is used, with oxygen flow of 15 l min^{-1}, entrained air flow is:

$$= \left(\frac{15 \times (1 - 0.6)}{0.6 - 0.2} \right)$$

$$= 15 \text{ l min}^{-1}$$

In this example, as the entrained flow is the same as the driving gas flow, the entrainment ratio is 1:1.

In certain settings, the Venturi device may be connected to a length of corrugated tubing or a reservoir bag. This acts as a sink of oxygen-enriched air, maximizing oxygen delivery during initial peak inspiration. Such devices are used commonly in Recovery areas for patients recovering from anaesthesia

The Venturi effect has been in use in nature far longer than even Mapleson's classification. Deep-water sea sponges contain small flagellae that can move tiny amounts of water, but a large sponge can filter its own mass in sea water every 2–3 minutes. This is possible due to the conical arrangement of the sea sponge, which allows water currents to flow over its apical opening. As a consequence of the resulting pressure drop, water is dragged through the feeding pores in the sponge's sides.

Non-invasive Respiratory Support

In some cases, oxygen enrichment alone may be insufficient to achieve the required oxygen delivery and/or carbon dioxide clearance. Continuous positive airway pressure (CPAP) devices deliver oxygen-enriched gas mixtures under greater-than-atmospheric pressures. These devices have utility in (but not exclusively):

- Management of the acutely hypoxic patient, either as a temporizing measure prior to intubation or as a means of management while appropriate medical therapy becomes effective
- Support of recently extubated patients in the intensive care setting
- Management of acute pulmonary oedema
- Management of obstructive sleep apnoea

Positive pressure has beneficial effects on the proximal airways, reducing collapse and obstruction, and on distal airways and alveoli by reducing atelectasis and collapse, thus increasing the functional residual capacity (FRC). CPAP is delivered by a sealed delivery interface with the patient's upper airway. This may take the form of a tight nasal mask, face mask, face shield or helmet.

These devices function in a similar way to Venturi masks. A high-pressure oxygen source, usually 4-bar pipeline oxygen, is connected to a CPAP manifold. Within the manifold is a Venturi injector with a variable orifice, allowing differing levels of oxygen enrichment. This may be digital or analogue in nature. A flow restrictor prevents delivery of excessive pressures to the patient inspiratory limb. The patient face mask is connected to a T-piece breathing system, with an expiratory and inspiratory limb. A variable resistance valve is then connected to the expiratory limb, providing resistance to flow in both inspiration and expiration, thus delivering continuous positive pressure to the airway. The gas flows provided by such systems are sufficiently high so as to exceed maximum inspiratory flows and preserve fractional oxygen enrichment (a true, fixed-performance device). Some devices may incorporate a reservoir to further augment this. Humidification can also be added to such systems to mitigate heat and moisture loss from the airway, prevent sputum inspissation and enhance patient comfort and compliance.

High-flow nasal oxygen (HFNO) devices work in a very similar manner to a CPAP machine, insomuch as they use a Venturi injector to deliver high-flow gas with a carefully regulated FiO_2. As well as being a fixed-performance oxygen delivery system, they also provide some degree of CPAP and FRC improvement on account of the high flows employed. In addition, the patient interface (nasal cannulae) is much better tolerated than a close-fitting mask, and humidification is much easier to deliver without skin irritation associated with these masks (or 'rain-out' as encountered with full-face masks and helmets). In some patients, HFNO can also wash alveolar gas from the anatomical dead space during the end-expiratory pause, thus reducing rebreathing and offering some improvement in carbon dioxide clearance.

The next level of complexity of non-invasive devices involves the provision of differential pressures in inspiration and expiration, so-called bi-level positive airway pressure (BiPAP). In modern settings, these devices are usually self-contained digital devices and use either a pipeline high-pressure supply or an air compressor as the gas source, the latter of these being more commonly used in a domiciliary setting.

Scenario 2

A 5-year-old boy presents to the emergency department with a high fever, stridor and drooling. He is flushed and unwell. On the basis of these features, and the fact that he has not had childhood vaccinations, a diagnosis of acute epiglottitis is made. A plan for gaseous induction in the operating theatre is made jointly between the anaesthetic and ENT consultants. An inhalational technique places a number of different demands on a breathing system. The patient is likely to transition from spontaneously breathing, to controlled ventilation and possibly back to a spontaneously breathing pattern. Requirements will initially be for a low-resistance breathing circuit, achieving maximum efficiency in a spontaneous pattern. Once established, the patient will then be mandatorily ventilated during the procedure, with different design requirements to ensure efficiency.

What makes an efficient breathing system for a spontaneously breathing patient? Why is the Mapleson D system more efficient in positive-pressure-ventilated patients? What are the advantages of a draw-over vaporizer in the military setting?

Breathing Systems Overview

A *breathing system* is a combination of tubes, valves and filters which receive anaesthetic agents and gases from the common gas outlet, and convey these to the patient. In addition to these components, most systems will also include a connection to a scavenging mechanism (see Chapter 10). At the opposite end to the scavenging port, they interface with the patient through either a mask or invasive airway device, such as a laryngeal mask or endotracheal tube. Breathing systems vary in complexity from a simple Hudson mask to the circle system, as found within most modern anaesthetic machines. To avoid ambiguity, it is important to avoid use of the term 'circuit' as this implies the circle system, which is obviously a very particular form of breathing system.

Anaesthetic systems can be classified according to several schemas. These include the rebreathing characteristics of the systems (open, semi-open, etc.) and the Mapleson system of classification.

When comparing different breathing systems, it is useful to consider each in terms of its approximation of the 'ideal' breathing system, which would have the following characteristics:

- Simple design
- Cheap
- Robust and lightweight
- Able to deliver mixed gases and anaesthetic agents
- Operate efficiently in spontaneous or controlled modes of ventilation
- Usable in all age groups
- Has minimal dead space
- Prevents application of barotrauma

- Permits scavenging
- Allows warming and humidification of inspired gases
- Effectively eliminates carbon dioxide
- Low resistance
- Disposable

Open, Semi-open, Semi-closed and Closed Systems

An open breathing system describes an arrangement in which the patient obtains their breathing gas from the atmosphere and which does not permit rebreathing of respiratory gases. A classic example is the Schimmelbusch anaesthetic mask, where the patient breathes fresh gas from the atmosphere and exhales gas to the atmosphere, with gradual addition of an anaesthetic agent, usually ether (diethyl ether).

Semi-open systems consist of any apparatus in which fresh gas is supplied from piped or cylinder supply (with or without anaesthetic vapour), but which does not permit safe recycling of exhaled gases. A semi-open system will also prevent rebreathing of these gases but only if sufficient fresh gas flow (FGF) is used, otherwise rebreathing will occur. This is the inclusion of exhaled gas (which includes carbon dioxide) in the subsequent tidal volume and can lead to carbon dioxide narcosis. By definition, the systems classified by Mapleson (see below) are all semi-open.

In a semi-closed system, the exhaled gases are allowed to circulate and be rebreathed by the patient. In order for this to occur safely, such systems incorporate a mechanism for removal of carbon dioxide. When managed in this way, rebreathing is advantageous as it permits efficiency of gas use; use of the term 'recycling' to make the distinction from rebreathing is perhaps advisable. The circle system is an example of a semi-closed system, but it can function as a closed system if the FGF is precisely matched to the patient's oxygen consumption rate so that there is no increase in the volume of gas within the system over time. To complete this configuration of the circle, the adjustable pressure-limiting (APL) valve must also be completely closed. As there should be no increase in gas volume within the system, the pressure will not increase despite the closed APL valve. All carbon dioxide will be consumed by the absorption media and so no gas is exhausted to the atmosphere. Although such a system represents the greatest degree of efficiency in terms of anaesthetic agent usage, this is difficult to truly accomplish in practical terms as the greater consumption of oxygen compared with carbon dioxide production would lead to a pressure drop within the system.

The Mapleson Classification of Breathing Systems

Professor William Wellesley Mapleson (1926–2018) obtained his BSc in physics from Durham University and went on to write his PhD on the electric fields associated with lightning. Following this, he spent much of his career modelling the actions of drugs such as pethidine, propofol and muscle relaxants. He is, of course, best known for his work with breathing systems, aiming to classify them by the conditions required of each to prevent or reduce the level of rebreathing. The systems in use at the time were all of semi-open type and the Mapleson classification system assigns each type of system a letter from A to E, depending on the arrangement of the various components. The system of classification reflects the different gas flows required for optimal operation under spontaneous and controlled ventilator modes.

The gases a patient exhales consist of a mixture of dead-space gas and alveolar gas. Dead space is the proportion of the tidal volume that does not participate in gas exchange at the blood–airspace interface. This is divided into the physiological dead space (consisting of alveolar and anatomical dead space) and equipment dead space. The latter is the volume of any part of the circuit between the patient's airway and the fresh gas flow (for example a face mask). As dead-space gas is, by composition, the same as fresh gas, system efficiency can be optimized by aiming to retain as much of this portion of the exhaled breath as possible to contribute to the next breath. Alveolar gas, on the other hand, contains carbon dioxide and must be vented from the system. Devising a system which recycles all dead-space gas and vents all alveolar gas, with the lowest possible flow of fresh gas into the system, is the central aim of breathing system design.

Mapleson A

The arrangement shown in Figure 9.1 is preserved for all Mapleson A systems however they are constructed, be that the traditional Magill or the coaxial Lack configuration. An understanding of the dynamic events in the inspiratory cycle is vital, as this is

Chapter 9: Ventilators and Breathing Systems

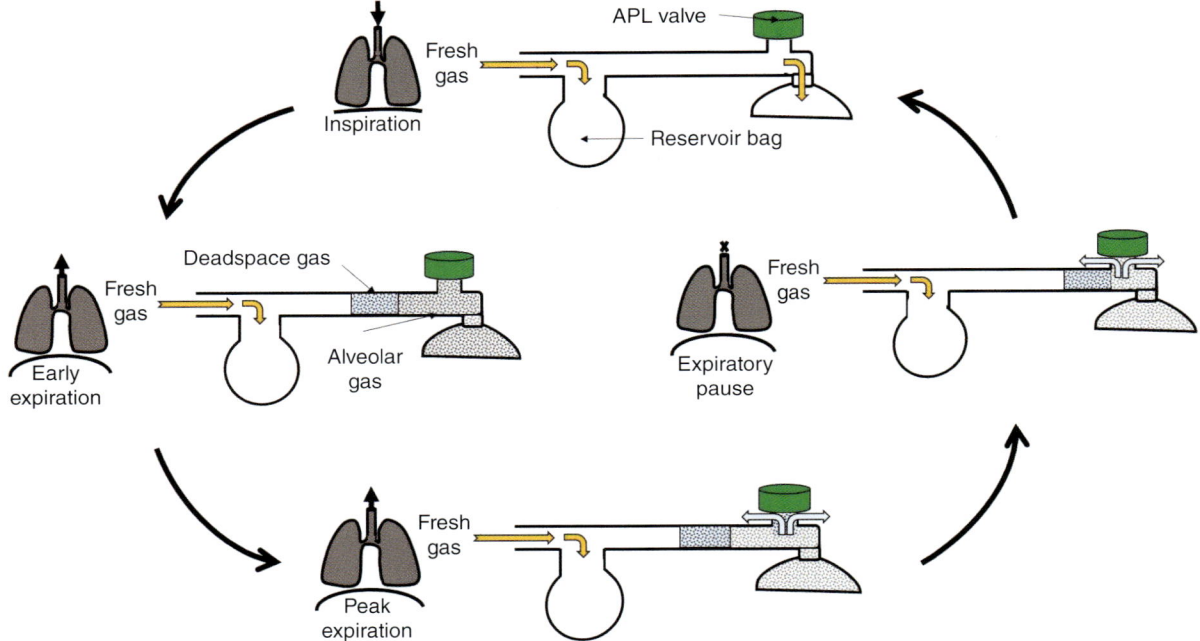

Figure 9.1 Workings of a Mapleson A system

fundamental to explain the differences in efficiency in spontaneous versus mandatory ventilation. In both cases, this system functions most efficiently in the spontaneous breathing patient, where the events during the respiratory cycle occur as follows:

1. Inspiration: the fresh gas flow has already been delivered to fill the system and reservoir bag. As the patient breathes in, the tubing and reservoir bag empty and the 'clean' gas flows into the patient.
2. Early expiration: the dead-space gas (containing minimal carbon dioxide), along with oxygen and anaesthetic agents, flows back into the system.
3. Peak expiration: the expiratory flow increases, resulting in increasing the pressure within the system. The reservoir bag and tubing will already contain fresh gas. As a consequence of the pressure increase, this gas will be vented to the atmosphere via the APL valve, whilst the flow of fresh gas will still be 'pushing' clean gas towards the APL. By the end of expiration, the only alveolar gas remaining is between the APL valve and the alveoli (this includes the volume of the patient's anatomical dead space and the volume of the breathing system distal to the APL valve).
4. Expiratory pause: fresh gas flow replaces all of the gas within the system, as far as the APL valve, with fresh gas from the anaesthetic machine.

As a consequence, there is minimal rebreathing of alveolar gas, and some of the dead-space gas is conserved. Mapleson A systems in spontaneously breathing patients can therefore operate with fresh gas flows less than the patient's alveolar minute volume.

If Mapleson A systems are used for controlled ventilation, squeezing of the reservoir bag results in the loss of a large proportion of the fresh gas flow via the APL valve, and the circuit empties. During the following expiration, the alveolar gas now fills the reservoir bag as it is not distended enough to increase system pressure and force the expiratory gases to escape through the APL valve. If nothing were changed, the patient would then rebreathe a significant amount of their expired gases. The only way to overcome this is to increase the fresh gas flow rate up to three times the minute volume.

Mapleson B

Mapleson B systems are no longer used in modern anaesthetic practice. This arrangement places the

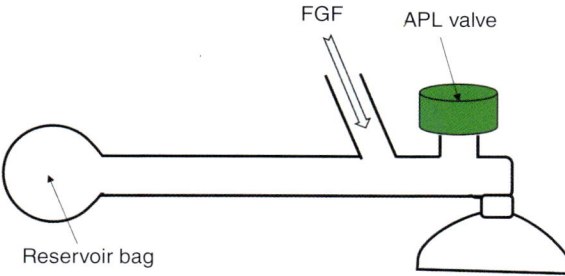

Figure 9.2 Mapleson B system

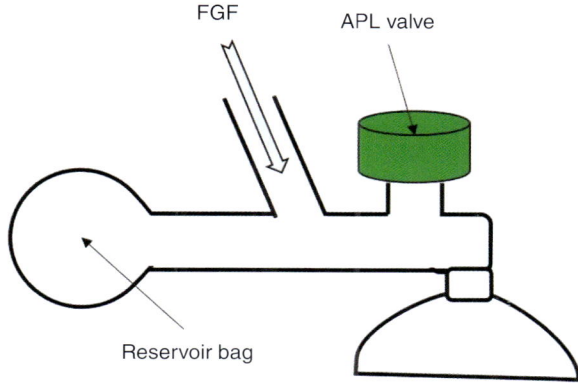

Figure 9.3 Mapleson C system

fresh gas close to the patient connection (Figure 9.2). As the patient exhales, they fill the system with alveolar gas, some of which vents to the atmosphere via the APL. During the expiratory pause, FGF fills the system from the inlet to the patient connection. There is minimal dilution of the previously exhaled anaesthetic gas within the reservoir bag. As such the system is inefficient in spontaneous ventilation, as the majority of the FGF during the longer expiratory phase vents to the atmosphere via the APL. During inspiration, the patient inhales the fresh gas between the connection and FGF input, along with a proportion of the reservoir bag containing mixed fresh and previously exhaled gases. The system is therefore inefficient in both modes of ventilation, requiring at least two and a half times the minute-volume FGF, and potentially more during spontaneous breathing.

Mapleson C

The operation of the Mapleson C system is broadly similar to that of the Mapleson B, with the exception of the volume of flexible tubing between the FGF inlet and the reservoir bag (Figure 9.3). Mapleson C systems are similarly inefficient in terms of FGF requirements in both spontaneous and controlled ventilation. They are no longer used in anaesthetic delivery. Previous examples included the Mapleson C system with a 'to and fro' carbon dioxide absorber. This system aimed to increase efficiency by safely allowing rebreathing and thus reducing FGF requirements. Problems occurred due to the bulky nature of the canister and its proximity to the patient connection, which meant a risk of dust inhalation.

The Water's bag (an example of a Mapleson C system) is commonly used in resuscitation, intensive care and recovery settings as a means of ventilating patients for short periods where adjustable inspiratory pressures are required.

Mapleson D

The Mapleson D, E and F systems are modified T-Piece systems, where the patient connection has two limbs: an afferent flow limb where the fresh gas emerges, and an efferent flow limb where the exhaled gases are exhausted. The most-commonly used Mapleson D system in modern practice is the Bain circuit, where the afferent and efferent limbs are arranged co-axially with the FGF limb running within the expiratory limb.

Mapleson D systems, in contrast to the Mapleson A, are efficient when used in controlled ventilation modes, and less efficient when used in spontaneously breathing patients. The respiratory cycle in a Mapleson D system runs slightly differently (Figure 9.4):

1. Expiratory pause: the FGF emerges from the T-piece and fills the system in the direction of the reservoir bag.
2. Inspiration (positive pressure): as the bag is squeezed, the fresh gases are directed into the patient – the tubing closest to the patient will contain freshly filled gas.
3. Expiration: as the patient breathes out, the dead-space gas fills the empty reservoir bag before the alveolar gas then fills the system. As the bag is already full, excess alveolar gas is vented via the APL. As expiration finishes, and the expiratory pause begins, this remaining alveolar gas is purged from the system by the incoming FGF.

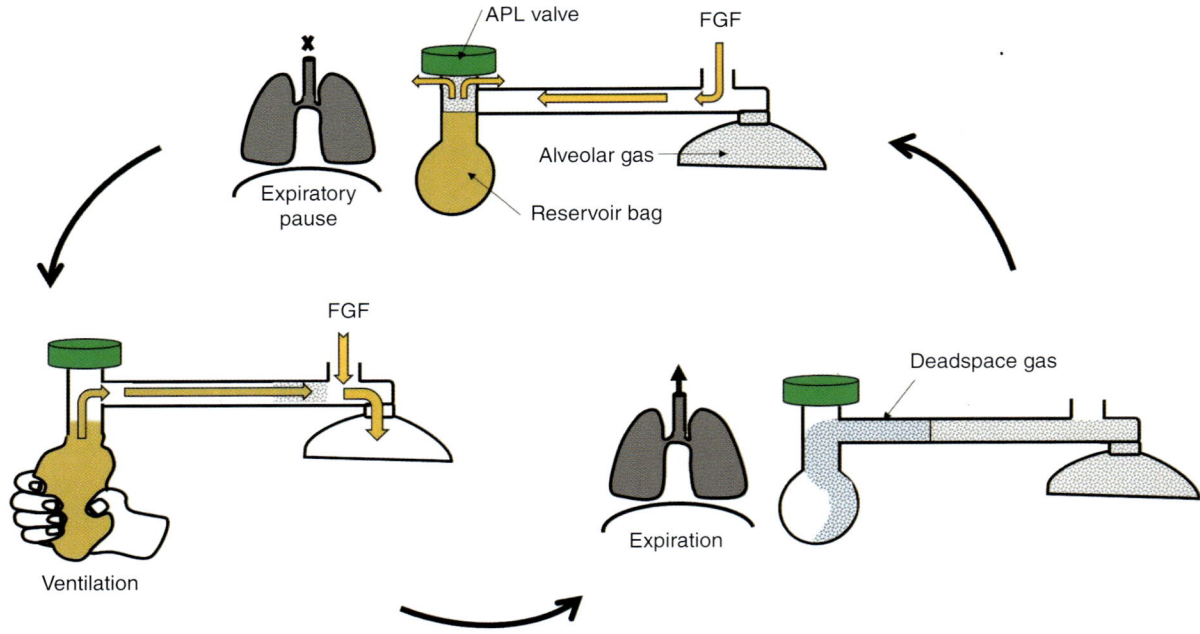

Figure 9.4 Workings of a non-coaxial Mapleson D system during controlled ventilation

During controlled ventilation, the expiratory pause allows the FGF to purge alveolar gas from the system, preventing rebreathing. When operated in this way, Mapleson D systems have been shown to require an FGF of as little as 0.7 times the minute volume to prevent significant rebreathing. If the patient breathes spontaneously, and the expiratory pause is reduced or eliminated, much higher flow rates are required to eliminate rebreathing, equating to three times the minute volume or higher.

One of the major advantages of the Mapleson D, E and F systems is that the FGF is introduced very close to the patient end. This means that these systems can be longer than a Mapleson A without increasing the dead space; indeed, one of the key advantages of the Bain system is it can be up to 2 m in length.

The Humphrey ADE system

The Humphrey ADE system is a hybrid apparatus, combining the advantages of Mapleson A, D and E systems to render the system maximally efficient in both spontaneous and controlled modes of ventilation. A control lever switches between an internal configuration equating to a Mapleson A or a T-piece (Mapleson D/E). In the D/E configuration, a ventilator can be connected via the exhaust gas port.

Circle Breathing System

The major advantage of the circle system over all of the systems described by Mapleson is the ability of the patient to rebreathe gas. In order for this to occur safely, the circle system incorporates a means of removing carbon dioxide from the exhaled gases. Allowing the patient to rebreathe exhaled gases means these can be recycled, and so overall gas consumption is substantially reduced. Indeed, once the patient has become saturated with anaesthetic volatile, the only addition required to the circuit is the patient's basal oxygen consumption (around 250 ml min^{-1}). In addition to conserving costly anaesthetic agents, the circle system also allows greater conservation of moisture and heat within the system.

A simple circle system incorporates a reservoir bag and FGF supply, and two unidirectional valves to ensure flow of all exhaled gas through the absorber (Figure 9.5). Inspiratory gas consists of a mixture of fresh gas and gases that have passed through the absorber back to the patient. The circuit also contains an APL valve and, in most cases, a ventilator which

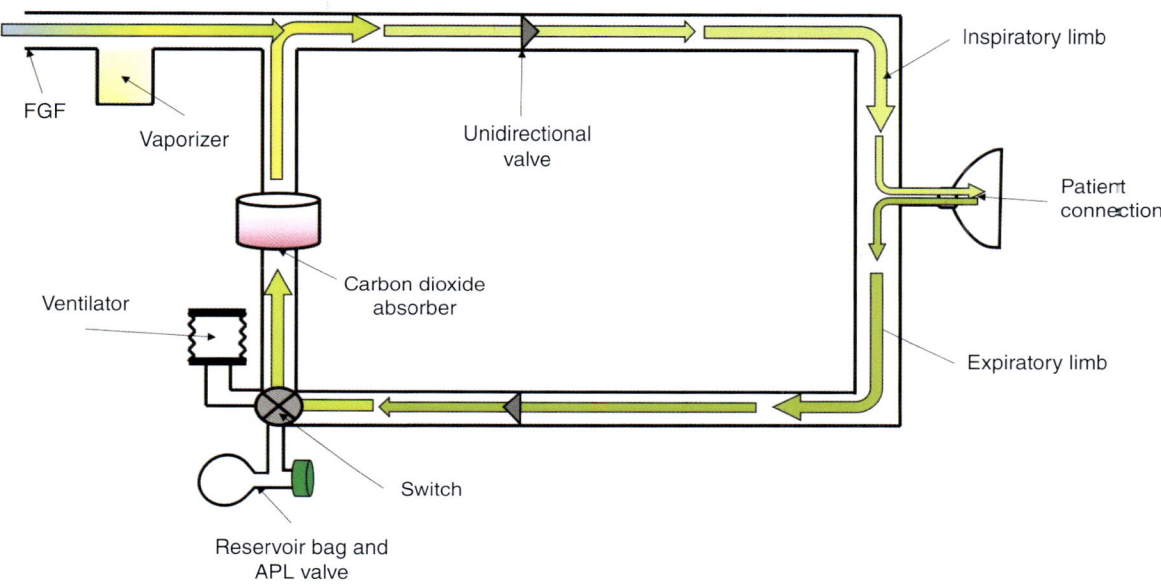

Figure 9.5 The circle breathing system

can be brought into the circuit via a switch. The circle system can be used with paediatric and adult patients. In the paediatric population, modifications to the delivery circuit are required to minimize dead space. Without these changes, the small tidal volumes generated may not be sufficient to open the valves, and excessive rebreathing may occur.

Vaporizers and the Circle System

Anaesthetic vaporizers can be positioned either within or outside the circle (see Chapter 8). The former arrangement is not commonly used in UK hospitals. Vaporizers within the circuit are of low resistance type as, in this position, they contribute to the resistance to flow in the spontaneously breathing patient. The low flows also make them comparatively inefficient and the vapour concentrations within the circuit take time to rise. Water vapour from the patient can also condense within the vaporizer, necessitating frequent drainage. In-circuit vaporizers have the advantage that they do not require pressurized gas supplies, and delivery of anaesthetic volatile can be demand-regulated.

More commonly, the vaporizer is placed outside the circuit. The amount of vapour added to the circuit is dependent on the FGF and the concentration dialled on the vaporizer. At low flows, equilibration will take considerably longer to be established.

Although we are used to the cumbersome nature of the rebreathing system in anaesthetic practice, compact versions have been created to replace traditional open-circuit scuba breathing apparatus for diving. Just as in anaesthetics, one of the major advantages of this is efficiency, with less wastage of gases and enhanced dive endurance. When we breathe air, either on land or via a standard open-scuba system, each exhaled breath contains 15% oxygen, 75% nitrogen and the remainder is carbon dioxide and other gases. For a diver, this means that only around 5% of the volume of the diver's tank ends up as oxygen in the bloodstream, the remaining 95% bubbling to the surface. A closed system, like an anaesthetic circuit, avoids this inefficiency. These systems are more comfortable to breathe due to the warming and humidifying effects of the carbon dioxide absorption process. In addition, the reduced loss of mass inherent in these systems means less ballast is required by the diver, as buoyancy remains constant, even over prolonged periods.

Mechanical Ventilation

Mechanical ventilators are a highly varied group of devices, used to support a patient's respiratory effort, or to replace it entirely. At a basic level, the outcome of this support is the enhanced movement of gases into and out of the lungs. The means by which this is achieved varies significantly and it is helpful to understand the mechanics of ventilation by classification into different modes of operation.

Negative Versus Positive Pressure Ventilation

In order for a gas mixture to move into the patient's lungs, a pressure gradient must exist. This can be accomplished either by lowering the pressure within the lungs relative to the atmosphere, or by raising the pressure within the atmosphere (or gas mixture) relative to the lungs. Negative pressure ventilators operate by the former of these modes of action; the classic example is the 'iron lung' that was employed to treat patients suffering from polio in the 1930s to 1950s. Of course, it is also the way we normally breathe in our daily life – the rib cage and diaphragm action causes an increase in thoracic volume, and hence a negative pressure gradient.

In negative-pressure-ventilation systems, a negative pressure is applied to the thorax and, in the iron lung, the abdomen as well. This causes an increase in the intrathoracic volume which, in turn, transmits the negative pressure to the intrapleural space causing expansion of the lungs and gas to be drawn in through the airway. Expiration occurs either by passive recoil or by active positive pressure to the thorax and abdomen. Negative pressure ventilation has the advantage that it does not necessitate endotracheal intubation, and the absence of high intrathoracic pressures results in a greater degree of cardiac stability. A modern example of this type of ventilator is the Hayek oscillator. This device consists of a rigid cuirass applied to the thorax, connected via a wide-bore, low-resistance tubing to a pump. The pump diaphragm then rapidly cycles the pressure within the cuirass about a baseline value to achieve alveolar ventilation.

Positive Pressure Ventilators

The majority of modern ventilation devices use positive pressure to deliver support. As a consequence of the variety of environments in which they are used, coupled with a wide variety of clinical conditions they can be used for, ventilator development has created many different models and types, with different modes of operation. This makes classification of ventilators challenging. However, it is useful to subdivide these various types according to the method of cycling, from inspiration to expiration and back again, and by the mode of application of positive pressure.

Classification by Cycling

Intermittent positive pressure ventilation (IPPV) of the lungs involves a phase of active application of positive pressure (inspiration) followed by passive lung emptying (expiration) – with or without the application of positive end-expiratory pressure (PEEP). The ventilator *cycles* between these two phases. Ventilator cycling can occur through a number of different mechanisms.

The dimensions of a breath can be controlled by adjusting the volume or pressure applied, and the duration of gas delivery. All of these influence the flow rate of gas into the patient. Any one of these can be used as the primary determinant for when inspiration ends and expiration begins, i.e. cycling.

1. Volume cycling

    In volume cycling, a flow sensor and a means of time measurement are connected within the ventilator, so that a given volume can be set (volume = flow/time). Once this volume has been achieved, the inspiratory flow is stopped and the ventilator cycles to expiration. Pressure is therefore a dependent variable.

2. Time cycling

    In a time-cycled mode, an electronic or mechanical timer determines the end of inspiration against the user-set value. The ventilator can then cycle to expiration immediately, or a pause can be programmed. Most modern ventilators incorporate such a pause, allowing for more even-filling across lung units with differing time constants, thus minimizing barotrauma and volutrauma in short time-constant lung units.

3. Pressure cycling

    In a pressure-cycled ventilator, airway pressure is sensed by the ventilator and the inspiratory phase terminated when a given pressure is reached. In this setting, volume becomes a dependent variable, and will fall if there is any decrease in compliance and vice versa.

Once the inspiratory phase is terminated, expiration occurs passively. The termination of expiration is dictated by the point in time at which the next inspiration is due (as determined by the respiratory rate – i.e. it is time-cycled). This is simple maths: a respiratory rate of 15 breaths a minute equates to a 4-second respiratory cycle (15 divides into 60 seconds four times). It is possible to influence the duration of

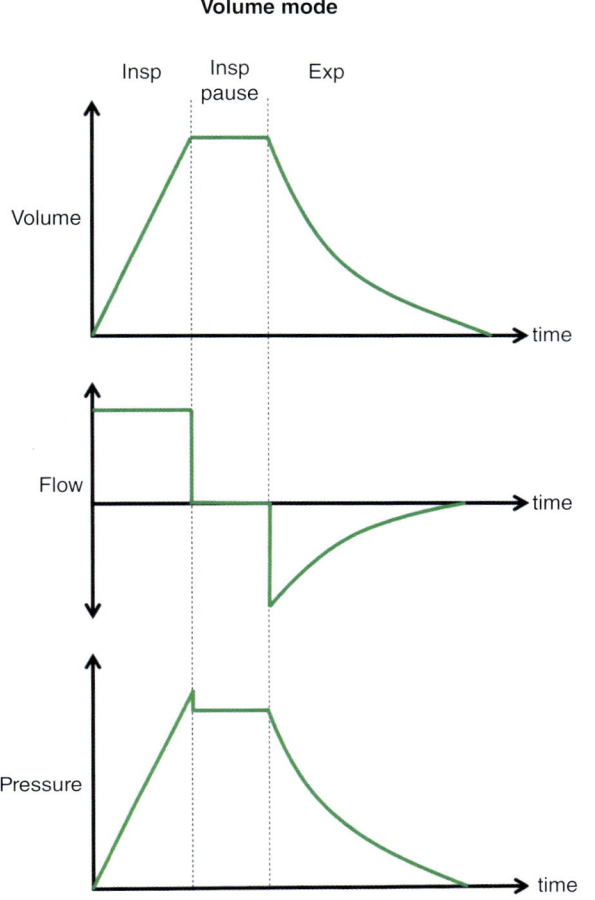
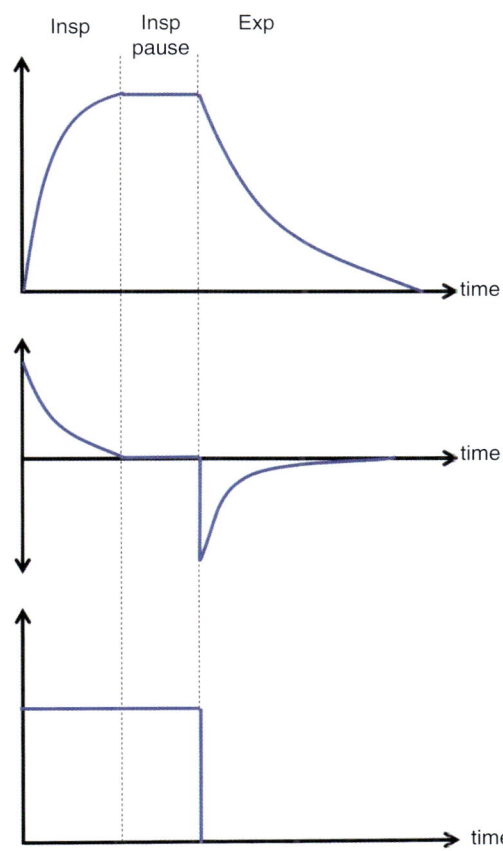

Figure 9.6 Pressure, volume and flow waveforms during ventilation

expiration as a proportion of that 4-second window: increasing or decreasing the inspiratory time reduces or increases the duration of the expiratory phase. The ratio of inspiratory to expiratory time is the I:E ratio. An I:E ratio of 1:3 in a 4-second cycle equates to an inspiratory period of 1 second, and an expiratory time of 3 seconds.

In synchronous or supported spontaneous modes, the end of expiration can also be flow- or pressure-cycled to co-ordinate with the patient making a spontaneous effort.

Modern ventilators may use a combination of any of the above to determine inspiratory and expiratory cycling, allowing for greater flexibility in optimizing ventilation and patient–ventilator synchrony. Any of these parameters may also have preset limits to add further safeguards against ventilator-induced lung injury.

Changes in pressure, volume and flow versus time have characteristic appearances depending on the method of ventilatory cycling (Figure 9.6).

Volume-Control Ventilation

In volume-control ventilation (VCV), a constant flow is delivered so as to achieve the volume target within the set inspiratory time. As a result, there is a gradual pressure rise observed as inspiration progresses from the PEEP value to the peak inspiratory pressure. The slope of this rise is dependent on patient compliance and airway resistance. Following inspiration, an inspiratory pause may be programmed where no further gas flow occurs. At this point the pressure declines to the plateau pressure as the lungs recoil. The plateau pressure is a key target when titrating to avoid barotrauma to the lung; it is the most accurate reflection of the pressure within the alveoli themselves. Most ventilators incorporate a pressure limit to prevent excessive peak pressures being applied during delivery of the specified tidal volume. The flow–time curve in VCV consists of a square wave during inspiration as fixed-rate flow occurs and then ceases. Expiratory flow follows a decelerating pattern as the lung empties passively.

Pressure-Control Ventilation

In pressure-control ventilation (PCV), a fixed pressure is rapidly achieved, creating a square wave on the pressure–time waveform. The flow–time curve, by contrast, shows high initial flow with subsequent flow deceleration as the lung fills and compliance decreases. In this circumstance, the peak pressure and plateau pressure are the same, as the slower inflation of the lung results in increased time for the lung to fill, and so there is minimal recoil when flow ceases. In circumstances where lung compliance is reduced, the tidal volume will thus be smaller for a given inspiratory pressure. The deceleration of the inspiratory flow has the advantage of more homogeneous flow distribution within the lung, with more favourable V/Q ratios as a result. This advantage is enhanced in the diseased lung where there is even greater heterogeneity of time constants throughout the lung.

Classification by mode of operation

Ventilators differ in the way in which they use mechanical power to deliver gases to the lungs. This variety allows different models to be used in different settings dependent on available resources and titrated to different patient populations and pathologies. Ventilators can be broadly classified into four categories depending on how they apply positive pressure:

1. 'Mechanical thumbs'

    Pressurized gas in medical settings is available from pipelines and cylinders. When this gas flow is connected to a patient's breathing system, a pressure is developed. This pressure can be used to drive positive pressure ventilation. The simplest form of this is best observed in the recovery or paediatric setting when a T-piece or Mapleson F system is intermittently occluded by placing a human thumb over the expiratory limb. As flow from the gas source is constant, an increase in pressure results. This pressure rise then leads to inspiratory flow, which then cycles to expiration when the anaesthetist removes the occlusion. This principle is applied in so-called 'mechanical thumb' ventilators, replacing the anaesthetist's hand with a mechanism.

    The Sechrist Bird VIP ventilator uses this principle; an electronically controlled solenoid is used to intermittently occlude the expiratory limb, with pressures, timing and volumes being independent variables depending on the model of ventilator. In this mode of ventilation, inspiratory flow is determined by available flow from the gas supply, making it more suitable for use in paediatric or neonatal settings; the tidal volumes can be achieved in less time, permitting the higher respiratory rates these patients require.

2. Minute-volume dividers

    Minute-volume dividers operate using a constant flow of driving gas, which becomes the effective minute volume; the entirety of the FGF is delivered to the patient, with the ventilator dividing this flow into fixed volumes depending on the required tidal volume. For example, a flow of 8 l min^{-1} may be set to be divided into 20 400-ml breaths.

    The fresh gas is delivered to a reservoir, which is compressed either by a weight, spring or as a result of its own elasticity. A valve operates between this reservoir and the patient, which, when opened, permits flow of gas. This valve is linked to another one on an expiratory limb, such that when the inspiratory valve opens, the expiratory valve closes, and vice versa. Such ventilators are not commonly used in modern practice due to the waste of the inspiratory gas flow and the high flows required.

    The classical example of this type of ventilator is the Manley MP3. In the Manley ventilator, prior to inspiration, the bellows fill with fresh gas to a predetermined point whereupon the inspiratory valve opens and a weight above the bellows causes them to empty into the inspiratory limb. The position of the weight above the bellows can be altered to change the inspiratory pressure supplied. The tidal volume is controlled by adjusting a catch that restricts the degree to which the bellows can fill. Whilst inspiration is occurring, the FGF is diverted to a second bellows. When these are full, a mechanical linkage causes the valve-opening sequence to reverse, resulting in onset of expiration.

3. Bag squeezers

   Most modern anaesthetic workstations employ a 'bag squeezer' ventilator. These consist of a set of bellows into which the FGF is directed. These are then compressed to deliver fresh gas to the patient. The compression can be driven by placing the bellows within a non-compliant container and feeding a pressurized driving gas around the bellows. The bellows can be arranged upright or inverted. In the latter case, the bellows have a weight attached and refill downwards in expiration. In descending bellows, there is less resistance to expiration; however, in the event of a leak, ascending bellows will collapse under their own weight, alerting to a problem and preventing a mixture of drive gas with fresh gas. This would obviously not occur in descending bellows, allowing the potential for dilution of fresh gas. The bellows may also be compressed by means of a piston or a crank, connected to an electric motor.

4. Intermittent blowers

   Most modern intensive care ventilators operate by this principle. In an intermittent blower, a pressurized gas source, usually at 400 kPa, is used. This flow is modulated by low-compliance resistors so as to regulate gas flow to generate a predetermined tidal volume and pressure. The control mechanisms can include complex digitally controlled valves as in ICU ventilators, or more simple but robust pneumatic oscillators as in portable ventilators of the Pneupac® ventiPAC™ type.

Portable Ventilators

Portable ventilators are utilized to support patients outside of the ICU or theatre. This may be in the emergency department as a temporary measure, during transportation for therapeutic or diagnostic procedures, or during transfers between ICUs and other sites. Such ventilators are necessarily smaller and more robust than ventilators used in the ITU so as to render them portable. Over recent years their complexity has increased, allowing patients to benefit from virtually the same ventilatory support in transit as they would receive in the ICU.

The characteristics of the ideal portable ventilator include:

- Small
- Lightweight
- Robust
- Low power consumption
- Low gas consumption
- Ability to provide ventilatory support identical to that in the ICU
- Simplicity of operation
- Able to operate over wider range of environmental conditions
- Ability to fail-safe in situations of power- or gas-supply failure

Portable ventilators in common usage in the UK include the Smiths ventiPAC™ series, Dräger Oxylog® and Hamilton T1 ventilators.

The ventiPAC™ ventilator is a simple time-cycled flow generator. It uses the energy from the pressurized gas supply, which is usually an oxygen cylinder at 137 bar (when full), to generate both flow and the energy to operate the cycling mechanisms. It can deliver 100% oxygen or, by means of Venturi entrainment, 50%, by entraining room air. It is important to note, however, that when the 50% concentration is selected, increased resistance from non-compliant airways results in decreased flow, and thus decreased tidal volume. This is not seen when 100% is selected. The use of pneumatic cycling obviates the need for electrical power, however, and thus the ventiPAC™ is extremely useful in resource-limited and remote locations.

The Hamilton T1 and Oxylog® ventilators use microprocessor-controlled software, and flow and pressure sensors within the breathing circuit, to provide more advanced levels of ventilatory support. In contrast to the ventiPAC™, these ventilators can more effectively support spontaneous breathing and thus reduce the need for ongoing paralysis during transfers.

When preparing for transfer using a portable ventilator, planning for consumption of gases and of power is necessary.

Oxygen consumption can be calculated using the equation:

$$\text{Oxygen consumption} = \left[(\text{Minute volume} + \text{Bias flow}) \times \left(\frac{FiO_2 - 0.2}{0.8}\right)\right] + \text{Cycling requirement}$$

So, for an Oxylog 3000, operating with a minute ventilation of 8 l min^{-1} and a FiO$_2$ of 1.0, the oxygen requirement would be (bias flow of 500 ml min^{-1}):

$$= \left[(8 + 0.5) \times \left(\frac{1 - 0.2}{0.8}\right)\right] + 0$$
$$= 8.5 \text{ l min}^{-1}$$

For a patient being transferred using the same settings and a respiratory rate of 15 min^{-1} with a ventiPAC^{TM} ventilator the consumption would be (bias flow 20 ml cycle^{-1}):

$$= \left[(8 + 0) \times \left(\frac{1 - 0.2}{0.8}\right)\right] + (15 \times 0.02)$$
$$= 8.3 \text{ l min}^{-1}$$

To plan a transfer safely, this minute consumption is then multiplied by the expected duration of the transfer in minutes, and then doubled as a contingency for delays. For further safety, and a considerable simplification of the calculations, it is easier to work on the assumption the patient will be on 100% oxygen throughout. This simplifies the calculation to:

Oxygen requirements = [(Minute volume + Bias flow) + Cycling requirements)] × 2

The Hamilton T1 is a turbine ventilator, which therefore does not require any pressurized gas to function except for the oxygen requirements of the patient. This also means it will continue to ventilate at whatever pressures the patient requires, should the oxygen run out (but the FiO$_2$ will be limited to 0.21). It does mean that a power failure would be just as catastrophic as an oxygen failure with one of the other ventilators. The only gas required for a transfer on a trip with a Hamilton T1 is the oxygen needed by the patient.

Portable ventilator circuits contain two limbs, one to carry gas to the patient and the other to exhaust it, via a PEEP valve if necessary, to the atmosphere. Often, these are configured in a co-axial manner to reduce bulk. The modern microprocessor-controlled ventilators incorporate PEEP valves within the ventilator, making the circuits less cumbersome.

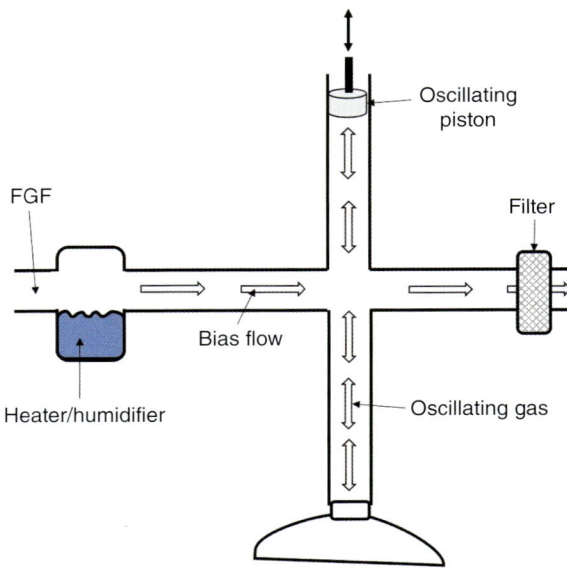

Figure 9.7 Oscillator ventilator schematic

Alternative Modes of Ventilation

The high-frequency oscillating ventilator (HFOV) produces respiratory rates far in excess of those seen in any other form of ventilation; between 2 and 10 cycles per second. The HFOV has much lower tidal volumes than those seen with conventional ventilation, thus minimizing volutrauma and atelectotrauma. It also consistently maintains higher mean airway pressures and so optimizes oxygenation.

In an oscillator, a flow of warmed, humidified gas is passed across the patient's endotracheal tube. This is the bias flow and is usually of the order of 20 l min^{-1}. This flow is oscillated by a gas-driven piston, which oscillates the gas at 2–10 Hz, leading to a respiratory rate of 120–600 breaths per minute (Figure 9.7). The amount of gas moving into and out of the lungs is determined by the frequency and amplitude of these oscillations. The amplitude is determined by the degree of excursion of the piston. This is scientifically assessed by observing the patient's 'wiggle factor'! When an optimal amplitude has been selected, visible movement should be observed from the chest down to mid-thigh. A reduction in the frequency of oscillation leads to an increase in amplitude, and thus an increase in carbon dioxide clearance. In addition to oscillation, some carbon dioxide clearance occurs through bulk flow down the airway, and some through the mixing of gas from short- to long-time-constant alveoli (Pendelluft ventilation). Oxygenation is determined by the FiO_2 and the mean airway pressure.

Randomized controlled trials early in the era of ventilation for ARDS showed that oscillatory ventilation was superior to conventional ventilation and caused less damage to the lung. However, the subsequent OSCAR trial, using lung-protective ventilation strategies, failed to replicate this benefit. As a consequence, oscillating ventilation has become less commonly used in adult ICUs in the UK.

APRV (airway pressure release ventilation), in contrast to HFOV, is a method of achieving open lung ventilation in ARDS, which is enjoying an upsurge in clinical interest. It can be delivered using a conventional ventilator with appropriate software. In APRV, the ventilator cycles between two pressures, the high pressure (P-high) and the lower pressure (P-low). The timing is configured such that the pressure is at P-high 85–95% of the time, and the remaining time is spent at P-low, which is usually set at 0 cmH_2O. The patient is able to take spontaneous breaths throughout the cycle. T-low is the time during which the ventilator reduces the pressure to P-low. This is titrated against expiratory flow so that, typically, the ventilator is set to cycle back to P-high once expiratory flow has reduced to around 40% (at most, to 25%) of peak expiratory flow.

Both APRV and HFOV theoretically allow a more lung-protective strategy and have been demonstrated to improve physiological variables in human and animal models. However, in both cases there are risks, including cardiovascular instability due to reduced venous return, lung barotrauma and risks of dynamic hyperinflation, potentially leading to pneumothorax. They have not yet been shown to improve patient outcomes, and so their use is currently less common.

ECMO and ECCO$_2$R

Extra-corporeal membranous oxygenation (ECMO) can be thought of as a modified cardiopulmonary bypass technology. Venous blood is drained into the ECMO circuit, oxygenated, and carbon dioxide is removed before rewarming, prior to return. ECMO allows for circulatory support, typically when there has been failure of conventional respiratory intensive care. It is a well-established therapy in neonates, and the technology has been refined over the last 40 years, with a decreasing morbidity and mortality. The procedure is not without its complications, which include bleeding, pneumothoraces, haemothoraces, pericardial tamponade, vascular tears, embolization, circuit failure, heart failure, pulmonary haemorrhage, pulmonary infarction, major haemorrhagic stroke and air emboli. As a result, and because of the cost of the equipment, the practice is restricted to specialist centres.

Types of ECMO

1. Veno-arterial (VA) ECMO

    In this version, deoxygenated blood is taken from a central vein or the right atrium, passed through the ECMO circuit and returned to a central artery. VA ECMO provides partial cardiac support (in addition to native cardiac output). It causes a significant reduction in right-ventricular afterload, a decreased cardiac workload and reduces cardiac oxygen consumption. The final oxygen content of the blood depends on a combination of ECMO and native patient blood flows (to the lungs). Patients cannot fully ambulate using this mode of ECMO due to the position of the cannulae.

2. Veno-veno (VV) ECMO

    In this configuration, deoxygenated blood is taken from a central vein or the right atrium, processed and then returned to a large vein. Because blood is being taken from and returned to the venous system, there is no change in central venous pressure or ventricular filling. Typically, pulmonary artery pressures fall in VV ECMO. Native cardiac output provides full systemic blood flow. VV ECMO is therefore used in situations where cardiac function is preserved (in spite of severe respiratory compromise).

3. Arterio-venous (AV) pumpless assist devices

    In this set-up, deoxygenated blood is typically taken from and returned to the femoral artery and vein, respectively. These devices can be thought of as pumpless membrane oxygenators. They allow a small amount of oxygenation, but predominantly offer carbon dioxide removal (extra-corporeal CO_2 removal – ECCO$_2$R). They also offer a mechanical approach to reducing RV afterload. AV pumpless assist devices are

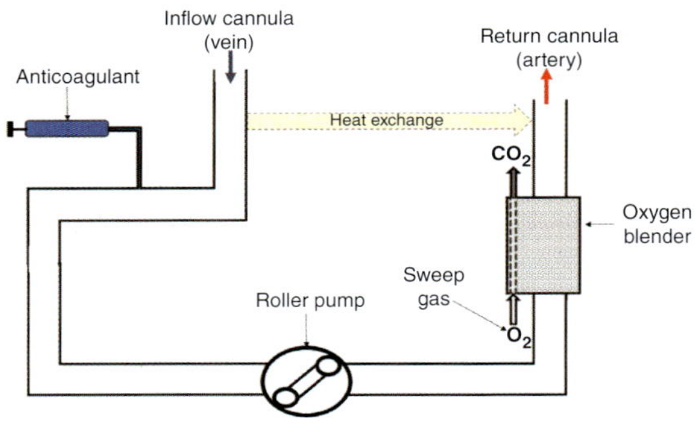

Figure 9.8 A typical ECMO circuit

dependent on native cardiac output, and require a cardiac index of at least 2.5 l min^{-1} m^{-2}. These devices are generally not suitable for oxygenation due to the relatively low blood flow across the device: they are predominantly used for ECCO$_2$R.

ECMO Circuit

All types of ECMO circuit contain the following components (Figure 9.8):
- Oxygenator – non-porous, hollow-fibre oxygenators are used
- Cannulae – the main limiter to flow in the circuit
- Pump – safety provided through regulation of negative pressure (stopping vessel wall damage, haemolysis and gas cavitation)
- Heat exchanger – to rewarm the blood prior to returning it to the patient
- Pressure transducers – for monitoring

For more details on the principles of these systems, refer to the discussions on cardiopulmonary bypass in Chapter 13.

As mentioned, ECMO is well established in neonates with a good evidence base. There have been several important trials in adult patients. The CESAR trial [1] showed an improved survival at 6 months (63% vs. 47%) in adults with severe acute respiratory failure using VV ECMO. That said, a systematic review of VV ECMO during the H1:N1 pandemic found insufficient evidence for its use in this patient population. ECMO has been used successfully in cardiac arrest and in retrieval medicine. Part of the reason the evidence supporting ECMO has been equivocal may lie in the nature of its provision. As a tertiary service delivered in a few specialized centres, ECMO concentrates expert opinion and dedicated multidisciplinary teams focused on respiratory care around the patient, and this may confer a substantial benefit, independent of the ECMO therapy itself. Patients demonstrating survival benefits in the CESAR study did not all receive ECMO, and part of the benefit may lie in the expertise of the centre they were referred to.

Summary

In this chapter, we have discussed clinical problems that are commonly encountered in the intensive care and anaesthetic environment as they relate to ventilation and anaesthetic gas delivery. We have examined potential responses to these problems and the physical principles governing their utility. In many cases, the delivery of ventilation and anaesthesia has become increasingly automated with computer-controlled anaesthetic workstations, and the principles underlying the operation of these systems can become distant. It is important to consider these principles despite this, so as to avoid the surprise and concern often experienced when faced with a Mapleson breathing system or when difficulties are encountered with modern workstations. This chapter provides an overview of these topics and should equip you with the grounding required for modern practice.

Questions

MCQs – select true or false for each response

1. Considering positive pressure ventilation using a time-cycled pressure control mode:
   (a) The inspiratory flow shows an exponential increase
   (b) The tidal volume produced is a product of the specified pressure and lung compliance
   (c) The peak pressure represents a good measure of lung compliance
   (d) Peak pressure and plateau pressure are very similar
   (e) Flow deceleration results in selective ventilation of short time-constant lung units
2. Regarding the Mapleson breathing systems:
   (a) Mapleson A breathing systems require high fresh gas flows to prevent rebreathing in the spontaneously breathing patient
   (b) In a Bain system, fresh gas flows equal to minute volume effectively prevent rebreathing when using spontaneous ventilation

(c) In traditional Mapleson A systems, the weight of the APL may drag on the airway
(d) In Mapleson A systems, the size of the patient mask has no effect on rebreathing
(e) Limitations in circuit length make the Bain system unsuitable for use in the MRI scanner

SBAs – select the single *best* answer

3. A 75-year-old man is admitted to the emergency department, acutely unwell. A blood gas is taken which shows a PaO_2 of 6.8 kPa, $PaCO_2$ of 7.5 kPa, bicarbonate of 29 mmol l^{-1} and pH of 7.36. He is breathing spontaneously with a GCS of 14/15 (E3, V5, M6). Which device is best suited to correct his hypoxaemia?
   (a) Venturi mask
   (b) Nasal prongs
   (c) Hudson mask
   (d) Commence non-invasive ventilation with supplemental oxygen
   (e) Reservoir mask and high-flow oxygen

4. A 14-month-old patient has been transferred to theatre and connected to a Jackson–Rees T-piece breathing system. Anaesthesia is being maintained with oxygen/nitrous oxide at 0.5 l min^{-1} for each gas and sevoflurane. The patient is being manually ventilated by squeezing the reservoir bag. The end-tidal carbon dioxide has begun to rise, the patient's temperature is 37.9 °C tympanic. The most appropriate initial action is:
   (a) Re-check the temperature
   (b) Change the soda lime canister
   (c) Abandon surgery and commence Dantrolene infusion
   (d) Increase fresh gas flow rate
   (e) Switch to a Mapleson A circuit.

Answers

1. FTFTF
   Inspiratory flow shows a near-instantaneous rise followed by an exponential decline. Peak pressure is controlled by the settings of the ventilator and is not dependent on compliance (cf. volume-control ventilation). Peak and plateau pressure are similar; the declining flow rate allows for more even spread across lung units of differing time constants, so there is less elastic recoil as flow returns to zero.

2. FFTFF
   Mapleson A systems require gas flows approximate to the minute volume in spontaneously ventilated patients and Mapleson D systems require similar gas flows in mandatorily ventilated patients. Traditional Mapleson A systems place the APL at the patient interface and its mass may displace the airway; co-axial systems eliminate this issue. The gas contained in the Mapleson A between the APL and the patient may be rebreathed, as such, a larger mask increases the rebreathing fraction. The Bain circuit has an inner tube within the outer tube. The gases do not mix until they emerge at the distal end of the circuit. Therefore, the length of the tube is not relevant in this context.

3. (a)
   Controlled oxygen therapy is essential in severe COPD and the Venturi mask is the only device capable of this accuracy (nasal prongs are affected by the size of the reservoir (the nasopharynx), the tidal volume and, in a mouth-breather, the peak inspiratory flow). There is presently no indication for NIV as the pH is normal and the patient has a good consciousness level. CPAP may be necessary depending on the underlying pathology, but this is not the first line therapy.

4. (d)
   A concern in a patient with a temperature and rising carbon dioxide may lead to concerns regarding rare reactions to volatile anaesthesia in paediatrics. However, common things are common; the fresh gas flow is sufficient when using a circle system with soda lime; however, this patient is being ventilated with a Jackson–Rees system, presumably on the auxiliary common gas outlet and so the absorber is not involved; changing it will not help. The fresh gas flow should be at least equal to the minute volume, and may need to be two to three times the minute volume to avoid rebreathing carbon dioxide. As the minute volume is likely to be 2.5–3 l min^{-1}, the fresh gas flow needs to be increased.

References

1. G. Peek, M. Mugford, R. Tiruvoipati, A. Wilson, E. Allen, M. Thalanany, C. Hibbert, A. Truesdale, F. Clemens, N. Cooper, R. Firmin, D. Elbourne. Efficacy and economic assessment of conventional ventilatory support versus extracorporeal membrane oxygenation for severe adult respiratory failure (CESAR): a multicentre randomised controlled trial. *The Lancet*, 374, 2009; 1351–1363.

Chapter 10

Safety in the Clinical Environment

Lauren Weekes and David Ashton-Cleary

Learning Objectives

- To describe the systems in place to remove waste gases from the operating theatre
- To appreciate the situations in anaesthesia which present a high risk for fires and explosions, including airway surgery. Explain the actions required to reduce these risks
- Understand the risks of electrical shock and describe the concepts of macroshock and microshock

Chapter Content

- Scavenging
- Fires and explosions
- Electrical safety
- Humidity and sparks

Scenario

Whilst providing anaesthesia for an emergency cardioversion in the operating theatre, the medical registrar tells you to remove the oxygen source from the endotracheal tube, and step away from the patient whilst defibrillation is undertaken. She also asks all theatre staff to step away from the patient.

How is the working environment protected from gases used in anaesthesia? How can the risk of combustion be reduced and what would be the correct course of action if combustion occurred? What safety measures are in place to protect staff and patients from unintentional electric shock?

Introduction

It is easy to think of the environmental hazards associated with anaesthesia as a historical artefact. After all, the first reported anaesthesia-associated fire was in 1850 as a result of ether (diethyl ether) combusting during facial surgery and we have all heard tall tales of the dangers of explosive cyclopropane. In reality, there continue to be incidents every year causing harm to patients from the theatre and critical care environments. In 2012, an oxygen cylinder placed on a patient's bed in an ICU caused a fire which spread rapidly to the bedding and curtains. This necessitated the evacuation of the unit and the unit was filled with thick black smoke. The patient suffered burns to the legs, and two staff were admitted overnight with smoke inhalation. It is therefore important to consider the safety implications of equipment and drugs we commonly use, as well as considering the wider safety set-up in the working environment.

Scavenging

Acceptable levels of anaesthetic gases in the theatre environment are regulated by Control of Substances Hazardous to Health (COSHH), part of UK law. Similar laws exist elsewhere, such as the Occupational Health and Safety Act (OHSA) in the United States (Table 10.1). This is due to concerns surrounding toxicity of anaesthetic agents, in particular nitrous oxide. This agent is a selective inhibitor of methionine synthase, with long-term use potentially leading to megaloblastic bone-marrow depression and neurological symptoms. There are also some potential links with fertility and increased risk of spontaneous abortion although these are not well established. Interestingly, desflurane and sevoflurane do not have specified limits under COSHH or OHSA as adequate safety data do not currently exist.

A time-weighted average allows assessment of the total exposure in a given period to be calculated, even though differing concentrations may be experienced for portions of that period. By convention, the standard 8-hour shift is used as an industry benchmark. For example, an anaesthetist may spend a total of an hour in the anaesthetic room doing paediatric

Table 10.1 COSHH and OHSA permitted limits for anaesthetic agents in the theatre environment [1, 2]

Substance	Permitted maximum in ppm as 8-hour time-weighted average (UK)	Permitted maximum in ppm as 8-hour time-weighted average (USA)
Nitrous oxide	100	25
Isoflurane	50	2
Enflurane	50	2
Halothane	10	2

gas inductions, using open-circuit techniques with exposure to nitrous oxide at 500-parts per million (ppm) concentrations. If the other 7 hours are spent in theatre using a circle system with theatre concentrations of 30 ppm, the time-weighted average can be calculated as follows:

$$\text{Time-weighted average} = \frac{(500 \times 1) + (30 \times 7)}{8}$$
$$= 88.75 \text{ ppm}$$

To minimize pollution of the theatre environment with waste anaesthetic agent and keep exposure within the set limits, modern anaesthesia breathing systems are connected to a scavenging system to remove the gases, to be safely disposed of. Scavenging systems may be either active, requiring energy to operate a pump system, or passive. Scavenging systems have the following components:

- Collecting system
- Transfer system
- Receiving system
- Disposal system
- Exterior port

Collecting System

This is most commonly a closed system, attached to the adjustable pressure-limiting (APL) or expiratory valve, but may also, rarely, consist of a funnel, positioned near to the patient's mouth. The latter is occasionally found in the context of dental anaesthesia where there may be difficulty in maintaining a close mask fit. Connectors for scavenging tubing are 30 mm, so as not to be confused with 15-mm breathing system connections.

Transfer System

This consists of wide-bore tubing, with 30-mm connectors as described. The system contains a pressure relief valve set at 10 cmH$_2$O to allow expiratory flow even if the system becomes blocked.

Receiving System

This protects the patient from both high and low pressures (−0.05 kPa to +5 kPa) and contains a reservoir to maximize efficiency in the presence of variable gas flow (between 0 l min^{-1} and 130 l min^{-1}). The reservoir is open-ended in active systems, and in passive systems consists of bags and valves.

Disposal System

Passive disposal systems vent the patient's waste gases directly to the atmosphere. This is fraught with difficulty, as excessively high winds outside the exhaust can generate potentially damaging negative pressures applied to the breathing system. Conversely, if the outlet is vertical then the weight of heavier anaesthetic agents can cause excessive positive pressure. Such systems are rarely used in the UK.

Charcoal canisters can be used to absorb volatile anaesthetics (although not nitrous oxide). However, they are inefficient and the charcoal needs to be changed after 12 hours of use.

Active scavenging utilizes a fan (low-pressure, wide-bore systems) or pump (higher-pressure, narrow-bore systems) to drive waste gases. The system should be capable of generating an extraction flow of up to 75 l min^{-1}. This will, however, produce an 'induced flow' whereby fresh gas is drawn out of the breathing system. The design of the system should be such to ensure the induced flow is no more than 0.05 l min^{-1}, otherwise low-flow anaesthesia techniques become very challenging to deliver safely. A low extraction flow reduces efficacy of the system but a high flow increases the induced flow.

Exterior Port

The waste gases are vented to the atmosphere unchanged.

Adjuncts To Scavenging

No scavenging system can completely remove all volatiles from the working atmosphere, so it remains important that the theatre complex air handling systems are capable of ensuring adequate air changes (15 exchanges per hour).

Fires and Explosions

Fire requires the following components:
- Ignition source
- Fuel
- Oxidizing agent

All three of these are readily available in the operating theatre and critical care environments. Despite the decline in use of flammable or explosive volatile agents (cyclopropane and diethyl ether) in the developed world, there are several remaining hazards of which the anaesthetist needs to be aware.

> Strictly speaking, an ignition source is not always necessary. Certain combinations of substances can burn or explode on contact with each other. These are referred to as hypergolic substances and are used as rocket propellant. Examples include monomethylhydrazine in combination with nitrogen tetroxide. Although a hypergolic rocket motor is simple (through lack of an ignition system), these propellants usually provide less energy per mass of propellant compared to conventional combinations such as hydrogen–oxygen. They are also extremely toxic and corrosive substances, which makes them very challenging to work with.

Flammable Gas Mixtures

In a flammable gas mixture there is a combination of fuel and oxidizing agent. The proportions of these will determine whether the mixture can ignite, explode, or cannot burn at all. Flammability limits are defined by the ratio of fuel to oxidizer, and if either the proportion of fuel or oxidizer is too great, it cannot burn. For example, cyclopropane in air has flammability limits of 2.5–10% cyclopropane concentration; outside of these concentrations, it will not ignite. In oxygen, those flammability limits are predictably widened: 2.5–63%.

An explosion is a reaction that occurs very rapidly, often more rapidly than the speed of sound, and it is associated with the generation of great heat and pressure (blast wave). Explosions of flammable gas mixtures may occur when they reach their stoichiometric concentrations; this term describes when the proportions of fuel and oxidizer are perfectly matched so all the fuel and all the oxidizer are consumed by the reaction. For cyclopropane in air, this is a 4.7% concentration. This is calculated by determining the equation for the reaction to give the molar proportions of the reactants which lead to a complete reaction:

$$4C_3H_6 + 18O_2 \rightarrow 12CO_2 + 12H_2O$$

From this we can see cyclopropane and oxygen react perfectly in a 4:18 (or 1:4.5) ratio. Because oxygen only makes up 21% of air, it will take a larger volume of air to supply enough oxygen molecules. The volume for air is calculated as follows:

$$\left(\frac{1}{0.21}\right) \times 4.5 = 21.4$$

So, the stoichiometric ratio for cyclopropane in air is 1:21.4, which is a cyclopropane concentration of 4.7%. If we take a step back to a pure oxygen mix (1:4.5 ratio), that equates to a 22.2% concentration; we have a lot more oxidizer, which means we can oxidize a much greater quantity of the fuel. If we have equal volumes of the two mixtures, clearly the 22.2% mixture contains nearly five times the number of molecules of cyclopropane to act as fuel in the reaction: a much bigger bang!

Ignition Sources

These are usually related to electrical equipment, such as electrosurgical tools, defibrillators and power sockets. Spark-ignition is most common when such equipment develops a fault. Static electricity has previously been considered an ignition risk in the presence of volatile agents such as cyclopropane. High-powered lasers (Class 4, i.e. >500 mW), including carbon dioxide lasers, produce enough energy to ignite flammable material. There are a specific set of precautions when the use of lasers is undertaken; some to reduce the risk of fire; and some to reduce risk to staff and patients from misdirected laser beams:

- Reduce FiO_2 to the lowest safe level
- Ensure appropriate laser-specific equipment is used, e.g. specialized endotracheal tubes
- Cover potentially flammable tissue with damp gauze when practicable
- Avoid spirit-based skin preparation
- Cover exposed hair with water-based lubricating gel
- Use blue-dyed saline in endotracheal tube cuffs for laser airway surgery so cuff rupture is immediately detectable

- For laser airway surgery, prefilled syringes of saline must be immediately available to extinguish airway fires
- All staff must wear laser goggles specific to the wavelength of laser in use
- Appropriate training for staff, including operators and laser safety officers

Medical electrical equipment, strictly speaking, may still have a rating of AP or APG (anaesthetic proof ± category G). This relates to the device representing an ignition source in the presence of flammable anaesthetics. Since these agents are no longer widely used, this is essentially of historical interest only. AP equipment is safe with an ether–air mix within 5–25 cm of escaping breathing gases so can safely reach 200 °C. APG can be used within 5 cm of escaping ether–oxygen mixes, and so must operate below 90 °C.

Fuel

A fuel is a substance that stores chemical potential energy that may be released as heat energy. Aside from the flammable anaesthetics, there are many other potential sources of fuel. Alcohol-based surgical skin preparation is associated with at least one reported incident per year in the UK, usually when it has not been allowed to dry and diathermy has been applied. Ethyl chloride ('cold spray'), intestinal gases such as methane and hydrogen, and combustible materials such as drapes, dressings and bed clothes may all be considered potential sources of fuel in the operating theatre.

Oxidizers

A source of oxygen must be present for a fire to propagate. In the medical setting, this may be from air, concentrated oxygen or nitrous oxide (or less commonly nitric oxide or hydrogen peroxide). In the presence of heat, nitrous oxide breaks down as follows:

$$2N_2O \rightarrow 2N_2 + O_2 + \text{Energy}$$

This gives a 33% oxygen mixture and produces additional thermal energy; nitrous oxide is thus both a fuel and an oxygen source.

Fires started in the presence of high concentrations of oxygen burn more violently and with greater release of heat than those burning in the presence of air. Safety precautions for the use of oxidizing agents include keeping oxygen and nitrous oxide cylinders free from grease and oil, ensuring they are regularly serviced and placing such cylinders in a proper bracket or trolley for transportation.

A pure oxygen atmosphere was used in early space flight to circumvent issues with nitrogen (risk of decompression sickness and relative hypoxic mixtures) but a launch-pad test of Apollo 1 ended in tragedy when an electrical spark led to a flash fire and explosion within the capsule. The overpressure of the event led to a partial rupture of the capsule when the cabin pressure reached 2 atm. All three astronauts died rapidly of carbon monoxide poisoning. The incident led to a compromise of a 60:40 oxygen–nitrogen atmosphere being adopted for the remainder of the Apollo programme.

Minimizing Risk of Fire

US data have shown that a number of factors are implicated in higher risks of surgical fires:
- Use of monopolar diathermy
- Use of lasers
- Procedures above the xiphisternum
- Open-source oxygen from face masks or nasal cannulae

Where several of these factors are present, it is suggested that explicit fire planning is performed before the start of surgery. The World Health Organization (WHO) Surgical Safety Checklist time-out is a logical time to address the fire risk. Where possible, alternatives to the above should be sought. For example, consider using bipolar diathermy or harmonic scalpels, performing sedation without supplemental oxygen or using a gas mixer to reduce the FiO_2 of gas mixtures delivered by face mask.

Management of Fire

It is clearly important to undertake regular fire safety training as well as to be familiar with local protocols in the area in which you work. It is also useful to drill evacuation plans for specific areas, for example, a fire in the ICU or in theatres.

Recognizing Fire

Fire may not always be immediately obvious; alcohol-based fires often do not burn with a visible flame.

There will be other clues to the presence of fire such as palpable heat, visible aura or evidence of drapes, bedding, etc. burning.

Attempts to Extinguish Fire

If there is fire involving the patient then emergency steps should be taken to extinguish the flames and minimize the subsequent impact. The sooner that burning material is removed from the patient, the lower the risk of serious burn injury. Saline or water can be used to douse flames, or non-flammable material, e.g. wet towels or packs, can be used to smother the fire. The flow of oxidizing anaesthetic gases to the patient should be immediately ceased and if ventilation is required, it should continue on room air.

If the fire is in the airway, the tracheal tube and other foreign bodies should be removed immediately and the fire extinguished with saline that should be immediately to hand. The patient's airway will need inspecting for evidence of burns and/or debris, preferably via rigid bronchoscopy. Consideration should be given to reintubation.

If simple techniques to extinguish a patient fire have been unsuccessful, or the fire does not involve the patient, the alarm should be raised. The procedure for this varies according to local protocol; commonly it involves the use of wall-based alarm bells or via a dedicated emergency line to switchboard. If it is safe and practical to do so, extinguishers can be used to tackle the fire. The ASA recommends the use of carbon dioxide extinguishers since these are less likely to cause harm to patients and staff or damage surgical equipment when compared to dry-powder extinguishers; they are still effective at extinguishing most types of operating theatre fire. Dry powder may be used as a 'last ditch' resort whilst planning or undertaking evacuation.

If the fire is spreading, the emergency shut-off device for the gas supply should be used (area valve service units (AVSUs) – Figure 10.1). These are in a panel outside the theatre. This should be done in conjunction with immediate evacuation of the area and preferably in consultation with local fire and rescue service commanders.

Evacuation of Fire-Affected Areas

The affected area should be evacuated of all staff and patients, as per the predesignated fire plan, which should give at least three options for evacuation routes. Fire doors should be shut as areas are left

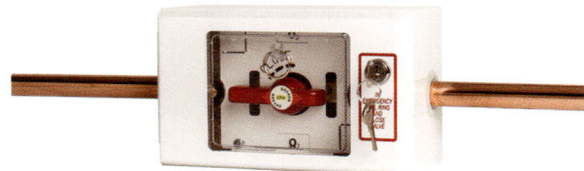

Figure 10.1 An AVSU: these valves isolate the medical air and vacuum supplies for one of the theatres (image courtesy of Precision UK)

and should not be opened again except by fire service personnel. The order of patient evacuation should be first, patients in imminent danger from the fire; second, ambulatory patients; then those who are non-ambulatory.

Electrical Safety

Physics of Electrical Safety

Electrical current is the flow of electrons through a conductor where there exists a potential difference (voltage, measured in volts, V). Current is measured in amperes (A). Resistance (measured in ohms, Ω) to the flow of electrons will reduce the current in a conductor. These relationships are delineated in Ohm's law:

$$V = IR$$

where I is current, V is potential difference and R is the resistance.

> Why is current represented by 'I'? The original phrase was *'intensité de courant'*.

Current may have a unidirectional flow, direct current (DC), or alternating forward and backwards flow, alternating current (AC). AC is the standard form for UK mains supply, at a frequency of 50 Hz. See Chapter 2 for more on the fundamentals of electricity.

Macroshock

For electricity to cause harm, the person needs to form part of a circuit. The current travels through the tissues with a magnitude determined by the impedance of the various tissues encountered along the electrical path. Current determines the likely clinical effect. Mains circuits in the UK carry 240 V of alternating current at 50 Hz, which is delivered from where it is generated via a live line. It also travels with a neutral line, which completes the circuit back to the generation source. A connection to earth is a mandatory safety feature in UK devices; it is the long pin on the UK three-pin plug. Earth is always at a lower potential than live, so electrons will travel from live to earth if a connection is made, particularly in case of faults. Should the current run to earth, it will usually cause a surge through the live line, sufficient to trip fuses or circuit-breakers, isolating the device from the live supply, rendering it safe until the fault is fixed. If human tissue contacts the circuit, forming an alternative route between live and earth, current will flow through it. This will also usually cause the circuit-breaker to activate but often not without significant energy transfer to tissues in the interim.

Determinants of clinical effect are:

1. Magnitude of current
2. Path of current through the body
3. Type of current (AC or DC)
4. Duration of current exposure

Table 10.2 gives an approximate guide to the effect of different currents on the human body.

Risk of harm is dependent on frequency in a U-shaped pattern, thus DC is safer than mains AC but high-frequency AC is least dangerous (Table 10.2). AC and DC produce differing effects when voluntary muscle control is lost; DC tends to produce a single muscular contraction, often throwing the victim clear. AC by contrast causes tetanic spasm, often rendering the victim unable to let go of the source of the shock.

The magnitude of the current flowing through the body is dependent, as mentioned, on the voltage but also the impedance (in the case of AC) or resistance (in the case of DC) of the tissues. This can vary dramatically. The resistance of dry skin is up to 100,000 Ω. When wet, this will be significantly reduced, perhaps down to 1,000 Ω. We can calculate the difference in resulting current (hence harm) associated with a 240-V mains shock with differing skin conditions:

$$V = IR$$
$$I = \frac{V}{R}$$
$$= \frac{240}{100,000}$$
$$= 2.4 \text{ mA (for dry skin – results in mild tingling)}$$

$$= \frac{240}{1,000}$$
$$= 240 \text{ mA (for wet skin – risks onset of VF)}$$

Once the skin resistance is reduced to 500 Ω, the electrical current will cause burning, and further reduce the resistance to current flow.

The body may form part of a circuit by two principal methods: resistive or capacitive coupling.

Resistive Coupling

This is where there is a direct connection between the patient, source of electricity and earth (either directly, or via an earthed object). The current may be supplied by faulty equipment or be a leakage current. A leakage current is a small current (<500 µA) generated as an inevitable consequence of the fact that all electrical equipment is at a higher potential than earth, and there is no perfect electrical insulation.

Table 10.2 Current thresholds (in mA) for various effects, depending on form of electrical energy delivered

Effect on body	DC	AC	
		50 Hz	10 kHz
Slight sensation	0.60–1.0	0.3	5–7
Clear perception	3.5–5.2	0.7–1.1	8–12
Pain (muscle control maintained)	40–60	6–9	35–55
Pain (loss of voluntary muscle control)	50–75	10–16	50–75
Severe pain, difficulty breathing	60–90	15–20	60–90
Ventricular fibrillation after 3 seconds	500	100	–

If you run your finger tip lightly over the metal case of a mobile phone while it is charging, you will likely feel a buzzing or tingling sensation. This is an everyday example of leakage current. This particular current is categorized as 'enclosure leakage current' – enclosure refers to the case of a device.

Capacitive Coupling

This is a scenario whereby there is no direct connection between the patient and the electrical source but instead the body becomes one plate of a capacitor. A capacitor allows the storage of electrical charge and consists of two conducting plates separated by an insulating material. When DC is applied to a capacitor, current only flows until the positive plate reaches the same potential as the source. However, when AC is applied to a capacitor, the plates alternate polarity at the same frequency as the source. This causes electrons to oscillate in the gap, effectively completing the circuit. The safety issue occurs when an item of electrical equipment, such as the operating lights, become one plate of a capacitor and the patient acts as the other:

$$\text{Impedance} = \frac{\text{Distance between plates}}{\text{Current frequency} \times \text{Surface area of plate}}$$

The relationship above shows that as the frequency increases and the distance between plates lessens, the impedance (roughly analogous to resistance in an AC circuit) lowers and thus the risk of shock becomes greater.

Microshock

Usually a reasonably large current is required to produce a clinically significant shock. However, if a very small current is applied directly to electrically sensitive cardiac tissue, it can produce ventricular fibrillation with a very small current (50–100 µA). This can occur when a medical device is in direct contact with such tissue, as in the case of a central line or pacemaker wire. Leakage currents are addressed further below.

Protection Against Shock

All medical devices are classified according to the degree of protection from shock that they offer. The International Electrotechnical Commission (IEC) regulates standards for medical electrical equipment and, for the sake of these regulations, divides the components into the power supply (Class I–III) and the 'applied parts' [3]. The applied parts are those which are designed to be, or may possibly become, directly connected to the patient, for example ECG leads, pulse-oximeter cables or defibrillator cables. These are classified into Type B, BF or CF and each of these may be subclassified as to whether they are defibrillator-proof.

Class I Equipment

Class I equipment is the most basic degree of protection from shock. There is insulation between the live parts and conductive parts such as the metal casing or chassis of the equipment. These metallic parts must, in turn, be connected to earth. Should a fault occur that might otherwise allow these parts to become live, a new low-resistance circuit (to earth) is generated, leading to a higher current that melts the fuse and breaks the circuit. The basic requirement for Class I equipment is that exposed metal parts cannot become inadvertently live as a result of one single fault. In other words, for the casing to become live and cause a macroshock hazard, at least two faults would have to occur, e.g. concurrent failure of the live-parts insulation and the earthing system.

Medical devices classified as Class I require fuses on the live and neutral supply at the equipment end of the power supply, as well as in the mains socket (to negate the effect of a malfunctioning socket or plug). Such fuses, circuit breakers or residual current devices (RCDs) are required to operate sufficiently quickly to prevent fibrillation in a user in contact with the device at the time when the fault develops: 250 ms at 40 mA or 50 ms at 200 mA. There is no agreed symbol in use to indicate that equipment is Class I and it is not mandatory to state on the equipment itself that it is Class I although it sometimes carries the symbol for a protective earth (Figure 10.2).

A functional earth (the same symbol as a protective earth but without the circle) is, as the name suggests, a design rather than a safety feature. It is used in some sensitive forms of electronic equipment, such as radio and telecommunications equipment which require an earth connection to dissipate sources of electrical interference. It may well be normal for a functional earth to have a small current through it in normal use. Some devices use the protective earth conductor as a functional earth connection. Just to complicate matters, some Class II equipment (which, by definition, lacks a protective earth) may have a functional earth.

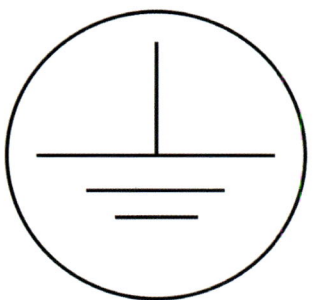

Figure 10.2 Symbol for protective earth, sometimes found on Class I equipment

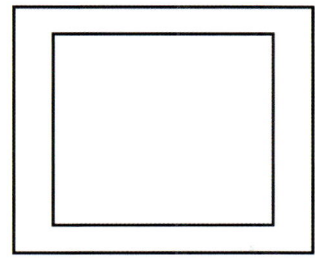

Figure 10.3 Symbol for Class II double-insulated equipment

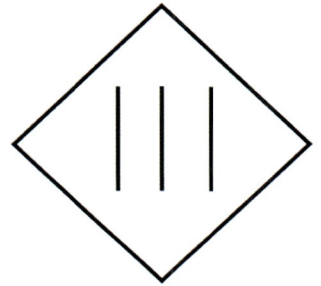

Figure 10.4 Symbol for Class III equipment

Class II Equipment

Class II devices have reinforced or double insulation, preventing any contact between live parts and conducting material. They do not require an earth but should, as a minimum, be fused at the equipment end. One tell-tale feature denoting Class II equipment is a plastic earth pin on the mains plug; as this class of equipment does not require an earth connection, the manufacturer can save weight and money by not using a brass earth pin on the plug. Class II is denoted by concentric squares (Figure 10.3).

Class III Equipment

Class III equipment features safety extra low voltage (SELV), either by being battery-powered or by including step-down transformers. SELV must not exceed 24 V AC or 60 V DC. The risk of macroshock is removed, but microshock is still possible. Current IEC standards relating to safety of medical electrical equipment do not recognize Class III equipment; if no connection to mains is possible, such devices are instead labelled as 'internally powered'. Class III equipment does have a recognized symbol (Figure 10.4) but, as this is not a safety standard approved for medical devices, you are unlikely to encounter it in clinical practice.

Type B

Type B are applied parts which provide a particular degree of protection against electric shock, with allowable leakage currents of up to 100 mA. This means that the part is acceptable for general clinical use, but not for direct cardiac connection. The various symbols for the types of applied parts are shown in Figure 10.5. These are self-explanatory to a large degree; the stick-person denotes the 'body' for Type B equipment, adding a box around it implies a floating circuit (e.g. BF or CF) and adding old-fashioned defibrillator paddles is defibrillator-proof. A defibrillator-proof rating means that the equipment will not be damaged by discharge of a defibrillator into the patient to which it is connected.

Type BF

Type BF parts are as Type B but with isolated or floating (F-type) circuits. A floating circuit is where the mains electricity supply is separated from the patient circuits by an isolating transformer. The mains side of the circuit has a coil to which AC is applied. This in turn induces a current via an electromagnetic field in a secondary coil on the patient side of the circuit. Although current flows in the patient-side circuits, there is no direct connection between this circuit and earth. This means that if the patient circuit is incomplete (i.e. switch in the off position) and a fault occurs, there cannot be a secondary circuit via the earth so this situation cannot result in a shock. An example of a device with a floating circuit is a defibrillator. The charging current is generated by a

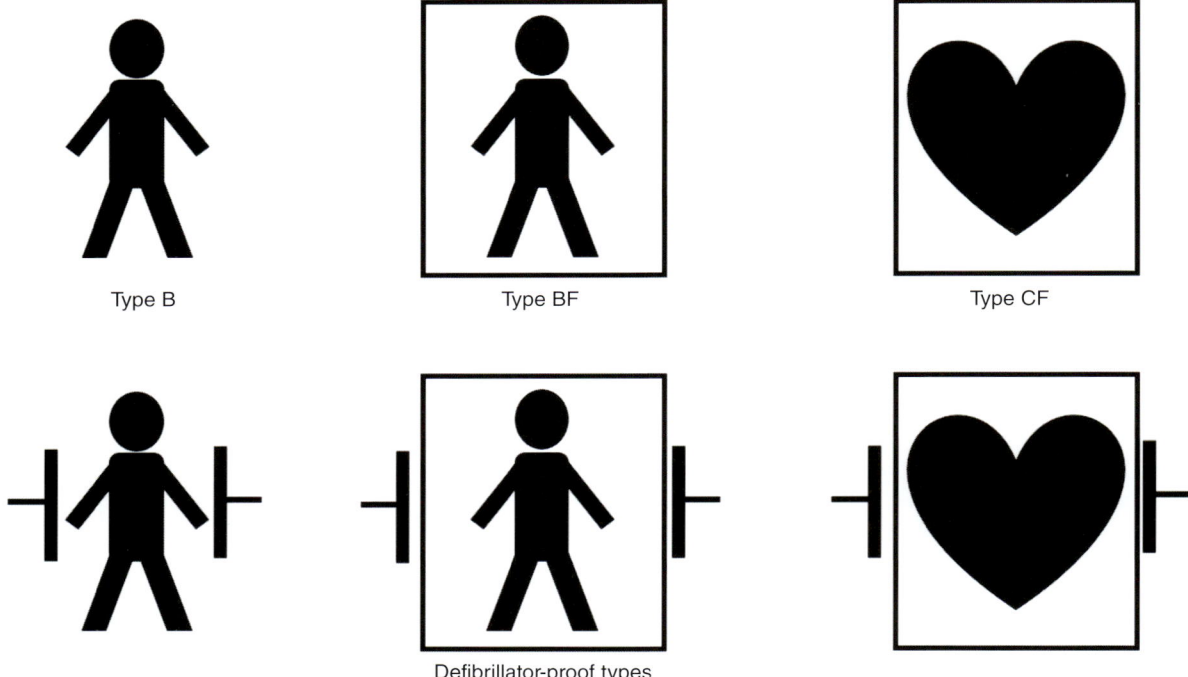

Figure 10.5 Symbols for applied part types

step-up transformer that isolates it from the mains supply (Figure 10.6).

Type CF

Type CF are applied parts with a leakage current of less than 0.05 mA to 0.01 mA per electrode. They are considered safe for direct cardiac connection, e.g. invasive pressure transducers. Incidentally, there is no 'Type A' equipment – the 'B' is for body and the 'C' is for cardiac. Similarly, there is no 'C' equipment; all equipment designed for direct cardiac connection requires a floating circuit as part of the protection and so there is only a Type CF category.

 This entire classification derives from the IEC standard 60601–1. These regulations also govern other crucial design features of medical electrical devices. Such aspects include their resistance to ingress of water or debris, method of sterilization, safety in an oxygen-rich environment and whether they are suitable for continuous or only intermittent use.

Equipotential Bonding

A further consideration is the range of potentials which may exist between the metal casings of various medical equipment in close proximity to the patient. This typically results from leakage current to the casing in the setting of poor earthing. Equally, a fault in one item may result in the casing being at mains voltage whilst another item, touched simultaneously, would have its case at earth potential: a current would flow, resulting in macroshock. To mitigate this, all these devices are often connected (bonded) together onto a single busbar which, in turn, has a high-quality connection to earth (Figure 10.7). This ensures that, at worst, all the casings are equipotential and ideally, provided the earth is good, this potential will be zero. Devices featuring such a connection usually have a metal post or a socket on the back to connect the bonding cable and have the symbol shown in Figure 10.8. With the system illustrated in Figure 10.7, if the diathermy develops a fault, even without the supplemental earth connection, the bonding would mean the theatre table would also be at 240 V. If the surgeon touches both, there will be no current flow through them between the two devices so they won't get a shock.

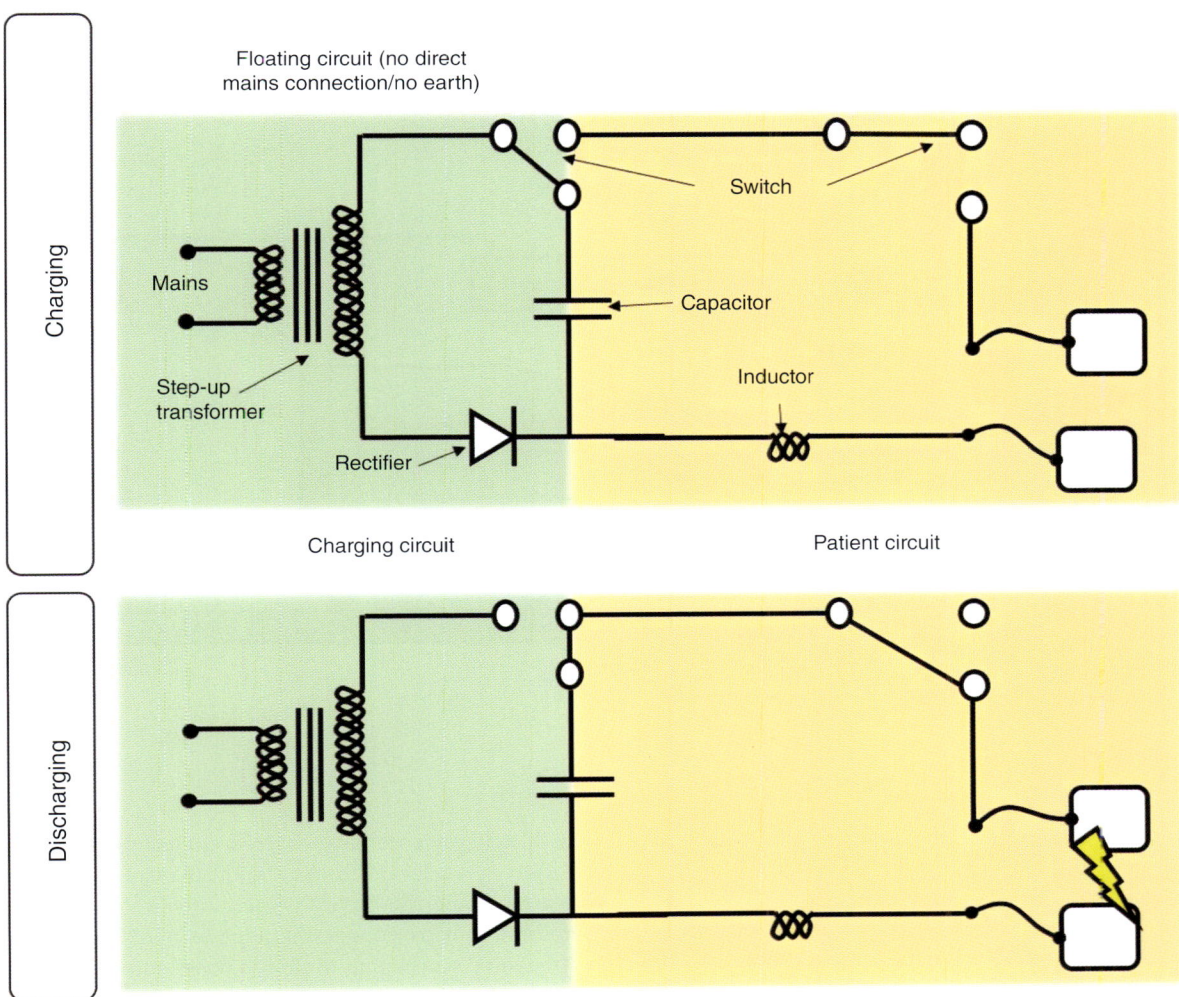

Figure 10.6 A defibrillator is an example of a device employing a floating circuit

You may also notice a yellow/green earth cable strapped to the metal gas or water main as they come into your home: have a look under the kitchen sink or by your gas meter. This is protective equipotential bonding in your home. All these metal pipes coming into your home may otherwise represent a more effective earth route than the earth connection to a faulty electrical appliance. Without bonding, if you touched a faulty bathroom water heater and the cold tap simultaneously, you may get a fatal shock. Bonding of the cold-water pipe to the earth connection at the fuse box means the potential difference between the faulty appliance and the copper pipe remains close to zero.

Humidity and Sparks

The principal safety reason for maintaining optimum humidity within an operating theatre environment is for the prevention of electrostatic shock. This was historically of even greater importance in the era of explosive anaesthetic agents such as cyclopropane but is still of relevance today when gases supporting combustion are in use. A relative humidity of greater than 40% is considered sufficient for prevention of electrostatic discharge (see Chapter 3). It is also more comfortable for staff and may help prevent excessive drying of the patient's mucus membranes or exposed organs.

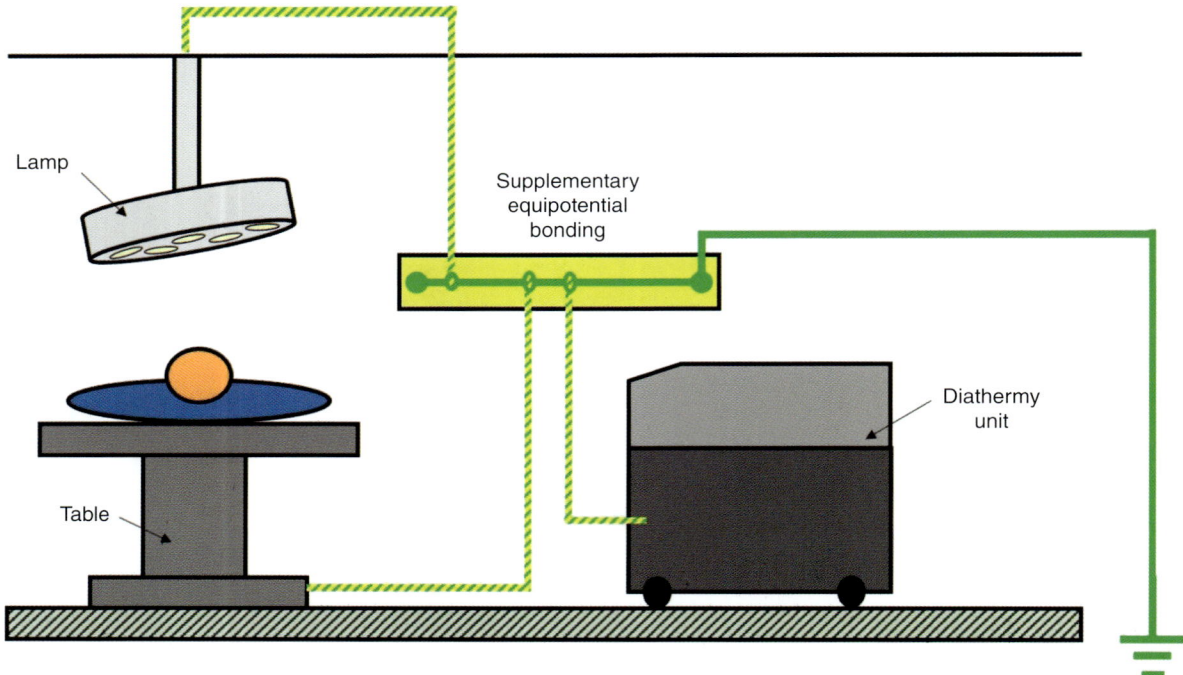

Figure 10.7 An equipotential bonding system in theatre

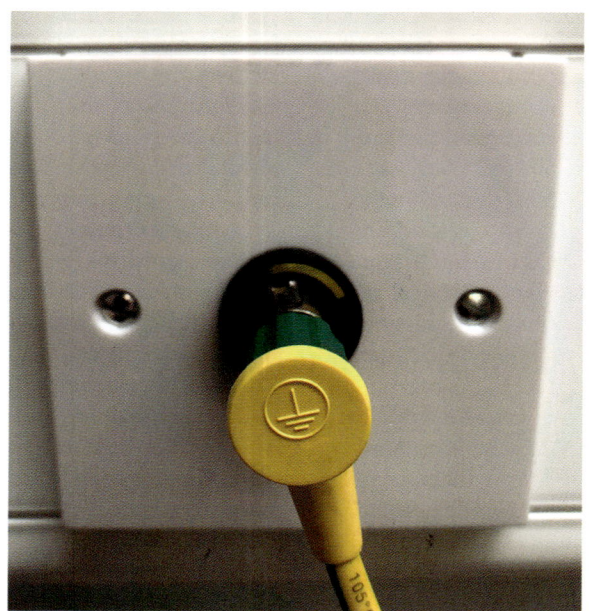

Figure 10.8 The equipotential bonding symbol (on a bonding cable plugged into a wall terminal for the equipotential bonding system)

Summary

In this chapter, we have covered environmental protection as is relevant to work in theatres and intensive care medicine. We have answered how we protect the environment from anaesthetic gases and vapours by discussing scavenging systems; these consist of collecting, transferring, receiving, disposal and exhaust components.

We have seen that there are several risks in the theatre from fire and explosion, although these are significantly less than in years past. Vigilance is required when the fire triad of fuel, oxidizer and heat are present in theatre; these risks can be reduced by adjustment of gas mixtures and reduced use of oxidizing gases, careful use of heat sources such as diathermy and laser, and minimizing availability of fuel, e.g. alcohol vapour in skin preparations. The importance of knowing your local fire protocols has been emphasized.

We have also looked in detail at electrical safety. The mechanism of electrical shock from malfunctioning devices, alongside the potential for harm or death, is related to current magnitude (including its relationship to skin impedance, which can vary widely), type of current, the path it travels through the recipient and exposure to current. We covered the rare circumstances of capacitive coupling, where the patient may form one plate of a capacitor, and microshock, where indwelling devices conduct leakage currents direct to the myocardium. In most countries, international standards which govern electrical safety are enshrined in legislation. There are particular specifications within these pertaining to medical equipment, classifying these devices as Class I, II or III according to protection from macroshock; and B, BF or CF relating to the degree of leakage currents.

Questions

MCQs – select true or false for each response

1. Regarding classification of electrical safety:
   (a) Class I equipment is the safest, having double insulation, double fusing and no connection between live and earth
   (b) Class II equipment only has double insulation and no earth
   (c) Class III is low voltage
   (d) Type B prevents microshock
   (e) Type C is the rating applied to devices in contact with the heart, e.g. pulmonary artery catheters

2. Regarding ignition of gas mixtures:
   (a) Flammability limits specify the concentration of oxidizer which will permit combustion of the fuel
   (b) Flammability limits differ for oxidation agents
   (c) Stoichiometric mixtures burn completely
   (d) The rate of energy released in an explosion is linearly related to the concentration of fuel in the mixture
   (e) Nitrous oxide is a fuel and oxygen source

3. When considering electric shock:
   (a) Macroshock relates to the scenario of body-surface contact with a live source and an earth
   (b) Microshock is specific to the phenomenon of leakage currents conducted direct to the body tissues including the heart
   (c) Microshock relates to electrical induction of VF and macroshock relates to non-cardiac features, such as muscular contraction and skin burns
   (d) Equipotential bonding ensures that, in the event of an earth fault, the live and neutral are at the same potential, reducing the risk of shock
   (e) Use of Class III (low-voltage) devices is the recognized standard to minimize microshock and macroshock

SBAs – select the single *best* response

4. When selecting a system to provide scavenging of gases for a volatile anaesthetic combination of sevoflurane in oxygen and nitrous oxide for a community dental service, the best option is:
   (a) A charcoal cannister to offer the best combination of simplicity and portability
   (b) An open-funnel system so as to permit scavenging from the mouth as the dentist works
   (c) A passive system with a vent to the theatre window
   (d) An active system with an extraction flow of 75 l min^{-1}
   (e) An active system with an extraction flow of 120 l min^{-1}

Answers

1. FTTFF

   Class I equipment is the most basic, but not necessarily the safest class of power supply. It does have double fusing (live and neutral) but does not have double insulation (that is Class II). No equipment has a connection between live and earth; that would result in a short to earth and no power reaching the working circuits. None of these standards will prevent microshock although they will reduce it to an acceptably low risk if used properly. There is no Type C rating – all cardiac-contacting applied parts must feature a floating circuit and so are designated CF.

2. FTTFT

   Whilst the flammability limits do describe a ratio of fuel and oxidizer, they are presented in terms of the percentage of fuel in oxidizer, not oxidizer in fuel. Flammability limits do therefore differ for oxidation agents; the stoichiometry for a fuel:air mix is different from that of a fuel:oxygen mixture, for example, on account of the inert nitrogen and other components of air. The energy released is not a linear relationship for two reasons. Firstly, above and below the flammability limits, no combustion occurs and so at these fuel concentrations, no energy is released. Secondly, between the flammability limits, varying degrees of incomplete combustion occur, with peak energy release only occurring at the stoichiometric concentration.

3. TFFFF

Microshock specifically relates to induction of VF/VT by small leakage currents. Macroshock can lead to cardiac arrythmias if the path of the current traverses the heart. The distinguishing feature of the two is principally the magnitude of current involved; microshock concerns seemingly trivial currents but which, on account of a more direct route to the heart, are able to cause cardiac dysfunction. Equipotential bonding ensures that the earth connections (and hence the conductive parts of the casing in Class I equipment) are at the same potential. A system inducing a live-neutral short would stop the device functioning in normal operation and would also not stop an electric shock resulting from a connection between the live and the casing of a device. Class III equipment does remove the risk of macroshock but microshock is certainly still possible. With respect to medical devices, the IEC does not recognize Class III as a standard.

4. (d)

In what may be seen as almost a 'pop-up' theatre set-up in a remote, community setting, a simple, portable system may seem appealing but answers (a) to (c) all represent significant compromise. A charcoal cannister is inefficient and will not last indefinitely. The question also specifies nitrous oxide in the mixture, the only agent being used which has statutory exposure limits and the only one which charcoal will not adsorb. Passive systems are inefficient and, if poorly designed, can be dangerous. The question stem suggests formal volatile general anaesthesia rather than nasal-mask nitrous oxide as encountered in 'chair dental' anaesthesia, a practice which, in any case, has been abandoned on safety grounds. This therefore excludes an open funnel as our patients will have some form of formal semi-open breathing system. Distinguishing option (d) from (e) requires an understanding that a very high extraction flow will result in a high induced flow. This is not compatible with modern, low-flow anaesthesia. As option (d) permits this form of best practice, it is the correct answer.

References

1. Health and Safety Executive. *EH40/2005 Workplace Exposure Limits.* The Stationery Office, 2018.
2. Occupational Safety and Health Administration. *Anesthetic Gases: Guidelines for Workplace Exposures.* OSHA, 2000.
3. International Electrotechnical Commission. *International Standard IEC 60601-1, Medical Electrical Equipment – Part 1: General Requirements for Basic Safety and Essential Performance*, 3rd edn. IEC, 2005.

Chapter 11

Blood Pressure Measurement

Laura Beard and David Ashton-Cleary

Learning Objectives

- To understand the meaning and definition of blood pressure, and its context in clinical medicine
- To understand how invasive and non-invasive blood pressure is measured
- To be aware of the potential sources of error in blood pressure measurement

Chapter Content

- What is blood pressure and why do we need to measure it?
- Blood pressure measurement terminology
- Non-invasive blood pressure measurement
- Invasive blood pressure measurement

Scenario

You are asked to anaesthetize a 44-year-old patient for gastric bypass surgery. She weighs 136 kg (a BMI of 47 kg m^{-2}), and is on medication for hypertension (150/90 mmHg), angina and arthritis. The patient reports that her exercise tolerance is limited and she is unable to walk up a flight of stairs, which she states is, in part, due to knee pain. The surgeons believe that the operation will take about 4 hours. What method of blood pressure measurement will you select intra-operatively and why? The surgeons require the operating table to be tilted head up; will this affect the accuracy of the blood pressure reading if an invasive method is used?

Introduction

In medicine, and particularly anaesthesia and critical care, the measurement and manipulation of blood pressure is vital. Many of the drugs used to induce or maintain anaesthesia can cause hypotension. Conversely, an inadequately anaesthetized or analgesed patient can have significant hypertension. Control of blood pressure and avoiding the complications associated with hyper- and hypotension is a key aim of modern anaesthesia.

The means by which blood pressure is measured perioperatively will depend on several factors, including co-morbidities, type of surgery and requirements for post-operative critical care. A detailed knowledge as to how invasive and non-invasive blood pressure systems function is essential to aid in the selection of the correct method of measurement for your patient. Awareness as to the potential sources of error is also vital to ensure that your patient's blood pressure is recorded accurately.

The debate as to what blood pressure is 'correct' during anaesthesia or on critical care, how this might vary between patients and what duration of deviation from this ideal might be harmful to an individual continues. However, in 2016, the AAGBI and British Hypertensive Society jointly released a guideline on 'The measurement of adult blood pressure and management of hypertension before elective surgery', with the aims of unifying the management of patients referred between primary and secondary care, improving outcomes and reducing day-of-surgery cancellation rates [1].

What is Blood Pressure and Why Do We Need to Measure It?

Pressure is defined as the force per unit area, the SI unit being the pascal (Pa). Blood pressure is commonly expressed in the manometric unit, millimeters of mercury (mmHg), which measures pressure from the height of a column of mercury in a manometer.

Systolic blood pressure is generated from the force of myocardial contraction. The heart is a series of curved surfaces, therefore the amount of pressure generated is most correctly defined by Laplace's law which states for a sphere:

$$P = \frac{2T}{R}$$

where P = pressure, T = tension and R = radius. In a normal heart, if the strength of myocardial contraction increases and the radius remains the same, the pressure increases proportionately. This explains the rise in left-ventricular pressure during systole up until the point where the aortic valve opens. This is the phase referred to as isovolumetric contraction. In patients where the heart becomes distended and the myocardium is unable to increase the strength of contraction, the pressure generated is significantly reduced due to this increase in radius. This is why dilated cardiomyopathy leads to heart failure.

Blood in the circulation is also affected by hydrostatic pressure. When a fluid is held in a column (such as a blood vessel) the pressure throughout that column is not constant. This is because of the effects of gravity on the fluid molecules, which result in the pressure at the bottom of the column being greater than the pressure at the top due to the weight of the fluid above. Therefore, when blood pressure is measured with a cuff, it is conventionally performed on the arm, which roughly equates to the level of the right atrium. This is referred to as the phlebostatic axis of the body and this defines the zero-pressure reference point relative to which the blood pressure is measured. This is of similar significance when positioning an invasive pressure transducer (see later).

Blood Pressure Measurement Terminology

When people talk about blood pressure they are commonly referring to systolic pressure, diastolic pressure and mean arterial pressure (MAP). Less commonly, right-sided pressures such as central venous pressure, pulmonary artery pressure and pulmonary capillary wedge pressure are also recorded on occasion.

The systolic blood pressure (SBP) refers to the impulse pressure which moves each stroke volume of blood into the circulation (pulmonary or systemic for right and left ventricles, respectively). It is generated by ventricular contraction (systole).

The diastolic blood pressure (DBP) is the pressure within the arterial system and is a consequence of the compliance and tone of the arterial vessels. It therefore exists throughout the cardiac cycle but with the systolic impulse superimposed upon it. It is measured as the lowest pressure during the cardiac cycle. It is no less important than systolic pressure as it is the main driving force for coronary blood flow, in particular.

The MAP is the average pressure throughout the cardiac cycle (diastole and systole). It is a key determinant of organ perfusion pressure, for example, cerebral and renal perfusion pressure.

$$\text{MAP} = \text{DBP} + \frac{1}{3}(\text{SBP} - \text{DBP})$$

In the above equation, the term (SBP − DBP) is referred to as the pulse pressure. A third of pulse pressure is used in the equation because, at typical resting heart rates, systole lasts for one-third of the cardiac cycle and diastole makes up the remaining two-thirds. This doesn't hold true at higher heart rates; diastolic time shortens to a greater extent than systolic time. Arterial pressure monitoring systems therefore calculate the MAP from mathematical analysis of the area under the arterial waveform instead.

Calculation of MAP is somewhat similar to Ohm's law ($V = IR$) for electrical circuits. Voltage (V) equates to the mean blood pressure, current (I) is analogous to cardiac output (CO) and resistance (R) represents the systemic vascular resistance (SVR).

$$\text{MAP} = \text{CO} \times \text{SVR}$$

Blood pressure can be measured in several different ways, which can be divided into invasive or non-invasive methods and intermittent or continuous measuring of blood pressure (Figure 11.1).

Non-invasive Blood Pressure Measurement

Intermittent Measurement

Sphygmomanometers are the most widely used piece of equipment for blood pressure measurement. They can be either manual or digital and can use the auscultatory or oscillometric method to measure the different components of arterial blood pressure. To measure blood pressure, the following elements are required:

1. Inflatable pneumatic cuff
2. Pressure release mechanism, e.g. adjustable valve
3. Pressure gauge, e.g. mercury or aneroid

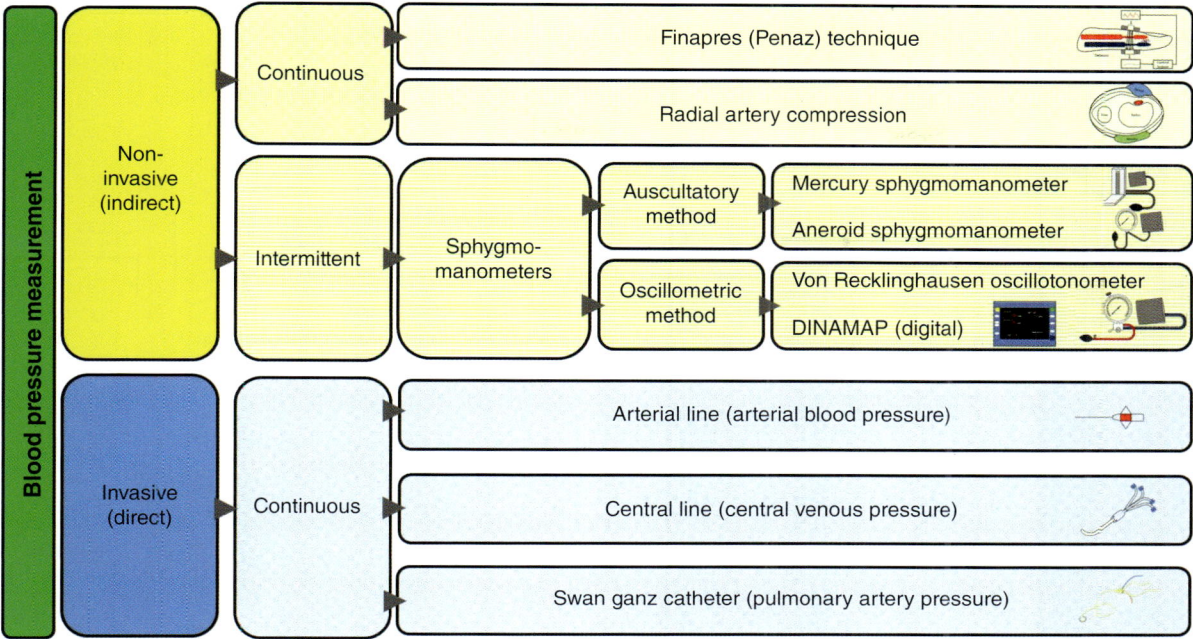

Figure 11.1 Classification of blood pressure measuring devices

4. Method for determining systolic and diastolic pressure, e.g. Korotkoff sounds or oscillations

Auscultatory Method

A stethoscope is placed over the brachial artery and the cuff inflated to a pressure above systolic pressure, temporarily obstructing blood flow within the artery. As the cuff deflates, pulsatile flow is gradually restored. The blood pressure is measured by auscultation of the Korotkoff sounds:

- Phase I = Initial tapping sounds (systolic pressure)
- Phase II = Sounds become softer
- Phase III = Sounds become more intense
- Phase IV = Sounds become muffled
- Phase V = Sounds disappear (diastolic pressure)

The systolic pressure is taken to be the pressure at which the first sound is heard (Phase I) and the diastolic pressure to be when the Korotkoff sounds disappear (Phase V). Previously, phase IV was taken to be the diastolic pressure but it was felt that using phase V was more reproducible. The MAP is then calculated from the measured systolic and diastolic pressures.

Oscillometric Method

Rather than listening for the appearance and disappearance of sounds at certain pressures to measure the systolic and diastolic pressures, the oscillometric method relies on observing the changing amplitude of oscillations:

- Systolic pressure corresponds to the onset of rapidly increasing oscillations
- Diastolic pressure is when the oscillations rapidly disappear
- MAP is the point of maximal oscillation

Other Methods

Manual palpation of the brachial artery for the appearance of pulsations can be used to measure the systolic pressure only, but it is not very accurate. A Doppler probe can also be used to measure flow (and so allow calculation of the systolic and diastolic pressures). However, this method relies on accurate placement of the probe and can be susceptible to interference, e.g. from diathermy.

Mercury Sphygmomanometer

Mercury sphygmomanometers use a manometer to measure pressure. A manometer consists of a column

Chapter 11: Blood Pressure Measurement

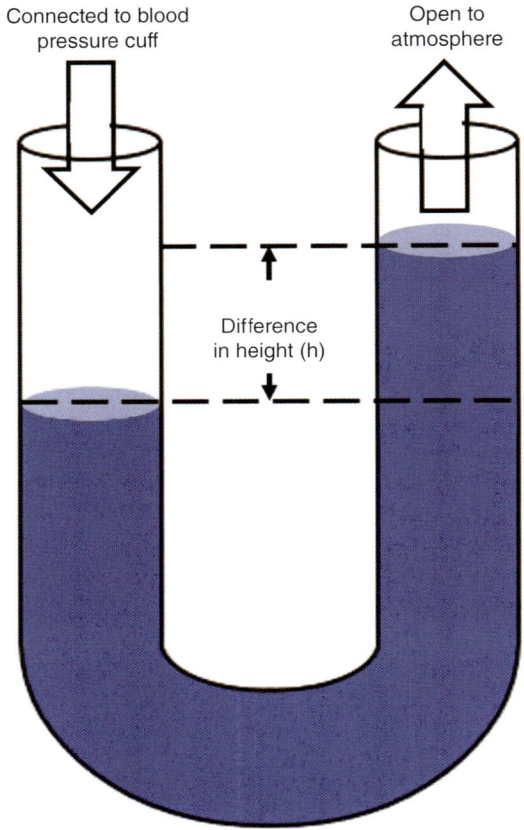

Figure 11.2 A manometer

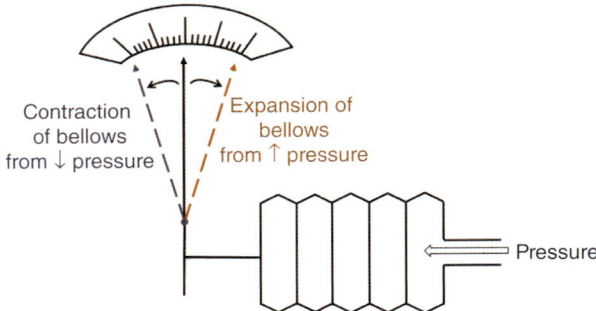

Figure 11.3 An aneroid sphygmomanometer

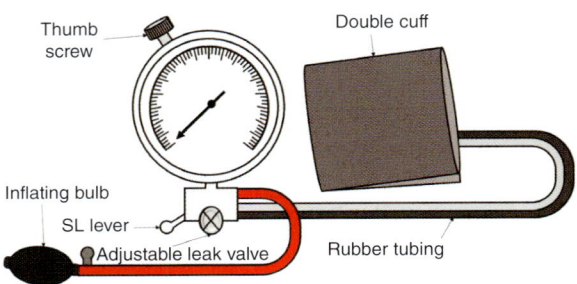

Figure 11.4 Von Recklinghausen oscillotonometer

of liquid in a U-tube (Figure 11.2). Incoming pressure from the cuff causes the liquid to be displaced around the tube. The pressure acts to overcome the effect of gravity, elevating the fluid level in the opposite limb of the tube. The resulting difference in height of the fluid levels in either limb of the tube relates directly to the pressure through the hydrostatic pressure equation:

P = Density × Acceleration due to gravity × Height

For blood pressure measurement, one end of the manometer is connected to the blood pressure cuff and the other end is open to atmospheric pressure. When pressure is introduced into the cuff this causes the column of fluid on the side open to atmospheric pressure to rise. The height of the fluid is then recorded and the pressure can be calculated using the equation above. Mercury is denser than water and so 1 kPa of pressure will support a 10.2-cm column of water or 7.5-mm column of mercury. It is for this reason that mercury is used in medical manometers because a more compact instrument can be designed with this differing scale.

Aneroid Sphygmomanometers

Aneroid sphygmomanometers were introduced due to safety concerns regarding the toxicity of mercury. Aneroid means 'without water' and the gauge consists of a capsule or bellows that expand or contract depending on the pressure within. The size of the bellows then causes a pointer to rotate and pressure is measured from a calibrated scale (Figure 11.3).

Von Recklinghausen Oscillotonometer

This blood pressure cuff uses the oscillometric method to measure blood pressure. The Von Recklinghausen oscillotonometer seen in Figure 11.4 has been known to make the occasional appearance in anaesthetic examinations!

Components:

- Double cuff – small 5-cm upper cuff (occluding cuff) and large 10-cm lower cuff (sensing cuff)

- Rubber tubing – connects the cuffs to the metal block
- Metal block containing a lever and valve
  (a) Sustained leak lever (SL)
  (b) An adjustable leak valve (the case valve – CV)
- Inflating bulb with an adjustable leak valve (the inflation valve – IV)
- Aneroid pressure gauge, dial and case
- Thumb screw to adjust needle to zero

How to use the Von Recklinghausen oscillotonometer:

1. Apply the cuff to the arm with the occluding cuff more proximal on the limb
2. Close the CV and IV, and inflate the cuffs with the inflating bulb until the pressure on the dial is above the expected systolic pressure for your patient
3. Open the CV to create a small leak; this valve is not adjusted again during the measurement – it allows air to leak slowly from both cuffs when the SL lever is held in the 'down' position
4. Hold the SL lever in the down position until needle oscillations increase, then release the SL lever back to the 'up' position; the dial indicates systolic pressure
5. Hold the SL lever in the down position once more; when the oscillations show a sudden decrease, release the lever – this is the diastolic pressure
6. The IV can now be opened to release any residual pressure remaining in the cuff

When the SL lever is in the up position the pressure in the occluding cuff is measured. When it is moved to the down position, pressure in the sensing cuff is measured and oscillations are seen. The MAP can also be measured and correlates to the point at which the oscillations are at their maximal amplitude. The most accurate measurements taken with the Von Recklinghausen oscillotonometer are of systolic pressure and MAP. The diastolic pressure is more susceptible to error, principally through problems of inter-observer disagreement.

Digital Sphygmomanometers

Digital sphygmomanometers are now commonly used in medical practice and by patients at home due to their reliability and ease of use. One commonly used device is the DINAMAP (device for indirect non-invasive automatic MAP). Such devices use the oscillometric method for blood pressure measurement but some machines can use the auscultatory method as a backup. The main difference from the other sphygmomanometers is the presence of a microprocessor and transducer. The microprocessor controls the inflation and deflation of the cuff. The cuff is automatically inflated 20–30 mmHg above the previous systolic pressure reading. The transducer senses pressure readings and is accurate to ±2%.

Special Considerations for Accurate Use of Sphygmomanometers

- For a manual system, ensure pressure in the cuff is released slowly at approximately 2 mmHg s^{-1} to allow accurate measurement
- The bladder of the cuff should sit over the brachial artery
- The width of the cuff should cover two-thirds that of the arm
- The width of the cuff's bladder should be 40% of the circumference of the arm.
- Fast inflation is required to reduce venous congestion
- The cuff should be around the limb at a point along the phlebostatic axis

The phlebostatic axis is an elaborate way of referring to the 'zero' line for blood pressure measurement. It is a line, parallel to the ground, which crosses the level of the right atrium. Conveniently, the arm lies on this line almost irrespective of the positioning of the patient. However, whilst placing a cuff on the leg or thigh of a patient who is supine would be perfectly acceptable, the reading would be erroneously high if the patient moved to a sitting or standing position.

Sources of error with non-invasive intermittent blood pressure measurement include:

- Incorrectly sized blood pressure cuff
  - Too small and the blood pressure is over-read
  - Too large and the blood pressure is under-read
- External pressure, e.g. from theatre table side-supports, surgeons leaning against the limb or the patient lying on the limb being measured
- Calcified vessels prevent compression of the artery, introducing inaccuracy

Additional sources of error with non-invasive digital blood pressure measurement are:

- Arrhythmias, e.g. atrial fibrillation may introduce inaccuracy or prevent a reading altogether
- Inaccurate at extremes of blood pressure, e.g. severe hypotension

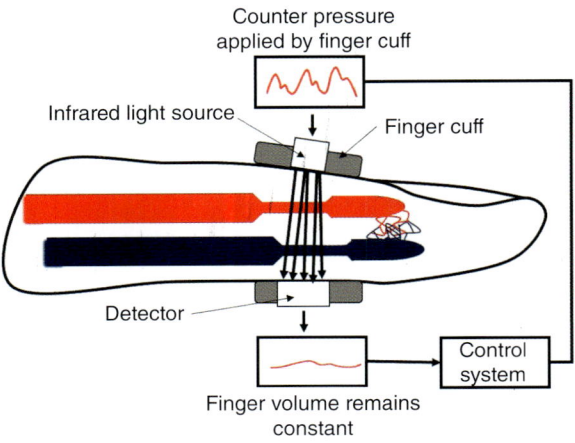

Figure 11.5 Finapres system

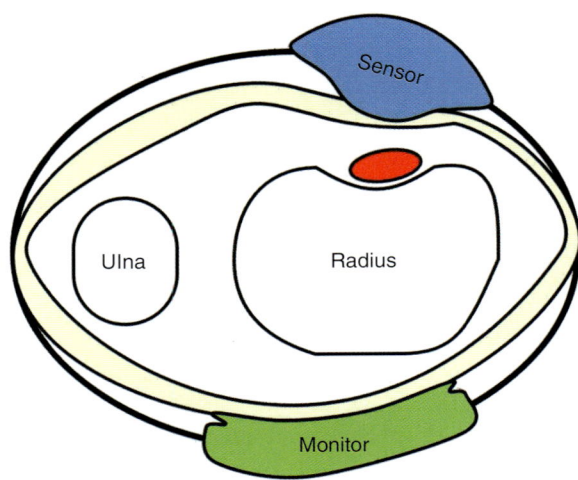

Figure 11.6 Cross-section of wrist demonstrating radial-artery compression device

Complications following repeated inflation and deflation for long procedures are:

- Nerve damage, e.g. neuropraxia
- Petechial haemorrhage
- Peripheral oedema
- Venous congestion of the limb

Continuous Measurement

There are two main techniques for the measurement of continuous non-invasive blood pressure measurement, the Finapres and radial artery compression.

Finapres

The Finapres uses the Penaz principle (also termed the volume–clamp method). It measures finger arterial pressure and consists of a finger cuff with an inflatable bladder and an infrared photoplethysmograph to measure blood volume in the finger (the underlying principle of this is very similar to a pulse oximeter – see Chapter 7) (Figure 11.5).

The photoplethysmograph measures the absorption of infrared light to determine the volume of blood under the finger cuff. The finger cuff then inflates and deflates to keep the volume of blood in the finger constant throughout the cardiac cycle. For example, during systole the volume of blood increases and so the cuff inflates to exert a pressure on the vessels to keep the blood volume constant. During diastole, the volume drops and therefore the pressure in the finger cuff reduces to maintain the constant volume. The finger cuff pressure changes in parallel with arterial pressure so that a continuous waveform of blood pressure is produced: a null-deflection philosophy. In essence, the blood pressure is determined by the amount of pressure the machine has to apply in order to keep the plethysmograph as a flat trace.

The pressure in the finger has to be calibrated at regular intervals during its use as haematocrit and smooth muscle tone will affect the readings. Newer machines are able to reconstruct the finger waveform and account for time delays and distortion in the signal so that a brachial pressure waveform can be constructed. Some Finapres machines also contain a brachial blood pressure cuff to calibrate readings.

The widespread use of this system is limited by concerns about the validity of the readings as it is affected by small changes in patient cuff position and tightness. Inaccuracies may also arise for patients with significant vascular disease or hypotension. Its clinical use is, for these reasons, relatively limited.

Radial-Artery Compression

A band comprised of a cuff and a pressure sensor is placed around the wrist over the radial artery (Figure 11.6). The pressure is increased until maximal oscillations are recorded (much like the intermittent oscillometric technique). An algorithm then analyzes the pulsations at this point to derive the systolic pressure, diastolic pressure and MAP. It is possible to display the blood pressure waveform, thus allowing continuous measurement. Accurate placement of the sensor over the radial artery is required to ensure reliable readings.

Invasive Blood Pressure Measurement

Invasive blood measurement is more accurate than non-invasive techniques and provides a continuous 'beat-to-beat' pressure waveform, enabling faster recognition and treatment of hypo- and hypertension. It is considered to be the 'gold standard' of blood pressure monitoring. Due to its complexity, it is generally confined to the theatre environment, critical care or coronary care settings.

> The Reverend Stephen Hales, an eighteenth-century clergyman, biologist and inventor, was the first to measure blood pressure invasively. He achieved this by inserting glass tubes into the arterial system of various animal species. The first subject was his 14-year-old mare who was dying of an abscess. The column of blood rose around 8 feet in a quarter-inch diameter tube and rose and fell 2–3 inches with each heartbeat. He later completed studies demonstrating the concepts of cardiac output (described as 'the time taken for an animal to expel a volume of blood equal in mass to its body weight') and distal systolic pulse amplification.

The measurement of invasive pressures, including central venous pressure and pulmonary artery pressure, are all based on the same technique using similar pieces of equipment (the catheter varies depending on the vessel being monitored). Table 11.1 lists considerations specific to systemic arterial pressure monitoring, namely indications, contraindications and some of the potential complications.

Arterial blood pressure is most commonly measured in the radial artery – this vessel is conveniently located and the hand also has collateral flow from the ulnar artery. Therefore, if the radial artery is blocked following insertion of the cannula, due to vasospasm or thrombus, the hand is still perfused. It is for this reason that Allen's test should be performed before radial-artery catheterization, to assess flow in the ulnar artery. The brachial artery can be used if

Table 11.1 Indications, contraindications and complications of invasive arterial monitoring

Indications	• Patients at risk of haemodynamic instability during anaesthesia or sedation, e.g. co-morbidities or particular surgical intervention
	• Requirement for cardiac output monitoring, e.g. PiCCO™
	• Long-term blood pressure monitoring (e.g. ICU) to avoid pressure injury associated with repetitive non-invasive cuff inflation
	• Requirement for frequent arterial blood sampling
	• Situations where non-invasive measurement is inaccurate or not possible, e.g. arrhythmias, extremes of blood pressure, obesity, non-pulsatile flow (e.g. cardiac bypass) or burns
Contraindications	• Infection, arterial insufficiency or tissue damage at selected site
	• Patient refusal
	• No suitable environment to care for arterial monitoring patients
Complications	• Ischaemia of limb secondary to vasospasm, arterial injury or thrombus
	• Infection
	• Inadvertent drug injection
	• Inaccurate readings, e.g. due to incorrect level of transducer, damping and resonance
	• Blood loss secondary to inadvertent disconnection
	• Blood sampling errors if saline not removed from line first

radial-artery catheterization is unsuccessful but it must be remembered that this artery has no collateral counterpart and ischaemia of the forearm and hand could result if the vessel is damaged. For this reason, the femoral artery is often selected as the second option after failed radial cannulation. This site has a higher rate of infective complications, however.

Components of Invasive Arterial Blood Pressure Measurement

1. **Flush solution** – Normally 500 ml of 0.9% saline, pressurized to 300 mmHg; in conjunction with a flow restrictor housed in the transducer apparatus, this ensures a constant flow of 4 ml h^{-1} through the system. This maintains patency of the connecting tubing by preventing reflux of arterial blood back into the system. This is connected to the transducer apparatus by a length of standard fluid tubing.
2. **Transducer** – Placed along the phlebostatic axis and requires calibration and zeroing. This converts pressure readings into an electronic signal for display as a waveform. The transducer housing is combined with the flow-restrictor, which controls the rate of continuous flush.
3. **Connection tubing** – The connection tubing between the transducer and the cannula in the patient is specifically designed to be relatively non-compliant to minimize damping: it is different from conventional intravenous fluid tubing. Three-way taps can be added to allow for blood sampling and zeroing. In many systems, the outside of the tubing is marked with a red tracer to distinguish the arterial system from the blue tracer of a central venous pressure line. This minimizes the chances of inadvertent accessing of the wrong system with, in particular, drugs.
4. **Intra-arterial cannula** – 20–22-gauge parallel-sided polyethylene or polytetrafluorethylene (PTFE otherwise known as Teflon™) cannula. These materials are selected as they reduce the risk of thrombus formation. The parallel sides ensure accurate pressure-wave transmission.
5. **Microprocessor, amplifier and display** – The electrical signal from the transducer is filtered, amplified and analyzed. It is displayed on the monitor as a wave with accompanying numerical read-outs of the blood pressure. Analysis of the waveform by additional systems can allow derivations of other values from the waveform such as cardiac output.

Blood pressure pulsations are transmitted from the arterial cannula up the connecting tubing to the transducer (Figure 11.7). This relies on hydraulic coupling: due to the incompressible nature of water, a pressure wave will pass through a column of fluid with little loss of energy. The transducer receives the incoming pressure waves and converts them into an electrical signal via the use of a strain gauge and Wheatstone bridge. The signal is then amplified and displayed on the monitor.

A transducer is any device that converts one form of energy into another. In this case, mechanical energy is converted into electrical energy. In most invasive blood pressure systems, a strain-gauge transducer is used (Figure 11.8). This consists of a diaphragm that separates the fluid system from a resistance wire. The wire is attached to the diaphragm, which moves when pressure changes in the arterial system. This alters the length and thickness of the wire, resulting in a change in the electrical resistance.

> In the strictest definition, the system for invasive pressure monitoring uses a pressure sensor not a transducer. The mechanical energy of the pulse alters the electrical characteristics of the strain gauge, altering the current so resulting in an electrical signal which the monitor can interpret. There is no direct conversion from mechanical to electrical energy, as the definition of a transducer would require. A motor converts electrical or chemical energy to mechanical energy, a bulb converts electrical to light energy; these are transducers. This is a medical misnomer which is, however, unlikely to change!

Most commonly, a Wheatstone bridge (Figure 11.9) is used to detect any changes in the electrical resistance of the strain gauge. The bridge consists of three known resistors (one of which is variable) and one unknown variable resistor (the strain gauge, in the case of a pressure transducer).

When the ratio of the known resistors (R_1/R_2) is equal to the ratio of the resistors on the other side of the bridge (R_v/R_u), the bridge is balanced and there is no potential difference to be detected by the galvanometer (G). However, when the pressure in the strain gauge changes, resulting in a change in resistance, the bridge becomes unbalanced, current flows and a potential difference is measured. This voltage is amplified and processed for display as a waveform on a digital monitor.

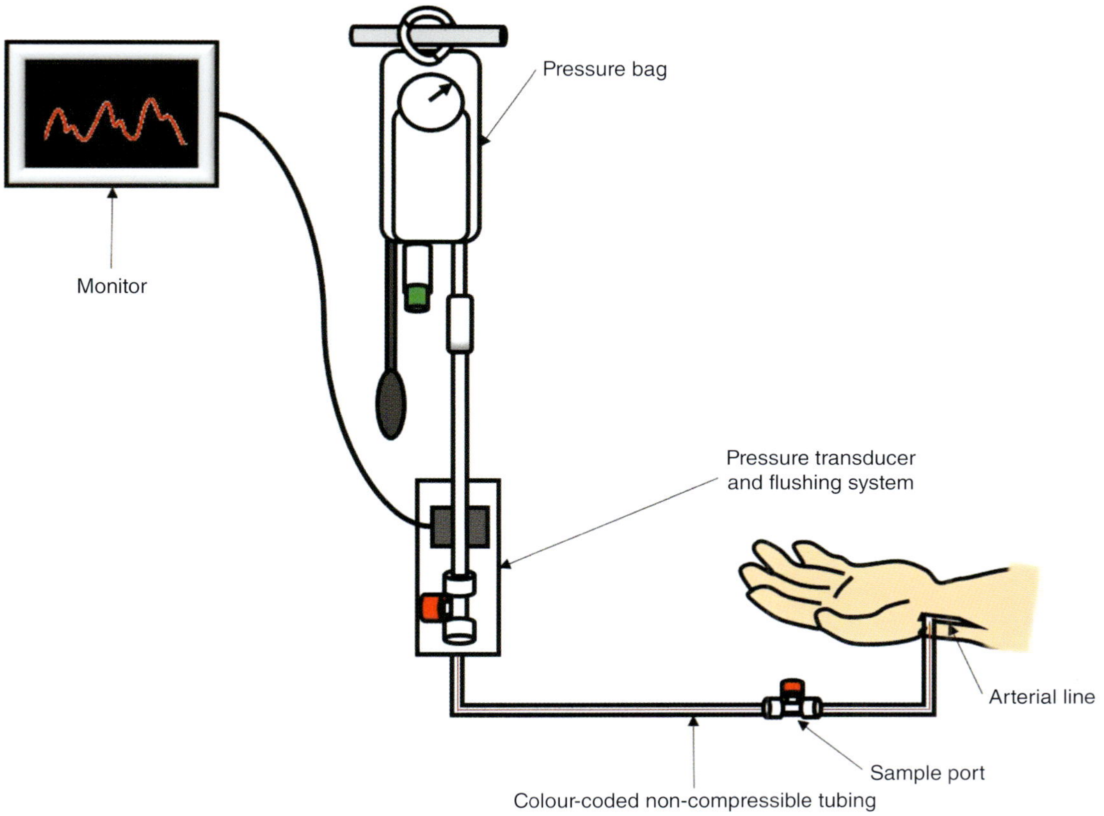

Chapter 11: Blood Pressure Measurement

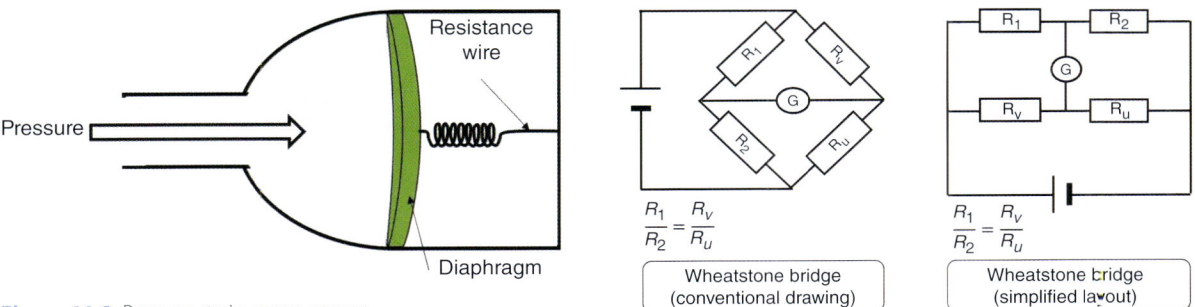

Figure 11.7 Set-up of intra-arterial blood pressure equipment

Figure 11.8 Pressure strain-gauge sensor

Figure 11.9 A Wheatstone bridge circuit

Newer versions of the Wheatstone bridge use four strain gauges in a different arrangement. When the transducer diaphragm moves, two of the resistors are stretched and two shortened. The sensitivity of this set-up is four times greater as all four strain gauges make up the Wheatstone bridge.

Errors Associated with Intra-Arterial Blood Pressure Measurement

1. Waveform Morphology

The morphology of the arterial pressure waves changes as you move away from the aorta due to

167

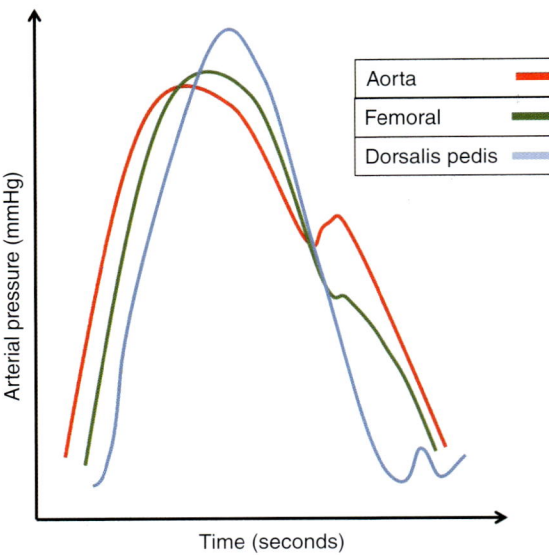

Figure 11.10 Distal systolic pulse amplification

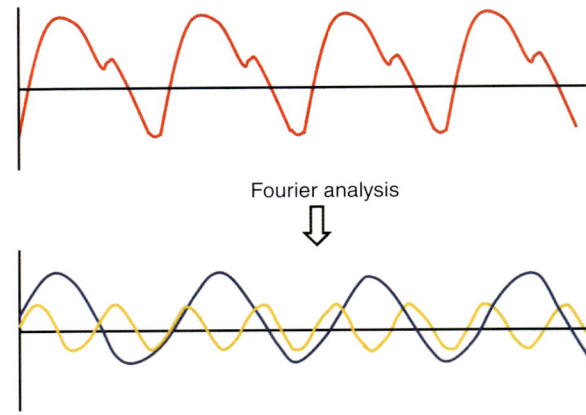

Figure 11.11 A simplistic Fourier analysis of an arterial pressure waveform

distal systolic pulse amplification (Figure 11.10). Reflected waves from the arteriolar bed interact constructively with the incoming systolic waveform. This results in an increase in the systolic pressure and decrease in the diastolic pressure (the MAP remains relatively unaffected). This phenomenon is more marked the more distal the vessel is from the aorta and explains why dorsalis pedis arterial lines read higher than aortic balloon pump transducers. Figure 11.10 demonstrates these changes in systolic and diastolic pressure and also identifies that the reflection wave can be seen in the distal dorsalis pedis arterial trace and is accompanied by almost complete loss of the dicrotic notch.

For the pressure waveform to be displayed it needs to be mathematically analyzed. This is done by the microprocessor. The waveform undergoes Fourier analysis: it is deconstructed into its component parts, the harmonic waves. The lowest-frequency sine wave is called the fundamental frequency or first harmonic and, for the arterial trace, equates to the pulse rate. The second harmonic is twice the frequency. The third, fourth and fifth harmonics are three, four and five times the frequency and so on. An arterial waveform is comprised of between 10 and 30 harmonics. The lower harmonics contribute most to the shape of the waveform as they have the largest amplitude. The more harmonics analyzed, the closer the mathematical model of the waveform is to the original arterial trace. Figure 11.11 demonstrates, very simplistically, how an arterial trace consists of multiple sine waves. The upper wave corresponds to the systolic pulse, the second harmonic roughly approximates, in this case, to the dicrotic notch (in reality, the notch is usually a combination of several of the higher harmonics).

2. Resonance

Resonance is a phenomenon in which an external force or frequency causes a system to oscillate at a greater amplitude. The frequency that causes the largest amount of oscillation is termed the 'resonant frequency'. The transfer of energy from one system to another is never 100% efficient and some losses do occur: this is called damping. When there is minimal damping, the resonant frequency often equates to the natural frequency of the object. In Figure 11.12, energy is applied to a system in a cyclical manner. As the frequency of energy input increases, there is a point where the amplitude of oscillations suddenly increases dramatically. This is the resonant frequency. As the frequency increases further, past the resonant frequency, the amplitude of the oscillations of the system again reduces. The natural frequency is the frequency at which a system oscillates freely once set in motion.

In clinical practice, resonance occurs when the frequency of the arterial waveform (i.e. the fundamental or any of its harmonics) approaches the natural/resonant frequency of the invasive blood pressure monitoring system. An increase in amplitude of the waveform oscillations will occur, causing over-reading of the systolic pressure and under-reading of the diastolic pressure (as with distal systolic pulse amplification, the MAP will be unaffected).

It is for this reason that an understanding of Fourier analysis is important. In order to avoid resonance effects in clinical practice, the design of the monitoring system must ensure the natural frequency of the device is higher than the frequency of the measured pressure waveform, its fundamental and harmonic waveforms. The fundamental frequency as mentioned before equates to pulse rate. At 60 beats per minute this is equal to 1 Hz and at 180 beats per minute it is equal to 3 Hz. The invasive blood pressure system therefore needs to have a natural or resonant frequency above the tenth harmonic which is between approximately 10 Hz and 30 Hz. Achieving these design specifications can, however, be difficult to achieve in clinical practice. To maximize the natural frequency of the arterial blood pressure system, short, wide and stiff (non-compliant) cannulae and tubing are used.

3. Damping

Damping is a result of energy losses in the system due to frictional or resistive losses. It reduces the effect of resonance and also prevents the invasive blood pressure system from approaching its natural frequency. Causes of damping in the invasive blood pressure system include:

- Three-way taps
- Air bubbles
- Clots
- Additional lengths of tubing
- Kinking of tubing/cannula

Over-damping results in an under-reading of the systolic pressure and over-reading of the diastolic pressure. The MAP is unaffected. Conversely, under-damping results in an over-reading of systclic pressure, under-reading of diastolic pressure and MAP is again unaffected (Figure 11.13).

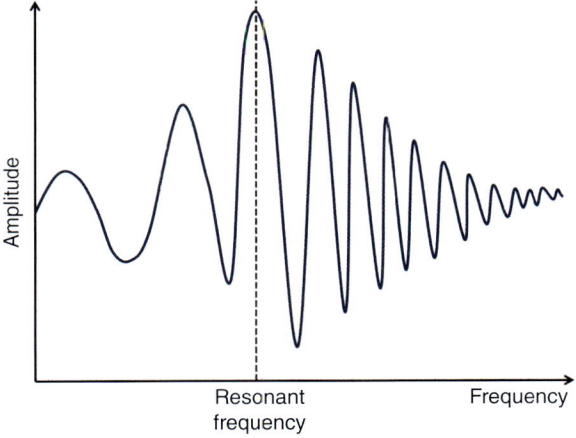

Figure 11.12 Identification of the resonant frequency of a system

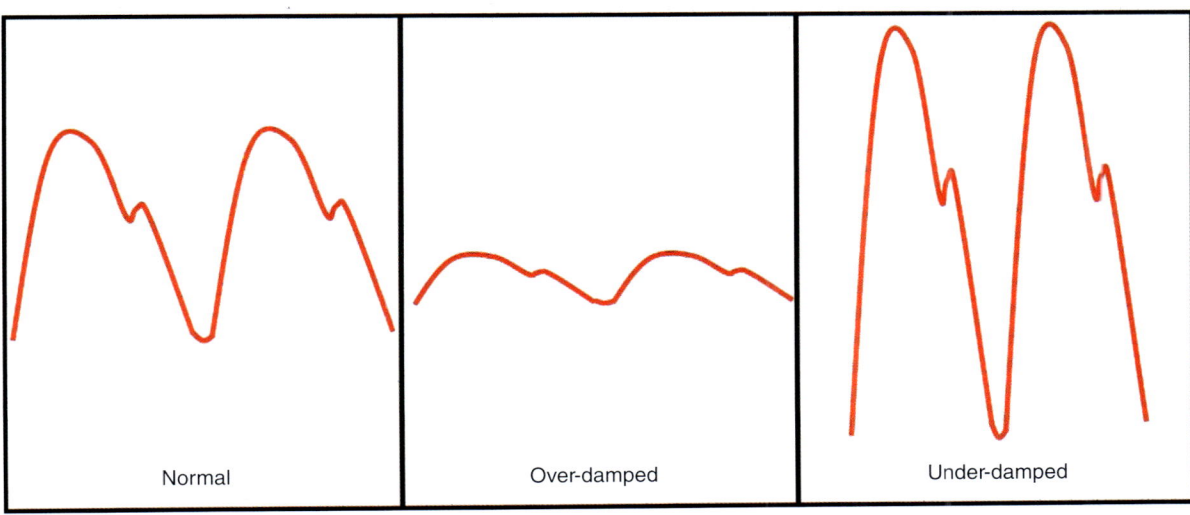

Figure 11.13 The effects of damping on the arterial waveform

Chapter 11: Blood Pressure Measurement

It is important that invasive blood pressure systems are able to respond quickly to changes in input; this is known as dynamic response. When there is zero damping, no energy is lost from the system so when a change occurs, the oscillations continue indefinitely. Therefore, some degree of damping is essential for invasive blood pressures to be rapidly and accurately displayed.

The damping coefficient (DC) is used to describe the degree of damping in a system, where 0 is no damping and 1, critical damping. Figure 11.14 demonstrates how the damping coefficient affects the response of the waveform to changes of input.

- Zero damping: DC = 0
- Under-damped: DC <0.64 – The system responds quickly but oscillates and overshoots; the systolic pressure is overestimated and diastolic pressure is underestimated
- Over-damped: DC >1 – The system does not oscillate freely and the response time is slow; the systolic pressure is underestimated and diastolic pressure is overestimated
- Critically damped: DC = 1 – There is no oscillation but the response time is slow
- Optimally damped: DC = 0.64 – There is a rapid response time with minimal overshoot

In clinical practice, the dynamic response of the monitoring system and degree of damping can be assessed with the fast-flush test. To perform the test:

1. Activate the flush device: this generates a square waveform on the monitor
2. Count the oscillations after the square waveform (Figure 11.15):

   a. In an optimally damped system, you should see one to two oscillations before returning to the baseline.
   b. In an under-damped system, there will be more than two oscillations before returning to the baseline.
   c. In an over-damped system, you will see one or no oscillations. Check for, and remove, any air bubbles, clots or additional lengths of tubing or three-way taps.

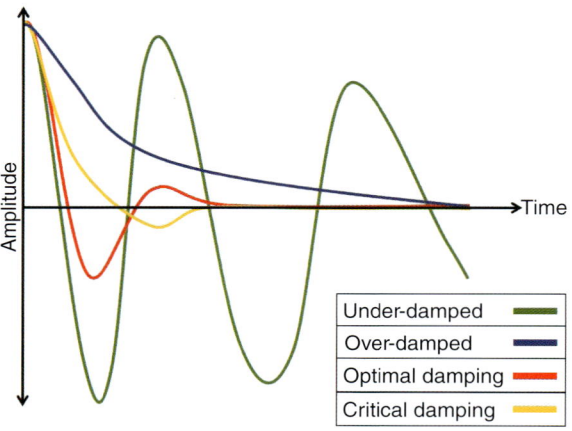

Figure 11.14 Effect of differing damping conditions

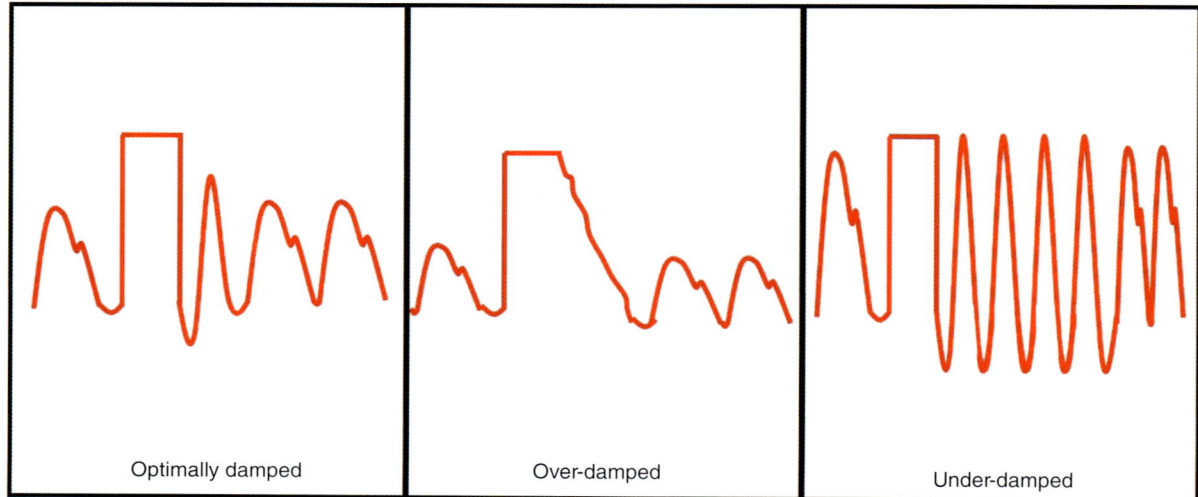

Figure 11.15 The fast-flush test in differing damping conditions

Chapter 11: Blood Pressure Measurement

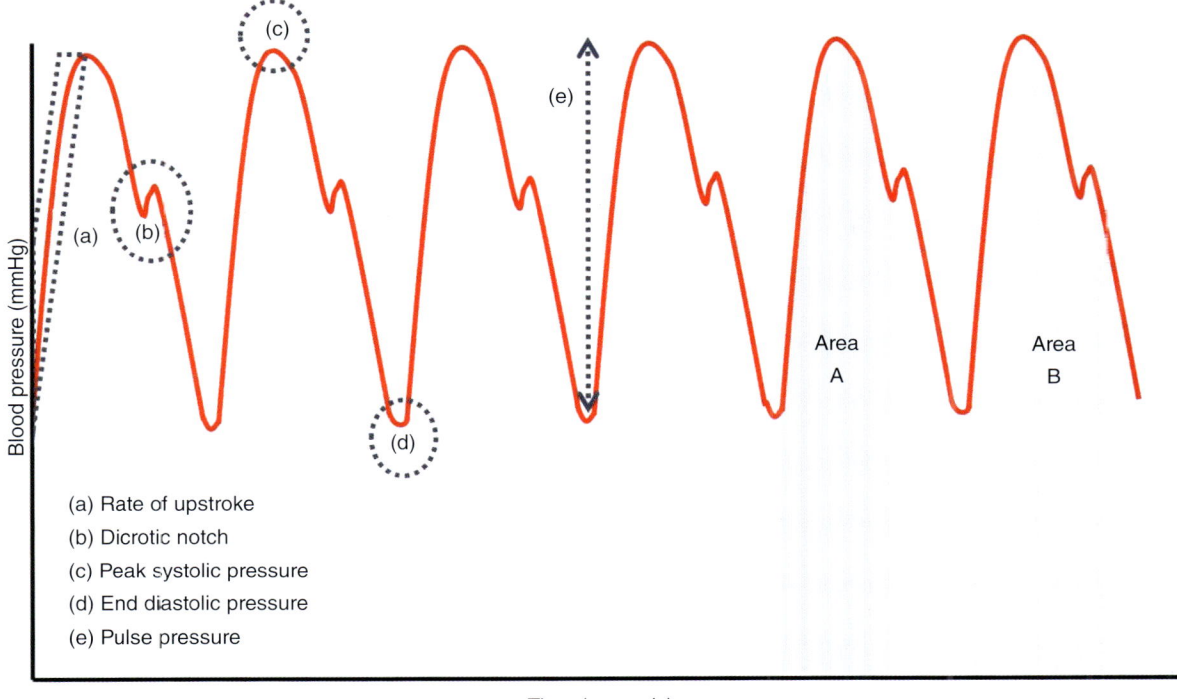

Figure 11.16 Additional information available from the morphology of the waveform

4. Zeroing

To measure blood pressure, atmospheric pressure must be discounted. The transducer should be exposed to atmospheric pressure and the pressure reading calibrated to zero. This can be done by turning the three-way tap next to the transducer 'off to the patient', removing the cap and pressing the 'zero' button on the monitor. The invasive pressure system should be calibrated to zero several times a day to exclude errors due to calibration drift within the system.

5. Levelling

As with a sphygmomanometer cuff, for accurate readings of blood pressure, the transducer should be placed along the phlebostatic axis. If the transducer falls on the floor, the pressure reading will be higher due to hydrostatic pressure. For example, if the transducer is 10 cm below the level of the heart, the blood pressure reading will be 7.5 mmHg higher than the true pressure. Similarly, if the transducer is 10 cm higher than the heart, then the blood pressure reading will be 7.5 mmHg lower than the actual value.

Additional Information from the Waveform

The waveform not only provides us with pressure readings but other important information (Figure 11.16):

- **Rate of upstroke** (dP/dt) reflects **myocardial contractility**
- The **dicrotic notch** represents closure of the aortic valve and its position on the downstroke is an indication of peripheral vascular resistance; in vasodilated patients the notch is lower down
- **Stroke volume** is estimated by measuring the area under the graph up to the dicrotic notch (area A in Figure 11.16)
- **Cardiac output** = Stroke volume × Heart rate
- **Pulse pressure**
- **Heart rate**
- **Stroke volume variability and/or pulse pressure variation** – an indicator of fluid responsiveness
- **MAP** is calculated as the area under the waveform (area B in Figure 11.16). By comparison, the method discussed earlier

(diastolic pressure + one-third of pulse pressure) is only an approximation:

$$\text{MAP} = \frac{\int_{t_1}^{t_2} P\,dt}{t_2 - t_1}$$

This is more simply expressed as:

$$\text{MAP} = \frac{\text{Area under pressure curve}}{\text{Duration of cardiac cycle}}$$

Summary

Blood pressure measurement and manipulation are central to what we do. For the most part, this concerns systemic arterial pressure, most frequently monitored by non-invasive methods. Blood pressure, as an overarching concept, also includes pulmonary arterial and central venous pressure and these, along with arterial systemic pressure, can be measured accurately via invasive means. Quantitative analysis of waveform data allows a wide gamut of haemodynamic data to be derived from the pressure waveform.

Now to come back to our initial scenario of the lady undergoing bariatric surgery. In selecting a blood pressure monitoring technique, there are both patient and surgical factors to consider which, on the balance of risk versus benefit, makes intra-arterial blood pressure monitoring the most appropriate method in this case. These factors are:

- Patient factors:
    (i) Obesity: may make non-invasive blood pressure recording difficult or impossible
    (ii) Co-morbidities, medications and poor exercise tolerance: high risk of haemodynamic instability, particularly on induction of anaesthesia; this can be most closely monitored with an intra-arterial blood pressure monitor
    (iii) Although not the main indication for intra-arterial blood pressure monitoring, it would allow for frequent blood sampling and monitoring of haemoglobin levels and $PaCO_2$ intra-operatively if required

- Surgical factors:
    (i) The surgery may take several hours, increasing the risk of peripheral oedema and neuropraxia with a sphygmomanometer cuff

The second issue concerned positioning of the patient intra-operatively. As we now know, provided the transducer is kept on the phlebostatic axis when the patient is moved, accuracy of the system ought to be maintained.

Questions

MCQs – select true or false for each response

1. The Von Recklinghausen oscillotonometer:
    (a) Uses Korotkoff sounds to measure systolic and diastolic blood pressure
    (b) Has a double blood pressure cuff
    (c) Most accurately records diastolic pressure
    (d) Is the most widely used non-invasive blood pressure measurement device in clinical practice
    (e) Has an integrated stethoscope
2. Regarding non-invasive measurement of blood pressure:
    (a) A blood pressure cuff that is too small records an artificially high blood pressure
    (b) Non-invasive measurements accurately record extremes of hyper- and hypotension
    (c) The bladder of the cuff should sit over the femoral artery
    (d) The cuff should cover two-thirds of the upper arm
    (e) Automated machines are inaccurate in the presence of atrial fibrillation
3. Concerning invasive blood pressure measurement:
    (a) The ulna artery is the commonest site of arterial cannula insertion
    (b) Is contraindicated in patients requiring cardiac bypass
    (c) Can cause ischaemia of the limb
    (d) Is always the best way to measure blood pressure
    (e) Can be used to determine right-ventricular performance
4. Regarding the physics of arterial blood pressure measurement:
    (a) Resonance causes an over-reading of systolic pressure and under-reading of diastolic pressure
    (b) An over-damped system is required to allow a rapid and accurate response to changes in input

(c) If the transducer is 10 cm below the level of the heart the blood pressure will read 7.5 mmHg less than the true value
(d) The arterial blood pressure system only needs to be 'zeroed' once
(e) A length of standard intravenous fluid tubing can be used to connect the saline bag to the transducer

SBAs – select the single *best* answer

5. A patient has an arterial blood pressure line inserted after induction of general anaesthesia. During the case you notice that the arterial pressure trace intermittently displays a flat trace, the patient's heart rate and capnography measurements are unaffected. The most likely cause of this is:
   (a) Over-damping of the arterial system
   (b) Resonance of the arterial system
   (c) Clots in the arterial cannula, causing intermittent obstruction
   (d) Automatic non-invasive cuff measurements on the same arm as the arterial cannula.
   (e) Intermittent loss of the patient's cardiac output

Answers

1. FTFFF

   This device uses a display of oscillations rather than the auscultatory method so does not use a stethoscope. It results in best estimations for systolic and mean pressures, not diastolic. Although automated non-invasive blood pressure machines use similar principles, the Von Recklinghausen device itself is no longer in common clinical practice.

2. TFFTT

   Non-invasive blood pressure measurements are least reliable at extremes of blood pressure and in the presence of arrhythmias such as atrial fibrillation. Cuffs are generally placed on the arm (over the brachial artery) or, occasionally, the leg or forearm. Use of a thigh cuff to occlude the femoral artery would not be feasible in adult practice.

3. FFTFT

   The commonest site for invasive cannulation is the radial artery. It will provide a non-pulsatile trace whilst on cardiopulmonary bypass but, far from being contraindicated, is routine practice in these patients: a non-invasive system will be unable to make any kind of measurement whilst on bypass. As for almost any clinical device, invasive blood pressure measurement has limitations and contraindications, meaning it is not always the best solution.

4. TFFFT

   The system should be optimally damped. A lowered transducer position will result in an over-reading not an under-reading. The system should be zeroed regularly to account for issues of drift. Standard tubing can be used between the flush bag and the transducer but the tubing from the transducer to the patient must be specifically designed for the task with appropriate length and compliance.

5. (d)

   The most likely cause is repeated inflation and deflation of the non-invasive cuff on the same arm, causing intermittent obstruction to blood flow, which is detected by the arterial line in the same limb. Although there is concern that a patient may have lost their cardiac output the fact that the capnography trace and heart rate are unaffected makes this rather less likely. Over-damping may diminish the responsiveness of the system but will not cause it to tend towards a total flat trace. Resonance will lead to increased oscillations. Clots are more likely to lead to a cumulative over-damping of the system, rather than a sporadic loss of the trace.

References

1. A. Hartle, T. McCormack, J. Carlisle, S. Anderson, A. Pichel, N. Beckett, T. Woodcock, A. Heagerty. The measurement of adult blood pressure and management of hypertension before elective surgery: Joint guidelines from the Association of Anaesthetists of Great Britain and Ireland and the British Hypertension Society. *Anaesthesia*, 71, 2016; 326–337.

Chapter 12

Cardiac Output Monitoring

Hozefa Ebrahim and Alistair Burns

Learning Objectives
- To appreciate the importance of monitoring cardiac output
- To understand the different methods employed in clinical practice to measure cardiac output
- To gain a practical understanding of the different parameters offered by cardiac output monitors
- To recognize the advantages and disadvantages of different monitors in practice

Chapter Content
- Washout curves
- Stewart–Hamilton equation
- Fick principle and dilutional methods of cardiac output monitoring
- Pulmonary artery catheter
- Lithium dilution methods
- Doppler ultrasound devices
- Analysis of the arterial waveform
- Non-invasive finger-cuff technology
- Visual echocardiography
- Bio-impedance
- Other methods

Scenario

A 64-year-old, obese patient is admitted to the critical care unit. He presents with hypotension and evidence of shock. He has pneumonia and acute-on-chronic renal disease. He has a history of ischaemic heart disease and had a pacemaker inserted following coronary angioplasty 2 years ago. He is also diabetic with known autonomic neuropathy.

With respect to managing his hypotension and poor organ perfusion, what investigative monitoring can you employ to determine whether he needs fluids, inotropes or vasopressors? How can one quantify cardiac output? What are the advantages and disadvantages of these different methods? What makes an ideal cardiac output monitor?

Introduction

Understanding an individual's cardiac output and organ perfusion is essential in managing them through a critical illness. It is also a core component of goal-directed fluid management in the perioperative journey. Whilst there is no substitute for clinical assessment, clinical signs alone are often inadequate when titrating inotropes and vasopressors. Therefore, there is a need for more precise mechanical methods of measuring cardiac output and associated variables. Moreover, the clinical culprit also changes with time; a patient who was dehydrated earlier may subsequently develop vasoplegia or even cardiogenic shock.

There are many different devices for measuring cardiac output. However, it is important to remember that all monitors measure parameters, which are used as surrogate markers for the truth! Whilst there is no perfect device at our disposal, attentive clinical application of mechanically generated numbers can lead to better outcomes in certain patients in anaesthesia and critical care. But beware – some mechanical devices can yield misleading numbers, especially under extreme physiological and anatomical conditions. Furthermore, incorrect interpretation of the measured variables can also do harm.

Some devices require the insertion of invasive cannulae such as venous and arterial lines. This can be associated with independent clinical risk. In addition, the location of the line can also be a source of error. Femoral arterial catheters often suggest a higher arterial blood pressure than radial lines. Studies have shown a reduction in vasopressor requirements by 30% by simply changing from radial to femoral arterial monitoring!

Whilst this is a physics textbook, it is worth mentioning some physiology. Blood flow and blood

Chapter 12: Cardiac Output Monitoring

Table 12.1 Comparison of different cardiac output monitors

Device	Cost	Invasiveness	Accuracy	Ease of use	Reproducibility
PAC	£££	Highly	+++	Difficult	+++
LiDCO™ (dilution)	££	Moderately	++	Moderate	+++
Doppler	£	Moderately	++	Moderate	+
Waveform analysis					
• Vigileo™	££	Minimally	++	Very easy	+++
• LiDCO rapide™	££	Minimally	++	Very easy	+++
• PiCCO™	££	Moderately	++	Easy	+++
Finger cuff	££	Non-invasive	+	Very easy	+++
Echocardiography	£££	Minimally	+++	Difficult	++
Bio-impedance	££	Non-invasive	+	Very easy	+++
Ultrasound velocity dilution	£££	Highly	+++	Difficult	+++
Magnetic resonance	££££	Minimally	+++	Difficult	+++

pressure mean different things. Interpreting the output of monitoring devices appropriately requires a sound understanding of the underlying physics principles. A machine is only as good as the person using it!

So, what is the ideal cardiac output monitor? There needs to be a balance between cost, invasiveness, usability, accuracy and reproducibility. Table 12.1 compares some of the machines on the market.

Washout Curves

An understanding of *washout curves* is fundamental to many methods of cardiac output monitoring. Therefore, we will explore this concept first.

Consider a beaker of water as illustrated in Figure 12.1.

The beaker contains a constant volume of 250 ml. A flow of water from a tap above enters at 50 ml min^{-1}. An overflow drain on the side of the beaker allows water to drain off at the same rate. As such, a constant volume of 250 ml remains in the beaker.

10 ml of red dye is introduced into the beaker whilst the fluid is stirred rapidly. The colour of the water changes almost instantly. However, as clear tap water continues to flow into the beaker, the dye is progressively diluted and the intensity of the colour washes away with time. Figure 12.2 shows colour intensity (concentration) plotted against time. As can be seen, the peak intensity is reached as soon as the dye is introduced. However, it diminishes exponentially with time.

Alternatively, consider the tap running at a flow rate of 100 ml min^{-1} instead. Figure 12.3 illustrates the effect this has on colour intensity. If the same amount of dye is introduced and stirred rapidly, the peak intensity of the dye remains the same in both experiments. However, the intensity of the colour in the beaker seems to be washed away faster as it becomes diluted.

The rate at which this dye is washed out is used to calculate cardiac output using the Stewart–Hamilton equation, but more about that shortly.

Now consider how this example is analogous to the right heart and pulmonary arteries. Let us replace the beaker with the pulmonary artery. The flow of tap water becomes the flow of blood through the pulmonary artery (aka cardiac output). The dye can be replaced with various marker substances such as biologically compatible dyes (e.g. indocyanine green) or iced saline. The challenge becomes designing a piece of equipment that can introduce a 'dye' and detect its intensity (or concentration) in a timely fashion.

Let us explore this further. To calculate the 'washout curve' more accurately, we need a method of measuring the concentration of dye in the blood at any one time. Let us imagine that our red dye is in fact radioactive. On the side of the beaker, we install a

Chapter 12: Cardiac Output Monitoring

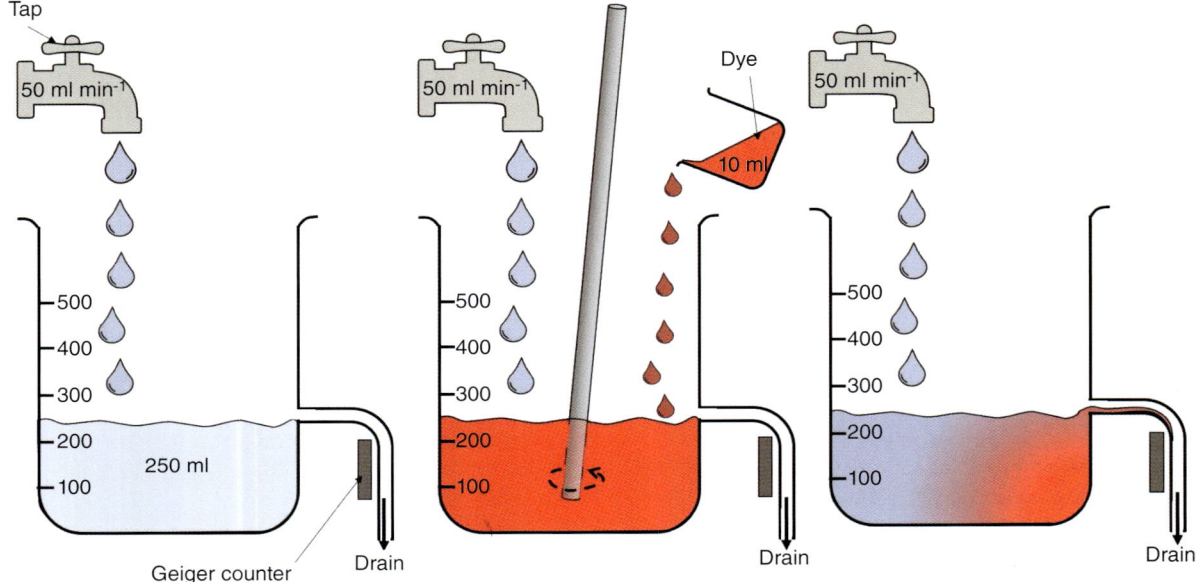

Figure 12.1 Schematic of the principle underlying the washout curve

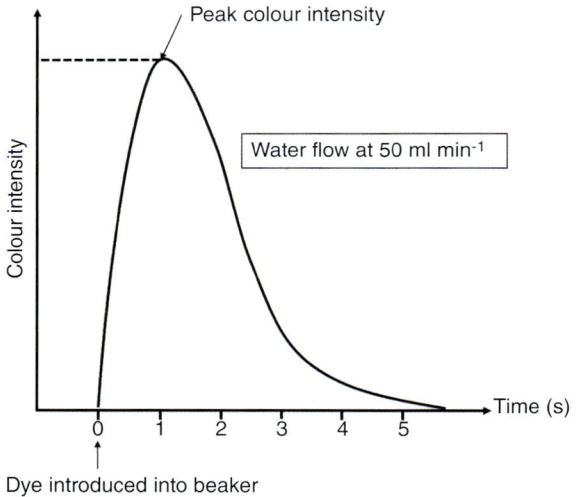

Figure 12.2 A graph demonstrating the relationship between colour intensity and time during an exponential washout process

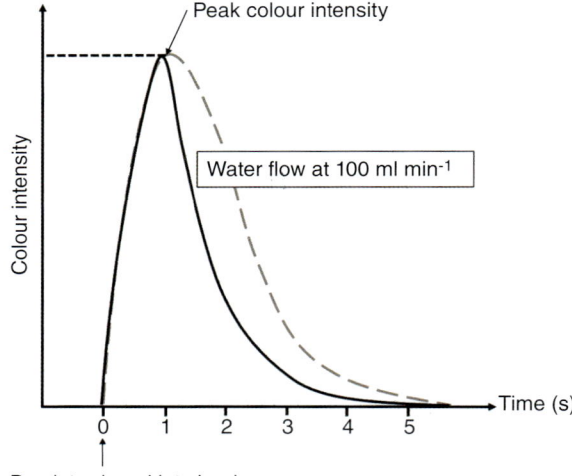

Figure 12.3 A graph demonstrating the relationship between colour intensity and time during an exponential washout process, but with a faster flow of water

Geiger counter, an instrument for measuring radio-activity. The Geiger counter records the level of radio-activity every 0.01 seconds, and gives us a reading in becquerels (Bq). Using our initial example, we can now produce an accurate washout graph.

In clinical practice, the dye or radioactive tracer can be replaced with many different markers, such as cold saline, lithium and various other markers.

Stewart–Hamilton Equation

The Stewart–Hamilton equation (Figure 12.6) employs the relatively simple mathematical equation to calculate the area under the curve (the shaded area). Since concentration is amount of dye per unit volume, the rate of flow can be subsequently calculated. Hence the calculation of cardiac output.

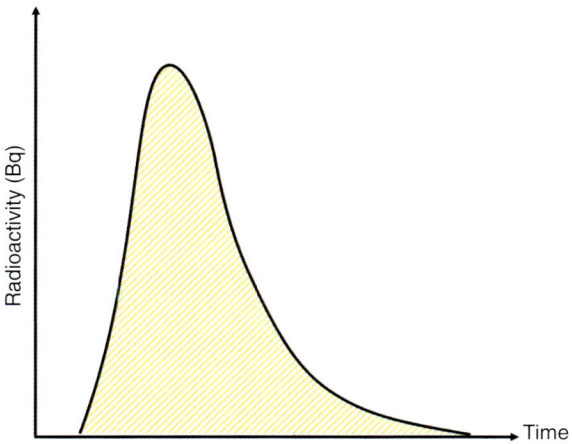

Figure 12.4 A graph demonstrating the relationship between radioactivity and time during an exponential washout process

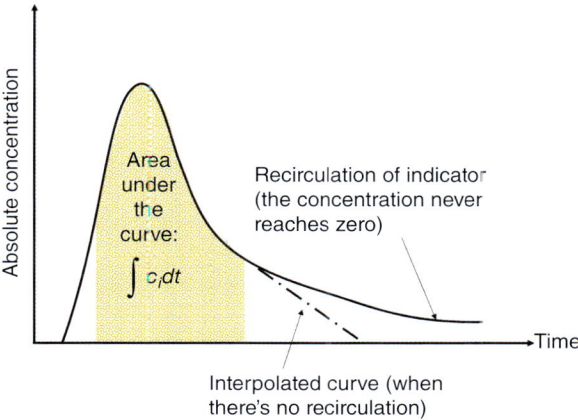

Figure 12.5 The Stewart–Hamilton equation is applied to the washout curve to calculate the rate of flow of blood, i.e. cardiac output

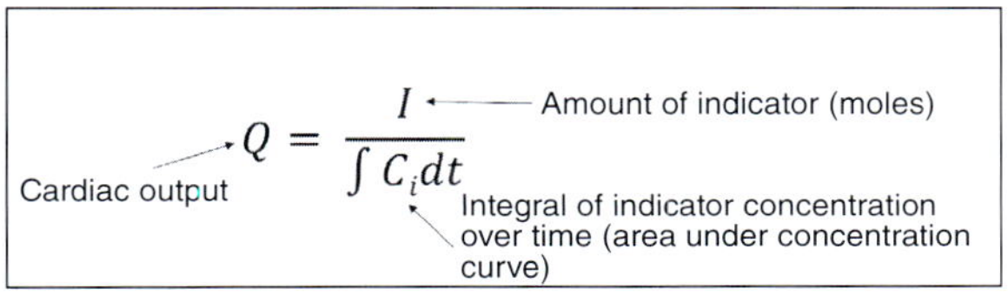

$$Q = \frac{I}{\int C_i dt}$$

- Q = Cardiac output
- I = Amount of indicator (moles)
- $\int C_i dt$ = Integral of indicator concentration over time (area under concentration curve)

Figure 12.6 The Stewart–Hamilton equation for indicator

The Stewart–Hamilton equation is often viewed as some vast array of unintelligible algebra, particularly if you never cared much for calculus at school, but it need not be as bewildering as all that. The term on the bottom of this equation means to take the total change in concentration of the indicator and multiply it by the time interval over which that change occurs (dt): this is the equivalent of 'counting squares'. To prove how we get from that to cardiac output (Q), we can first rationalize the equation to what the units are for each term:

$$\text{Volume per unit time} = \frac{\text{moles}}{\frac{\text{moles}}{\text{volume}} \times \text{time}}$$

To simplify further, we can first sort out the 'double divide by volume' on the right by bringing the volume term to the top line of the equation. After that, the next step is to cancel any similar terms above and below the line:

$$= \text{volume} \times \frac{\cancel{\text{moles}}}{\cancel{\text{moles}} \times \text{time}}$$

This leaves us with matching terms on both sides of the equation. In other words, we have proven that the relatively complex mathematics to the right of the equation all boils down to the same terms as on the left, allowing us to calculate Q.

$$\text{Volume per unit time} = \frac{\text{volume}}{\text{time}}$$

Fick Principle and Dilutional Methods of Cardiac Output Monitoring

Adolf Eugen Fick, born in 1829, was a German-born physician and physiologist. His initial interest in maths and physics turned into a love of medicine. He graduated in 1851 and, by 1870, he had demonstrated the measurement of cardiac output using a technique that we now call the Fick principle.

The basic principle is that blood flow to an organ can be calculated if certain information is known:

- The amount of a substance taken up by the organ per unit time
- Concentration of the substance in the arterial blood supplying the organ
- Concentration of the substance in the vein leaving the organ

In Fick's original work, the 'organ' was the whole body, and the marker substance was oxygen. However, this theory can apply to different organs and different markers. Various gases, chemicals or temperature can be used as the marker substance.

Chapter 12: Cardiac Output Monitoring

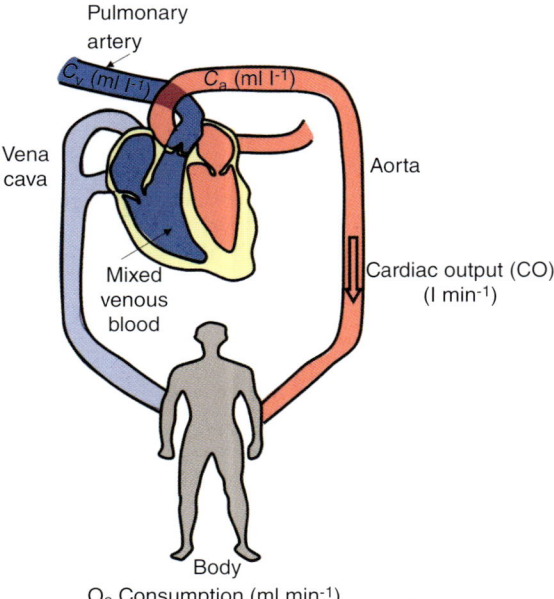

Figure 12.7 The Fick principle

This is an important concept that many devices are based upon.

Consider the schematic shown in Figure 12.7. The cardiac output is the flow of blood in the aorta. This is equal to the flow of blood back through the caval system and ultimately into the pulmonary artery. The blood, by the time it reaches the pulmonary artery, is referred to as mixed venous blood: it is a combination of blood from the superior and inferior vena cavae, the coronary sinus and the Thebesian veins (small veins draining the endocardium directly into the ventricles). The oxygen concentration is measured in millilitres per litre of blood.

The human body consumes a certain amount of oxygen in a minute, which we usually measure in millilitres per minute. By definition, this must equal the amount of oxygen leaving the heart, minus the amount of oxygen returning to the heart. The amount of oxygen leaving the heart is equal to the cardiac output (in volume) multiplied by the concentration of oxygen in the aorta. The amount of oxygen returning to the heart is equal to the cardiac output multiplied by the concentration of oxygen in the pulmonary artery.

Mathematically this is displayed as:

$$\dot{V}O_2 = (CO \times C_a) - (CO \times C_v)$$

where $\dot{V}O_2$ = oxygen consumption, CO = cardiac output, C_a = oxygen concentration of aortic blood and C_v = oxygen concentration of mixed venous blood. Rearranging the equation allows us to solve for cardiac output:

$$CO = \frac{\dot{V}O_2}{C_a - C_v}$$

The term $C_a - C_v$ is referred to as the arteriovenous oxygen difference.

The concentration in aortic and mixed venous blood can be measured via conventional blood gas machines. However, radial arterial blood is often substituted for an aortic sample for obvious, practical reasons (unless the patient has an aortic balloon pump *in situ*). Central venous blood is sometimes substituted for mixed venous blood. Strictly speaking, both of these substitutions mean the eventual result is slightly inaccurate.

To calculate oxygen content in blood, we use the equation:

$$O_2 \text{ content} = Hb \times 1.36 \times SpO_2 + 0.0032 \times PO_2$$

Measurement of oxygen consumption is much harder, and may be measured using a spirometer within a closed rebreathing circuit incorporating a carbon dioxide absorber. This is clinically very difficult, and therefore the Fick principle method of cardiac output monitoring is not commonplace.

The assumed Fick determination technique makes an assumption that the resting oxygen consumption is approximately 125 ml min^{-1} m^{-2} body surface area. This can give an approximation of cardiac output trends.

Pulmonary Artery Catheter

The pulmonary artery catheter (PAC) is an invasive, but accurate, method of cardiac output monitoring. It is widely regarded as the gold standard in the field. As the name suggests, it involves placing a catheter in the pulmonary artery.

The PAC is often referred to as a Swan–Ganz catheter, after two of its proponents: Jeremy Swan and William Ganz. Swan designed the catheter, whilst Ganz offered the idea of a tip-thermistor as a method of measuring thermodilution.

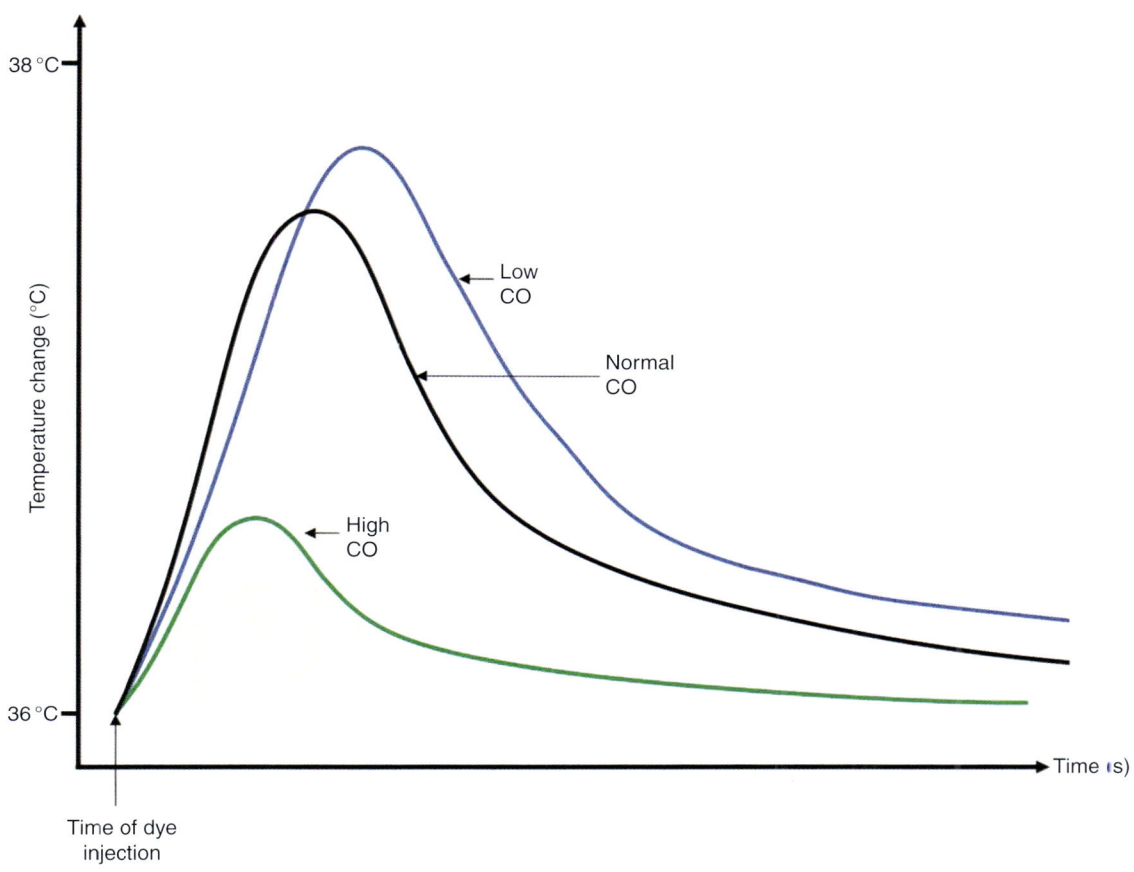

Figure 12.8 Temperature change during cardiac output measurement trial using a PAC with a heating element

The PAC is most commonly inserted through a sheath, placed in the right internal jugular vein. Usually measuring approximately 110 cm, the PAC is passed down the central veins to the right atrium. A balloon on the tip of the catheter is inflated, and the normal flow of blood through the heart guides the catheter as the user gradually advances more and more catheter into the patient. The balloon floats the tip through the right atrium, through the right ventricle and into the pulmonary artery. After passing along the pulmonary artery, it advances and becomes 'wedged' in the pulmonary capillaries. The balloon is then deflated to ensure blood can continue to flow past the catheter to the lung.

PACs utilize a thermodilution technique for measuring cardiac output whereby a change in temperature serves as the indicator. See above for an explanation of the washout method of calculating cardiac output.

Traditionally, a small volume of ice-cold saline is injected through a proximal port on the PAC, and the change in temperature of the blood flowing past the thermistor on the distal end of the PAC is measured continuously. However, using ice-cold saline is cumbersome. Therefore, newer PACs now have a heating element a few centimetres proximal to the thermistor thermometer. The heating element delivers a fixed amount of energy, creating a bolus of warmed blood in the right atrium to act as the *dye* as it flows downstream to the thermistor.

The data produced from the thermistor can be represented as a washout curve as discussed earlier. The curves are the same shape, irrespective of whether iced saline or a warming element is used; you just need to look at the direction of the *y*-axis to determine which it was. Figure 12.8 demonstrates a series of 'cooling curves' (the heater-element version of the

PAC has been used) rather than warming curves. In a high cardiac output state, rapid flow of blood through the right heart quickly dissipates the heat of the warmed blood. By the time it reaches the thermistor, the temperature really shows very little of a peak above body temperature. In a low cardiac output state, flow is so sluggish that two features of the curve are seen. Firstly, the peak is delayed in time because it takes more time for the heart to shuffle the warmed blood along to the thermistor. Secondly, the peak is higher than for the normal cardiac output curve. Again, this relates to sluggish flow failing to introduce enough body-temperature venous blood into the warmed bolus to drop its temperature significantly.

Lithium Dilution Methods

Understanding the maths behind washout curves and their uses, we can extrapolate the science to work for any type of 'dye'. We have discussed red food colouring and cold saline. However, other markers may be used, such as carbon monoxide and lithium. This is the basis behind the lithium chloride dilution device for cardiac output monitoring.

Lithium dilution techniques had gained popularity in the 1990s and 2000s, with some studies showing good correlation with PACs in clinical trials, in a wide range of haemodynamic circumstances.

The technique uses small boluses of lithium injected into a central vein. A typical bolus is 0.5–2.0 ml (0.15 mmol ml^{-1}) lithium chloride. Detection of lithium is through a radial arterial catheter, sampling blood at a rate of 4 ml min^{-1}, and the lithium concentration measured against time. A washout curve is produced as per previous examples, and the cardiac output calculated.

For increased functionality, many lithium dilution monitors use this technique to calibrate a device that ultimately uses analysis of the arterial waveform to give continuous, beat-to-beat information – but more about this later.

Doppler Ultrasound Devices

These devices use the principle of the *change* in frequency of ultrasound waves bouncing off blood cells as they flow through the aorta. They can provide continuous, minimally invasive data of cardiac output.

The science behind Doppler shift as a means to measure velocity has been around for over 150 years. However, the use of this science to determine cardiac output probably only stretches back about 25 years.

In 1842, Christian Doppler presented a paper in Salzburg, in which he stated that the shift in frequency of a reflected wave was proportional to velocity of the moving object. The scientific fraternity initially used this finding to ascertain velocities and distances in outer space, and only later used it to analyze the flow of blood through the body.

This is the same principle explaining how the pitch of a sound wave emitted by an ambulance siren moving towards you will increase, but decrease as it moves away (Figure 12.9). The very same principle is applied by road traffic police attempting to catch speeding motorists.

An ultrasound Doppler probe is inserted into the mid-oesophagus in order to measure the velocity of blood in the (almost) parallel descending aorta.

The principle of using a fixed waveform to measure velocity can be described mathematically by:

$$f_D = \frac{f_T 2v \cos \theta}{c}$$

Rearranged to solve for v, the velocity of the target (red blood cells in the aorta, in this case) is:

$$v = \frac{f_D \times c}{2f_T \times \cos \theta}$$

where f_D is the Doppler shift (which is measured), f_T is the transmitted frequency (which is fixed), θ is the angle of incidence (or insonation) between the path of the probe and the receiver and is assumed to be 45°, and c is the velocity of the wave in the medium. The angle of incidence refers to the angle that is formed between the descending thoracic aortic blood and the direction of the ultrasound beam (Figure 12.10). This angle has to be estimated in commercial devices, and is assumed to be 45° (the tip of the probe is manufactured with a 45°-angled tip to get as close to this assumption as possible). Clearly, this introduces an error into the estimation of velocities. At 90°, the Doppler effect cannot be practically observed because the equation above uses the cosine of this angle and the cosine of 90° results in multiplying the whole equation by zero!

The probe of the oesophageal Doppler monitor (ODM) system is placed within the mid-oesophagus. An ultrasonic waveform is pulsed towards the descending aortic blood, and the reflected signal is measured. The frequency of the transmitted pulse is typically in the region of 4 MHz. The measured Doppler shift is subsequently utilized by the bedside waveform analyzer to determine blood velocity, using the equation given above.

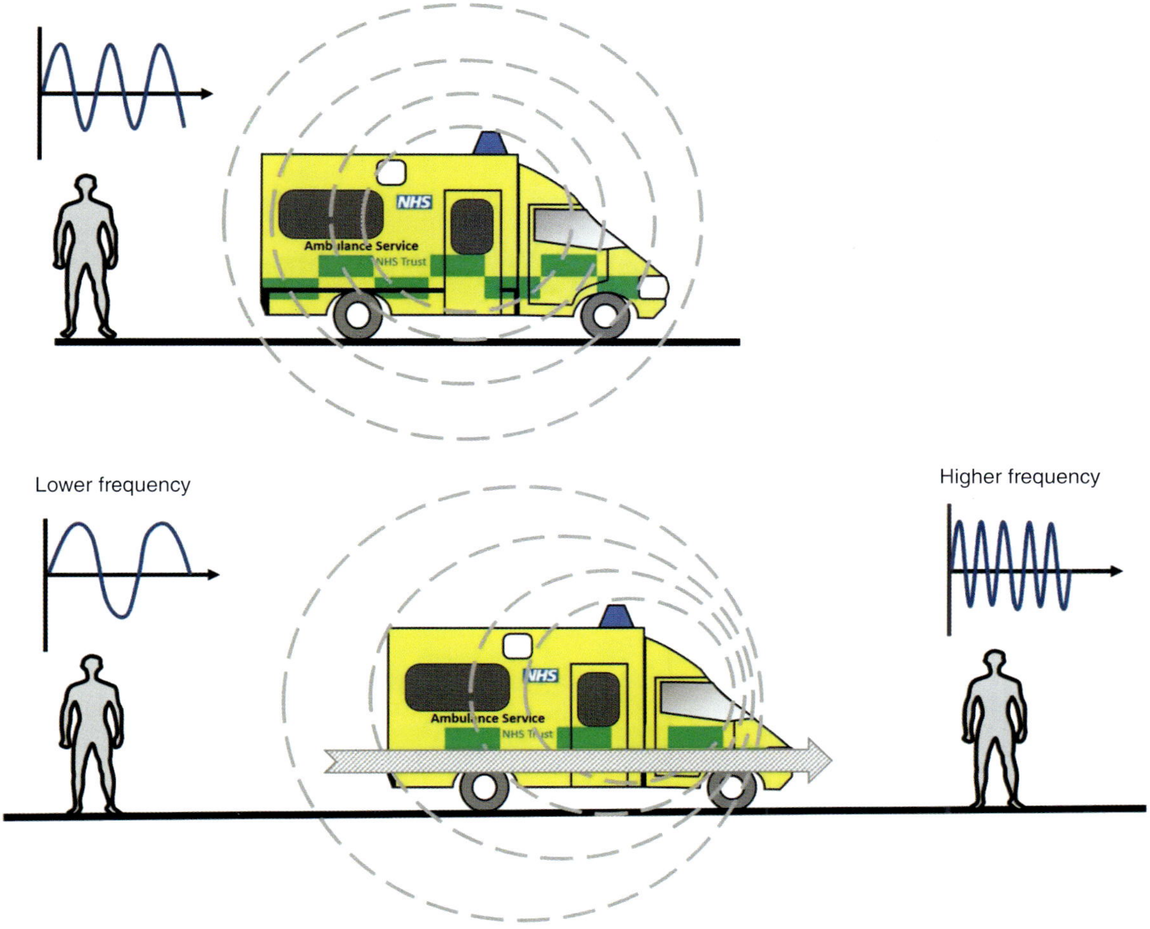

Chapter 12: Cardiac Output Monitoring

Figure 12.9 A moving vehicle relative to a standing person sounds like a changing pitch

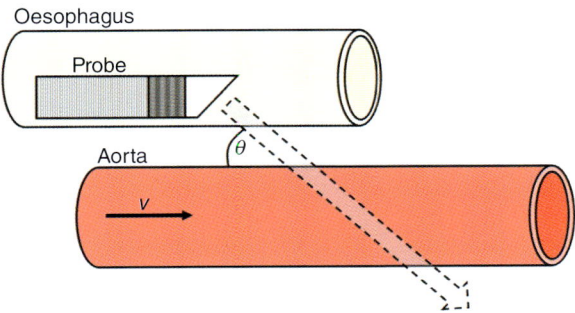

Figure 12.10 Angle of incidence of the oesophageal Doppler probe

Unlike a police officer measuring the speed of an individual car, we are not interested in measuring the velocity of an individual blood cell. Analyzing the geometric shape of the measured waveform gives us some basic information: the peak velocity of the aortic blood; the mean acceleration and velocity of the blood flow; and the average distance travelled by the blood cells during each cardiac beat, known as the stroke distance (Figure 12.11). The stroke distance is the key parameter which allows cardiac output to be derived using Doppler technology. It is derived from analyzing the area under the velocity–time curve. Moving one step forward, if one knows the average velocity of the blood cells, the time each heartbeat takes (also measured directly from the flow curve and known as the flow time) and estimates the cross-sectional area of the aorta, it is easy to calculate the stroke volume. Comparing these measured stroke volumes over time gives an accurate calculation of stroke volume variation (SVV), a good marker of fluid responsiveness. The flow time, in turn, can be used as a composite

181

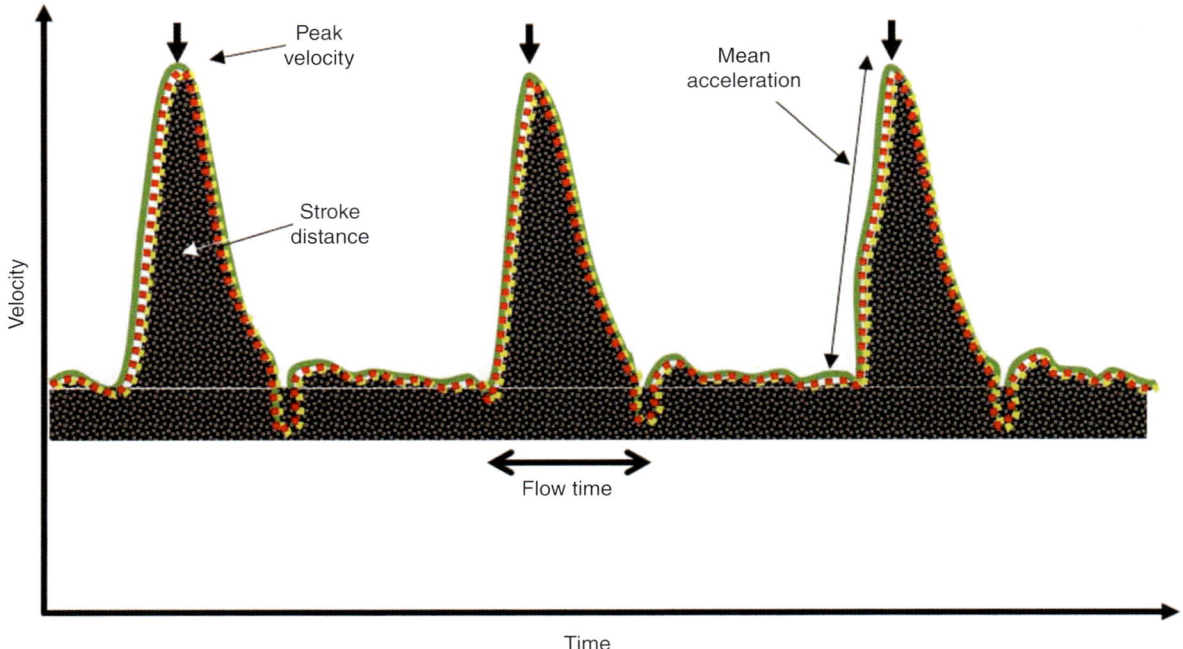

Figure 12.11 Typical velocity–time waveform generated by the ODM and some of the measurements obtained

marker of filling status and systemic vasoconstriction (although the ODM also calculates a value for systemic vascular resistance as well, if the central venous pressure and mean arterial pressure are known).

Some modern devices use Doppler technology to calibrate the device, and then analyze the arterial waveform to provide continuous data – see below.

Analysis of the Arterial Waveform

Analysis of the arterial waveform to determine cardiac output is currently being extensively studied. In recent years it has shown great potential.

The concept that cardiac output is related to pulse pressure was first described in 1904 by Erlanger and Hooker. They postulated that analysis of the arterial pressure contour could be used to determine cardiac output. However, devices with algorithms to electronically calculate such parameters have only recently been developed. These algorithms are often closely guarded industrial secrets, but all algorithms analyze the amplitude, width, rate and shape of the pulse to determine an estimate of cardiac output.

There are numerous methods by which analysis of the arterial waveform is used to estimate cardiac output. Some initially use an alternative technology for self-calibration, and then utilize waveform analysis for continuous measurement.

Examples currently on the market include PiCCO^{TM} (Pulsion Medical Systems, Munich, Germany), FlowTrac/Vigileo^{TM} (Edwards Lifesciences, Irvine, CA, USA) and LiDCO^{TM} (Cambridge, UK).

Non-Invasive Finger-Cuff Technology

Non-invasive finger-cuff technology utilizes the principle of waveform analysis, combined with a non-invasive method of estimating the arterial waveform to calculate cardiac output.

In 1967, Jan Penaz, a Czech scientist, invented a volume–clamp method for continuous blood pressure measurement (see Chapter 11 for a comprehensive description of this technology). The principle is to use an external cuff on the finger (or other specific anatomical locations) to induce a constantly adjusting pressure to equal that of the artery beneath. When the volume of the finger-cuff system is kept constant, the intra-arterial pressures are translated to the cuff, and therefore monitored.

The change in pressure recorded (arterial waveform) is then analyzed using proprietary algorithms. Using generalized data for age, weight, height and sex, an accurate estimation for cardiac output can be made. When combined with data for central venous pressure (if available), further estimations are made for systemic vascular resistance.

As significant variations from the norm can occur in patients with severe vasoplegia (sepsis) or vasoconstriction, the data obtained in such patients should be interpreted with caution. Although not in common clinical practice, the devices are still used with some success.

Visual Echocardiography

Echocardiography can be used in various settings as a means of cardiac output monitoring. Transoesophageal echocardiography (TOE) provides optimal views and in most large centres is readily accessible to the anaesthetist during surgery. However, in the ICU, transthoracic echocardiography is increasingly being performed at the bedside by critical care staff.

Cardiac output is derived mathematically as follows, forming the basis for clinical measurement:

Cardiac output = Stroke volume × Heart rate

The heart rate is easily ascertained from clinical assessment or patient monitoring; hence the primary role of echo is to estimate the stroke volume. Two main methods are utilized for this. The descriptions below focus on the left ventricle but may be adapted for the right.

Doppler-Derived Velocities

The most commonly employed method in the scenario described is to estimate the volume of blood passing a given point during each cardiac cycle, using Doppler-derived velocities.

Consider a hosepipe. If the pipe has a diameter of 4 cm and water flows at a velocity of 5 cm s^{-1} we can calculate the volume of water passing a given point in a 2-s interval by visualizing it as a cylinder (Figure 12.12).

The cross-sectional area of the hose:

$$\text{Area} = \frac{\pi \times \text{Diameter}^2}{4}$$

$$= \frac{3.142 \times 4^2}{4}$$

$$= 12.6 \, \text{cm}^2$$

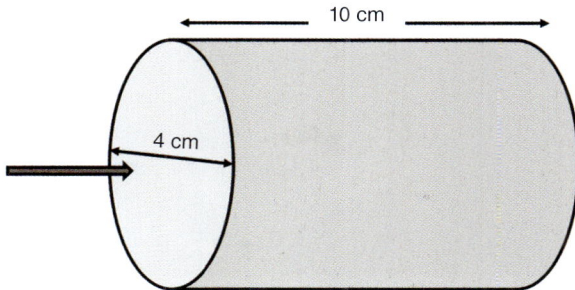

Figure 12.12 Cylinder of water which flows past a point in a 4-cm-diameter hose in 2 seconds (with a water velocity of 5 cm s^{-1})

As the water has a mean velocity of 5 cm s^{-1} then, after 2 s, a cylinder 10 cm long will have formed:

$$\text{Volume} = \text{Area} \times \text{Length}$$

$$= 12.6 \times 10$$

$$= 126 \, \text{cm}^3 \text{ or a flow rate of } 63 \, \text{cm}^3 \, \text{s}^{-1}$$

The shape of the myocardium is not uniform and changes throughout the cardiac cycle, which makes taking measurements challenging. The left-ventricular outflow tract (LVOT), however, is circular and remains roughly constant throughout the cardiac cycle. The diameter can be readily measured via TOE and the cross-sectional area estimated. Doppler measurements can then be used to calculate flow velocity in order to estimate a cylinder as above (Figure 12.13).

Unlike the hose example, the blood velocity is not constant and also varies throughout the cardiac cycle. To address this, the Doppler waveform is analyzed. The waveform represents a velocity/time graph; the area under the curve therefore provides the velocity–time integral, in essence a reading of the distance travelled by the observed volume of blood during one cardiac cycle. This may be employed in a modified equation:

Volume = Cross-sectional area × Velocity–time integral

As the volume calculated is that ejected every cardiac cycle, it provides an estimate of stroke volume. When combined with the patient's heart rate, this gives an estimation of cardiac output.

Although calculations are based upon the assumptions that the LVOT is round with a consistent diameter, there is some variation and hence error within

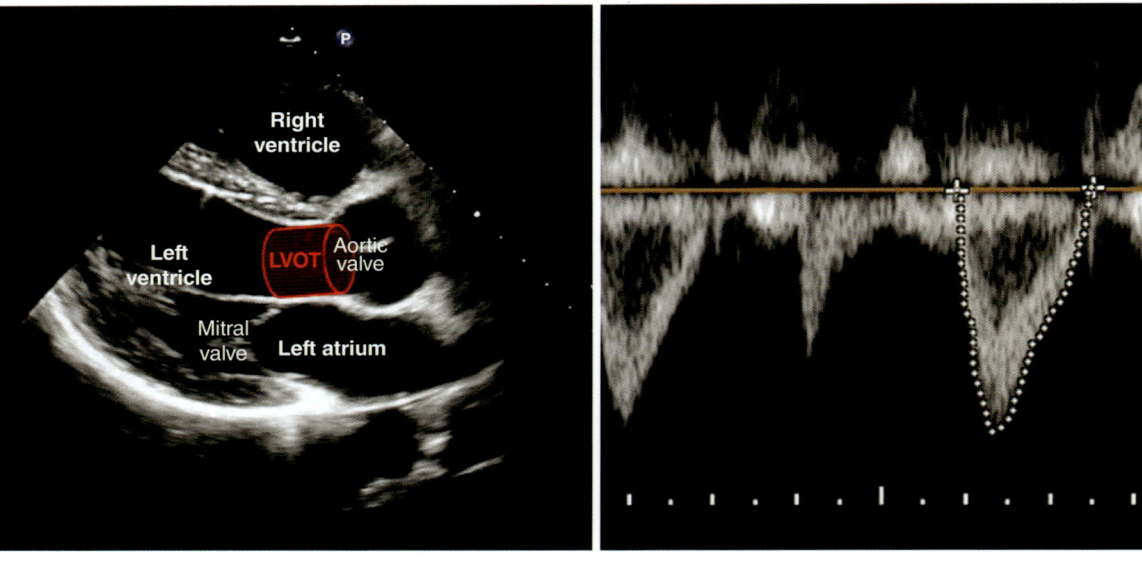

Figure 12.13 Parasternal long-axis echo view (left), demonstrating the position of the LVOT, and the resulting Doppler velocity–time integral (right), which is obtained for cardiac output measurement (Adapted from original images reproduced with permission of Dr B. Scrace)

these estimations. Despite this, a good correlation is achieved when compared to traditional thermodilution techniques.

Left-Ventricular Volumes

The alternative method is to directly measure the volume of the ventricle at its fullest and emptiest and calculate the change in volume. These are the end-diastolic volume (EDV) and the end-systolic volume (ESV), respectively. Hence for the left ventricle (LV):

$$LVSV = LVEDV - LVESV$$

The modified Simpson's rule allows these volumes to be estimated. Two two-dimensional longitudinal views are taken of the ventricle at right angles to each other at end systole. The border of the ventricle is traced and a computer model utilizes the two two-dimensional outlines to produce a series of elliptical discs, representing the three-dimensional ventricle. The individual volumes of the discs are calculated and the overall volume is derived from adding them together (Figure 12.14). The process is repeated at end diastole.

This detailed technique, typically performed during formal transthoracic echocardiography, also offers additional information about ventricular structure and function.

Bio-Impedance

This technology relies on the principle that the electrical impedance of the thorax varies in response to changes in intrathoracic fluid volume. Transthoracic electrical bio-impedance decreases as fluid volume increases. By analyzing the changes in impedance correlated to the cardiac cycle, certain inferences can be made with regard to the cardiac output, systemic vascular resistance and stroke volume.

Six electrodes are placed on the chest wall, and electrical resistance is measured from the outer electrodes towards the innermost. Proprietary algorithms are used to calculate estimates for cardiac output, systemic vascular resistance and stroke volume. These rely on generic assumptions regarding weight, height, gender and age.

In addition to errors introduced by these assumptions, clinical inaccuracies are commonplace due to diathermy currents, movement and arrhythmias, and this technology has not gained popularity yet.

Other Methods

Numerous other methods of cardiac output monitoring are available on the market in differing contexts and environments.

Ultrasound velocity dilution techniques are used more commonly in haemodialysis and extra-corporeal

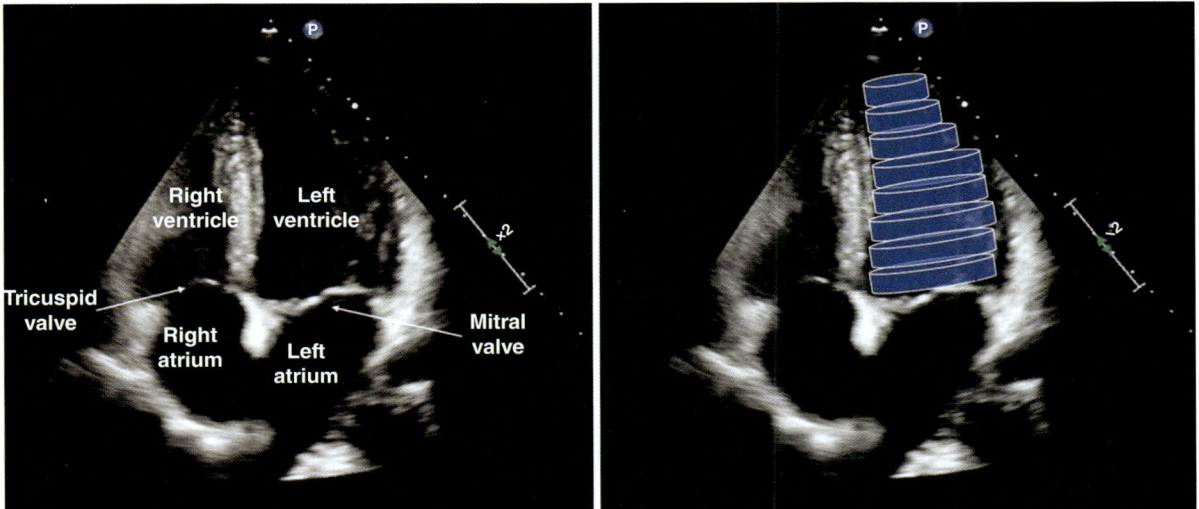

Figure 12.14 Two-dimensional image of the left ventricle (left), and representation of the elliptical discs produced during the combination of an orthogonal image for the modified Simpson's method (right) (Adapted from original images reproduced with permission of Dr B. Scrace)

machines to measure blood flow. The physical properties of blood determine the velocity of ultrasound waves within it. When 0.9% saline is injected into the system, a sensor can be used to measure changes in the ultrasound waveform from which the flow of the blood can be accurately determined. This method is not commonly used in standard ICU or theatre settings.

Magnetic resonance techniques for measuring cardiac output are based on the principle that the resonance properties of a proton are dependent on its velocity. Magnetic resonance is an accurate method of directly measuring cardiac output, but is limited by cost and access to equipment.

Summary

The importance of measurement of cardiac output in the clinical setting is becoming increasingly recognized. There are numerous technological methods for performing such measurements, in addition to good clinical examination. We are yet to discover the perfect machine, and one has to choose the equipment carefully.

The clinical scenario presented at the beginning of the chapter is by no means unusual. In such patients, it is often notoriously difficult to determine whether they need fluids, vasopressors or inotropes.

Indeed, their requirements change with time. The correct use of cardiac output monitors can guide the clinician.

In the most basic analysis of haemodynamic function, the SVV will give an indication of fluid requirement. A high SVV is associated with low preload. However, cardiac arrhythmias can render these investigatory values inaccurate. A low systemic vascular resistance is associated with low vascular tone, and suggests the clinical need for a vasopressor, such as noradrenaline. A low cardiac output (or low stroke volume) suggests a need for inotropic support. It must be remembered, however, that in the real clinical setting, more than one agent is required and, indeed, requirements may change over time.

Table 12.1 will help compare and contrast some of the different machines available.

Questions

MCQs – select true or false for each response

1. Regarding a pulmonary artery catheter (PAC):
   (a) Standard adult lines are 50 cm in length
   (b) A thermistor lies at the distal tip of the catheter

(c) 1.5 ml of air is required to inflate the balloon tip
   (d) Newer PACs do not require the injection of cold saline
   (e) The proximal lumen point may lie outside the heart
2. Which of the following are true regarding cardiac output monitors?
   (a) Magnetic resonance methods of monitoring are impractical due to the invasiveness of the technology
   (b) PACs are used less in modern practice due to inaccuracies with measurement
   (c) Oesophageal Doppler instruments have a good inter-user reliability
   (d) Pulse-contour devices are currently the most commonly used cardiac output devices in Europe
   (e) The use of finger-cuff technology is on the increase due to the value of perioperative goal-directed therapy

SBAs – select the single *best* answer

3. Which of the following statements is the most accurate regarding the use of cardiac output monitoring?
   (a) The use of PACs is decreasing nationally because they are expensive
   (b) Pulse waveform analysis instruments are being increasingly used because they are relatively cheap and minimally invasive
   (c) Finger-cuff technology is the cheapest method available on the market
   (d) Magnetic resonance technology is not used frequently in clinical practice because of the problems associated with sourcing magnetic resonance-safe ventilators and pumps
   (e) The use of bio-impedance has a promising future

Answers

1. FFTTT
   In spite of having many disadvantages, the PAC is still considered as the gold standard method of cardiac output monitoring. A line which was only 50 cm long would be far too short, and the standard adult line is 110 cm. A thermistor usually lies about 3.7 cm from the tip, not at the tip itself.
2. FFFTT
   Magnetic resonance methods of measuring cardiac output are indeed impractical, although not due to their invasiveness. MRI is expensive and the technology requires a lot of room. The reason PACs are used less in modern practice is due largely to the increased complications associated with their insertion and use. However, they are still regarded as one of the most accurate methods of measurement. ODMs have a tendency to be inaccurate due to even the slightest repositioning of the probe. Pulse-contour devices are indeed currently the most commonly used devices in the UK due to their relative non-invasiveness, ease of use and reasonable pricing. Intra-operative goal-directed fluid therapy has been shown to reduce the length of stay and post-operative complications, and in some centres finger-cuff technology is on the increase due to its non-invasiveness.
3. (b)
   All the statements in the question are true to an extent. However, the reason that PAC use is on the decline is multifactorial. Rather than cost, the reasons include the complication rate and the lack of familiarity of the equipment. Finger-cuff technology is relatively cheap, but the cost is comparable to other pulse-contour instruments, as well as Doppler. The actual costs depend on local contracts. Magnetic resonance technology for cardiac output monitoring is impractical and resource-consuming. This is a more valid reason for the lack of use in clinical practice. Bio-impedance technology is still in its infancy. If reliable, accurate and cost-effective instruments can be manufactured, the future may indeed be promising.

Chapter 13

Cardiac Support Equipment

Katie Ramm and Laura May

Learning Objectives

- To explain the principles of blood conservation and red-cell salvage
- To understand and describe the principles of temporary and permanent cardiac pacemakers
- To recall pacemaker classification and implications for anaesthesia
- To understand the electrical principles behind cardiac defibrillators; importance of components of the defibrillator circuit, capacitor function, monophasic and biphasic waveforms
- To understand and explain the principles of cardiopulmonary bypass
- To describe the principles of action, and the uses of, intra-aortic balloon counter-pulsation and other assist devices

Chapter Content

- Cell salvage
- Cardiac pacing and internal cardioverter defibrillators
- Defibrillators
- Cardiopulmonary bypass
- Intra-aortic balloon pumps
- Cardiac assist devices

Scenario

A 72-year-old patient is undergoing major urological surgery. He has a VF cardiac arrest during the case, with return of spontaneous circulation achieved after three shocks. He develops complete heart block for which he undergoes temporary pacing and insertion of an intra-aortic balloon pump to support cardiac function. He subsequently has a permanent pacemaker inserted.

What methods are available to minimize the need for an allogenic blood transfusion perioperatively? Can you give a brief outline of the stages involved in cell salvage? How does a defibrillator work? Think about the circuit diagram for the defibrillator: what are the key components? What methods are available for temporary pacing and what are the anaesthetic implications for a patient with a permanent pacing system? What is an intra-aortic balloon pump, how is it inserted and what is its mechanism of action?

Introduction

Throughout history, few organs have received as much attention in art and literature as the heart. Yet it is only in recent years that procedures to support and operate on the failing heart have been explored. Until the late 1800s the heart was considered untouchable by the surgical community. During a meeting of the Vienna Medical Society in 1881, Theodor Billroth, one of the most innovative surgeons of the time, was reported to have expressed the commonly held belief that, 'No surgeon who wished to preserve the respect of his colleagues would ever attempt to suture a wound of the heart' [1].

The first reported case series of cardiac surgeries were cardiac wound repairs, published in 1906, with survival rates of 40%. At the time, such surgical survival rates were deemed a success and paved the way for simple, elective cardiac procedures to be developed. It was not until the 1950s that innovations in technology and surgical techniques allowed more complex and open-heart procedures to be performed; hypothermia was first described for atrial septal defect repairs, and cardiopulmonary bypass was under development. Some of the earliest cardiopulmonary bypass patients were children undergoing repair of congenital heart defects, using a technique known as controlled cross-circulation. Here, the child's blood was directed from their vena cava to an adult-relative's femoral vein. Oxygenated blood was returned from the adult's femoral artery to the

Chapter 13: Cardiac Support Equipment

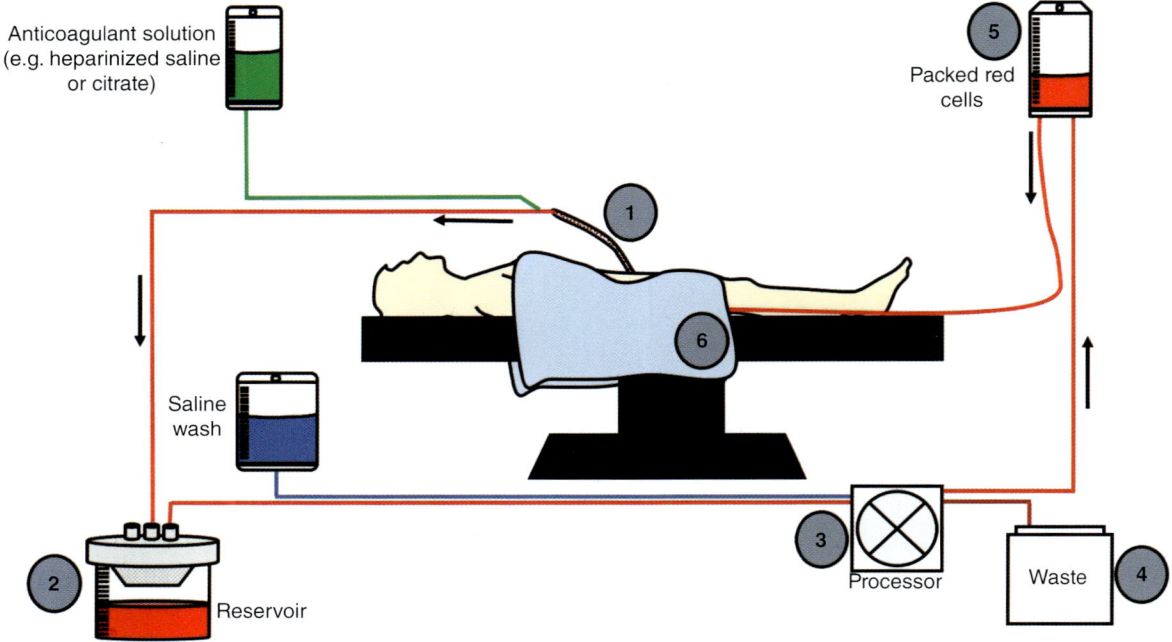

Figure 13.1 Schematic of a cell-salvage circuit

patient's carotid artery. The first open-heart procedures using heart–lung machines had mortality rates of around 50%, but nevertheless provided the encouragement needed to develop the machines which make today's procedures possible.

Having developed ways to correct congenital cardiac defects and techniques of coronary artery bypass grafting, surgeons of the 1960s turned their attention to cardiac transplantation and, in 1967, Christiaan Barnard performed the first human-to-human cardiac transplantation. However, this success gave rise to the need for new technologies as the demand for cardiac transplantation was greater than the supply of hearts to transplant. Ventricular assist devices were duly developed as a bridging therapy for those awaiting transplantation.

As with early forms of cardiopulmonary bypass, cardiac defibrillation and pacing techniques have evolved since the hand-cranked Hyman pacemaker of the 1930s. Attitudes and technology have changed dramatically since the days of Billroth and his contemporaries. It is important that the modern anaesthetist has an understanding of the physical principles behind the equipment used in surgery and support of the failing heart. The following pages will discuss some of the most common equipment encountered.

Cell Salvage

Blood was first transfused in animals in the seventeenth century, but it was not until 1818 that British obstetrician James Blundell performed the first successful human blood transfusion to treat postpartum haemorrhage. Today, around 1.8 million units of blood components are transfused in the UK each year, but less than 4% of adults are currently donors.

Allogenic red-cell transfusion is expensive: testing and processing costs are increasing, and the donor pool is decreasing. It is, also, not without risk. Complications can include febrile, anaphylactic or acute haemolytic transfusion reactions, transfusion-related acute lung injury or circulatory overload. Very rarely, blood may be contaminated with bacteria, viruses, prions or parasites.

Autologous erythrocyte salvage, or 'cell salvage' (Figure 13.1), was developed in the 1970s and is now well established in medical practice, reducing the need for allogeneic blood. Blood is collected from the surgical site, filtered, washed, reconstituted and returned to the patient. This can be a continuous or intermittent process, collected at the time of surgery or from surgical drains post-operatively. Many surgical specialities use cell salvage. Indications include anticipated blood loss >1,000 ml or more than 20% of estimated starting blood volume, preoperative anaemia or patients at a particular risk of bleeding. It can also be considered if a patient refuses an allogenic blood transfusion or has multiple antibodies or rare blood types.

The cell-salvage process can be outlined by the following six stages (Figure 13.1):

1. **Suction:** blood is suctioned from the surgical field to a reservoir via a wide-bore, low-pressure system to minimize haemolysis. The tip of the suction catheter should be fully submerged in a pool of blood to reduce the mixing of blood with air ('skimming'). Skimming will create air bubbles, increasing the surface area of the air–fluid interface, which is where haemolysis tends to occur. Double-lumen tubing is used to allow the delivery of an anticoagulant to the distal end of the catheter to mix immediately with the blood at the point of collection.
2. **Filtration:** the collection reservoir contains a 40–150-μm filter to remove debris and microaggregates from the suction material.
3. **Washing:** the filtered product is centrifuged and washed with sterile isotonic saline. The denser red blood cells move to the outer wall of the centrifuge whilst the less dense plasma collects in the centre. This allows separation and collection of the red cells, although up to one-third of red-cell volume can be lost during this process due to red-cell trauma and lysis.
4. **Disposal:** waste products, which include plasma, white blood cells, platelets, clotting factors, complement, fat, free haemoglobin and anticoagulant, are collected in a bag for disposal.
5. **Cell salvage:** the washed and resuspended red blood cells are collected in a bag ready for reinfusion.
6. **Reinfusion:** the red cells must be reinfused within 4 hours of processing if kept at room temperature. A standard 200-μm blood-giving set is required. As an alternative, a leucodepletion filter can be used (7–10-μm pores), which removes white cells which are implicated in febrile transfusion reactions, alloimmunization and transmission of some viral infections. Anywhere from 50% to 95% of the collected red blood cells are reinfused, depending on the efficiency of the processing. The reinfused solution has a haematocrit between 50% and 70%.

Advantages:
- Reduced need for allogenic blood and its associated risks
- Provides a method of transfusion if the patient has rare blood groups or antibodies
- May be acceptable to some religious groups where allogenic blood may be refused
- No preoperative patient preparation required, therefore useful in emergencies
- Reinfused at room temperature, thus reducing chance of hypothermia and its sequelae
- 2,3-Diphosphoglycerate levels are near-normal compared to stored blood, with consequent improvement in oxygen-carrying capacity
- Cell-salvaged red blood cells have a longer intravascular survival than stored blood
- Reduced long-term costs

Disadvantages:
- High initial costs (machine purchase)
- Cost of disposables
- Requires trained staff
- Time required for collection and processing
- Risk of bacterial contamination
- Risk of air, fat or microembolism
- Coagulopathy – cell-salvaged blood contains no platelets or clotting factors
- Salvaged blood syndrome – acute lung injury and renal failure
- Red-cell lysis during collection and processing – 'skimming'

Cardiac Pacing and Internal Cardioverter Defibrillators

Cardiac pacemakers stimulate the myocardium directly, with the capacity to treat both tachy- and bradyarrhythmias. Both temporary and permanent pacemaker systems are used regularly in clinical practice. External pacing, via specialist defibrillator systems, also has an occasional role in the emergency setting.

Temporary Cardiac Pacing

Temporary cardiac pacing is indicated in a wide array of situations. It can be used in emergency support of a patient with a haemodynamically compromising dysrhythmia. Patients with underlying atrio-ventricular

(AV) block undergoing non-cardiac surgery may have prophylactic pacing in case of progression to complete heart block. Similarly, certain cardiac surgical procedures have a high perioperative risk of high-grade AV block, necessitating backup pacing.

The most common mode of temporary cardiac pacing is trans-venous pacing. Using fluoroscopic guidance, a pacing wire is inserted into the right atrium or ventricle via the internal jugular, subclavian or femoral veins. Once in position, pulses of electric current are transmitted through the electrode to stimulate the heart. Pulses are less than 1 ms in duration and the current required is usually less than 20 mA for atrial and 25 mA for ventricular leads. The pacemaker will sense impedance through the pacing leads and automatically vary the voltage. This ensures that the current delivered to the myocardium matches that set by the operator.

Temporary trans-venous pacemakers also sense myocardial activity and their sensitivity to myocardial activity is set for each patient. Pacemaker sensitivity is the minimum voltage generated by the myocardium that the pacemaker will interpret as a P or an R wave. Usual ranges are 0.4–10 mV for atria and 0.8–20 mV for ventricles. The greater the sensitivity (the lower the value), the more likely it is that interference will be incorrectly interpreted as myocardial depolarization: depending on the pacemaker mode this could lead to inappropriate pacing or inhibition of pacing.

External transthoracic pacing uses a defibrillator with a pacing function to deliver energy via standard defibrillator pads. This is used in emergency situations, often whilst trans-venous pacing is being established. Even though the current is much lower than for defibrillation, it is uncomfortable for the patient as the muscles of the chest wall also contract with every impulse transmitted.

In the conscious patient, trans-oesophageal pacing is better tolerated than external pacing. An electrode is placed in the mid-to-lower oesophagus for atrial pacing, or the fundus of the stomach for ventricular stimulation. However, trans-oesophageal pacing is less commonly used, due to the relative complexity of passing the electrode down the oesophagus, compared to applying external adhesive pads.

Epicardial pacing requires pacing leads to be attached directly to the epicardium, therefore this is a method of pacing used after open cardiac surgery.

Permanent Cardiac Pacing

Cardiac pacemakers are highly sophisticated electronic implants that monitor and respond to intrinsic electrical signals, sensed within the heart. The first pacemaker was implanted in 1958 and now there are an estimated 900,000 patients who receive pacemaker therapy worldwide every year. The most common indication for long-term cardiac pacing in the UK is for those forms of acquired AV block with a high-risk of asystole: third-degree heart block or symptomatic second-degree heart block.

Permanent pacemakers are usually inserted by cardiologists under local anaesthesia. They consist of a pacing box (otherwise referred to as the pulse generator) and one or more leads. Pacing boxes, made of titanium or a titanium alloy, are impermeable to air and water and are smaller than the average matchbox. They are often embedded in the pre-pectoral fascia, just below the clavicle. Also, they can be inserted in the axilla, or the abdomen, for femoral venous insertions. The pulse generator is the control hub of the pacemaker system and contains a battery, usually lithium iodide, as well as the circuits that control the pacemaker's functions. The battery life is anywhere from 5 years to 11 years, depending on the degree of sophistication of the pacemaker and its use.

One or more electrode leads exit the pacemaker casing and travel intravenously to the heart, attaching to the endocardium. Pacemakers are either single-chamber, dual-chamber or biventricular, with leads terminating in the right atrium, right ventricle or coronary sinus (for left-ventricular pacing). Note that the term biventricular does not mean an electrode is placed in the left ventricle itself. The pacing leads transmit electrical impulses to and from the heart and pacemaker. All modern pacemakers can also communicate with an external programming device via radiofrequency communication.

The electrode leads are small, insulated, flexible wires. The pacemaker system (or 'PPM') is either unipolar or, more frequently, bipolar (Figure 13.2). In a unipolar system, a single electrode in the heart forms the cathode. The pacing box forms the anode, completing the circuit. In a bipolar system, both the anode and cathode are within the heart. Usually, both electrodes are combined in a single coaxial trans-venous wire, with the exposed conducting elements a short distance apart at the end of the wire. The most

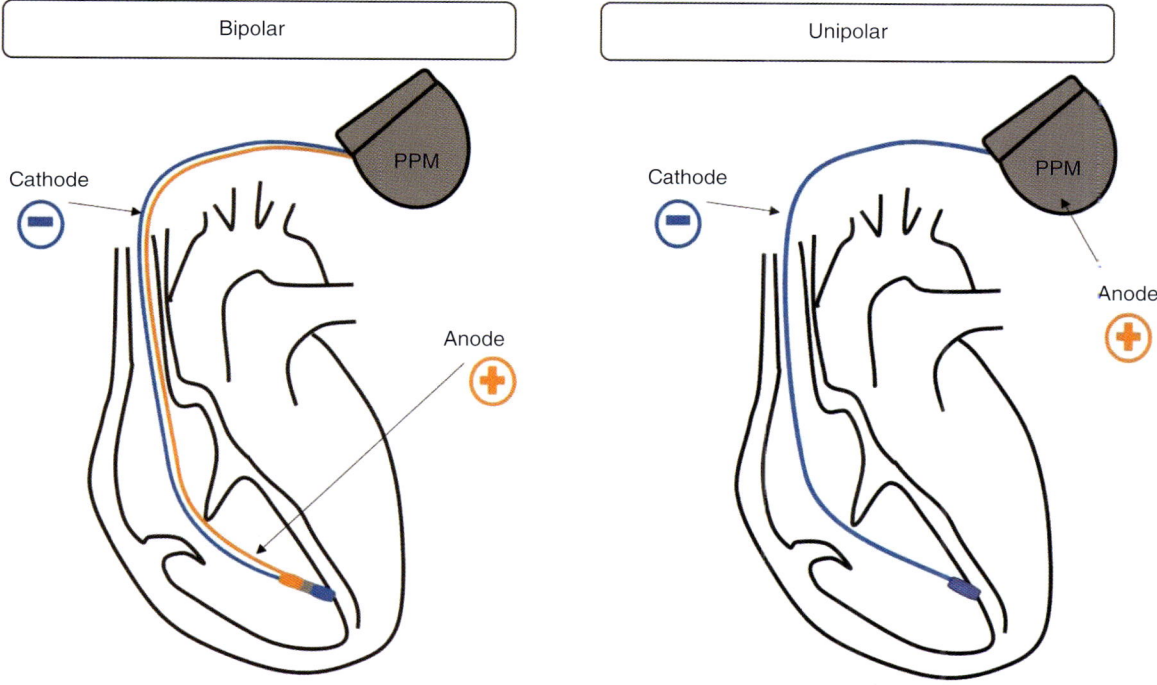

Figure 13.2 Schematic of bipolar and unipolar implanted pacemaker systems

common configuration for a bipolar lead is of a tip electrode on the end of the wire, complemented by a ring electrode, about 2 cm proximal to this. As the name suggests, a ring electrode is simply a portion of the conductor which is circumferentially exposed through the insulating material of the lead.

Unipolar leads are simpler, thicker, stronger and cheaper to manufacture. They are more sensitive than bipolar leads as they pick up signals over a more extensive length at the end of the wire, but this means more interference and a greater potential for malfunction. Bipolar leads therefore have a better signal-to-noise ratio and so these systems are more selective in when they pace. The pacing 'spike' from a bipolar system is usually much smaller on the surface ECG than with a unipolar system, as only a small volume of myocardium between the anode and cathode is depolarized. Note also that the term 'bipolar' only refers to the design of the lead, not to which chambers are involved.

The electrodes are made of platinum, titanium, silver, stainless steel, or various alloys. They either screw into the myocardium (active fixation) or anchor onto the surface of the heart (passive fixation). Fibrosis then occurs around the electrodes over the following months, thus reinforcing the fixation. The pacemaker generates an electrical current for a duration of approximately 1 ms. The pulse travels down the lead(s) causing myocardial depolarization and contraction if the energy applied is greater than the excitation threshold of the local cells. The lowest voltage to cause depolarization is used; this is known as the pacing threshold and is typically around 4–5 V. Many factors can affect the pacing threshold, including hypoxia, hypercarbia, acidosis, deranged electrolytes and altered temperature, together with many drugs and medications, particularly anti-arrhythmic agents. These factors are, of course, the same factors which alter the threshold potential for native myocardial depolarization. It is important to realize that many of these may be deranged in the acutely unwell patient, with consequent risk of pacemaker dysfunction.

As with temporary trans-venous pacing, the intrinsic myocardial activity is also sensed by the pacemaker leads. The atrial lead senses the P waves,

Table 13.1 Generic pacemaker codes (Adapted from The Revised NASPE/BPEG Generic Code for Antibradycardia, Adaptive-Rate, and Multisite Pacing [2])

Letter 1	Letter 2	Letter 3	Letter 4	Letter 5
Chamber paced	Chamber sensed	Response to sensed impulse	Program options	Anti-tachycardia response
O – None A – Atrium V – Ventricle D – Dual	O – None A – Atrium V – Ventricle D – Dual	O – None I – Inhibited T – Triggered D – Dual	O – None P – Programmable M – Multiprogram C – Communicating R – Rate modulation	O – None P – Paces S – Shocks D – Dual

and the ventricular lead the QRS complex. A pacemaker can be programmed to inhibit or trigger pacing if intrinsic activity is sensed.

Pacemaker Codes

Pacemakers are classified according to their mode of pacing. The North American Society of Pacing and Electrophysiology (NASPE) and the British Pacing and Electrophysiology Group (BPEG) produced a generic lettering code of up to five letters to define pacemakers. The first three letters of the code relate to the anti-bradycardia functions; the first letter indicates the chamber(s) paced, the second chamber(s) sensed, and the third describes the response to the sensed electrical activity. The fourth letter represents programmability, and the fifth, anti-tachycardia features. This is summarized in Table 13.1.

For example:

- VVI – Ventricle paced, ventricle sensed, pacing inhibited if a beat sensed, i.e. demand pacing
- VVIR – Demand ventricular pacing with a physiologic response to exercise
- DDD – Atria and ventricle can both be paced, atrium and ventricle are both sensed, pacing triggered in each chamber if no beat sensed

Leadless Pacemakers

In 2013, the first leadless, retrievable, permanent pacemaker was inserted in a patient. The device consists of a metal cylinder, a few centimetres in length, which is inserted via the femoral vein into the heart. This should be safer and more comfortable for patients. There will be no visible pacemaker device under the patient's skin and no incision scar. The infection risk associated with the leads and the risk of lead dysfunction are eliminated. The whole device is fully retrievable unlike the leads of existing pacemakers, which require surgical removal.

Implantable Cardioverter Defibrillators

Since the first implantable cardioverter defibrillator (ICD) was inserted in 1980, The National Institute for Health and Clinical Excellence (NICE) has issued guidance on increasing implantation rates. The UK is now averaging rates close to 50 insertions per million population per year. The indications for ICD insertion are for patients with severe left-ventricular dysfunction, those at risk of ventricular tachycardia (VT) or ventricular fibrillation (VF) (primary prevention), those with a history of syncopal VT, or following a VF/VT arrest (secondary prevention).

Much like an implanted pacemaker, the ICD pulse generator has several components: a lithium iodide battery, a capacitor, a microprocessor (which manages the defibrillator function) and an event recorder. An ICD can also be dual-function, operating as both a defibrillator and a permanent pacemaker. The pulse generator needs changing every 5–9 years. The ICD constantly monitors the intrinsic rhythm. When a ventricular arrhythmia is sensed, the ICD either delivers a shock or uses anti-tachycardia pacing to override the rhythm, followed by a shock if this is unsuccessful.

More recently, a subcutaneous ICD (S-ICD) has been developed. This device can deliver sufficient energy to defibrillate the heart without the need for leads. This therefore removes the risks and complications associated with leads and their insertion.

The NASPE/BPEG defibrillator code uses four letters to describe the features of the ICD. The first letter indicates the shock chamber and the second the chamber where anti-tachycardia pacing is delivered. The third letter indicates how tachyarrhythmias are detected, either by the intracardiac electrogram alone or with haemodynamic detection as well. The fourth letter may be replaced with the pacemaker code. For example, a ventricular defibrillator with haemodynamic or ECG tachyarrhythmia detection and with rate-modulating ventricular anti-bradycardia pacing would be labelled VOH-VVIR.

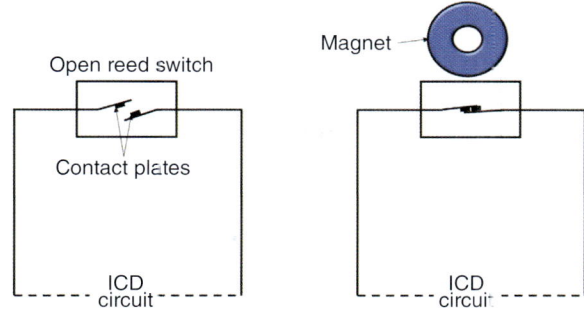

Figure 13.3 Magnet-operated reed switch in an ICD

Implications for Anaesthesia

Patients with implanted pacemakers and ICDs are provided with a registration card or 'passport', with essential details regarding the device *in situ*, including:

- Device manufacturer, model and serial number
- Date of implant
- Implanting hospital and follow-up hospital
- Indication

Prior to surgery, the information on this card should be reviewed, as well as determining the date of the last device check (ideally within the last 3 months), the remaining battery life, the degree of pacemaker dependency and information about cardiac function.

Most modern pacemakers work on-demand and have a rate-responsive feature allowing an appropriate rate adjustment in response to a physiological stress. This rate-responsive feature should be deactivated prior to anaesthesia as shivering, fasciculations, warming and movement can all cause unwanted tachycardia. The device may have a programmed sleeping period, with a lower intrinsic or paced rate at night, which may require deactivation, e.g. for out-of-hours surgery or a critical care patient. There are several types of sensor in use, the most common being activity sensors. These sense muscular activity by utilizing piezoelectric-based sensors or an accelerometer to detect changes in posture and movement. Other systems involve evaluation of the QT interval or changes in minute ventilation (measuring changes in transthoracic impedance), via the pacemaker leads. Micro-accelerometers placed in the tip of a unipolar pacing lead can also be used to detect vibration around the pacing box to create a rate-adaptive response.

Pacemakers and ICDs have a high degree of tolerance to electromagnetic interference and contain filters to reduce the effects of such radiation. However, high-intensity sources may still affect their function. In the operating theatre, electrosurgical equipment, especially diathermy, can cause interference. This interference can be misinterpreted as cardiac activity and cause pacing inhibition. Overwhelming background noise can be sensed and trigger spontaneous reprogramming of the device, for example from DDD to VOO. This could cause haemodynamic instability, even VF or asystole. Leads can become overheated, damaged or even dislodged, resulting in loss of capture. Bipolar diathermy is safer but, if monopolar must be used, the diathermy plate should be placed as far away from the pacemaker as possible, and the minimum effective current used in short bursts. If an ICD is *in situ*, defibrillation and anti-tachycardia functions should be deactivated in case of adverse responses to interference.

MRI in patients with a permanent pacemaker is relatively contraindicated. Devices can be damaged or reprogrammed, or pacing can be inhibited or inappropriately triggered. Local heating can also cause discomfort. However, MRI-compatible pacemakers are being developed and may become standard in years to come.

Pacemakers contain a magnet-operated reed switch (Figure 13.3). This is a very simple arrangement of two thin metal plates. The switch usually sits open but when a magnetic field is applied directly over the switch the reeds are attracted by the field and brought together. When the contact plates are opposed, the circuit is completed (Figure 13.3). The effect of closing this circuit depends on the pacemaker manufacturer, model and the remaining battery level. Placing a magnet over the pacemaker may cause no apparent change, may induce fixed pacing or may cause transient or continuous loss of pacing, with potentially catastrophic results. Patients with pacemakers should therefore avoid sources of strong electromagnetic interference. When a magnet is placed over an ICD, shock therapy may be inhibited whilst the magnet remains over the device, but only if programmed to do so. A magnet can therefore be placed over some devices for the duration of surgery. Any subsequent arrhythmias should be treated using external defibrillation equipment. Wherever the situation allows, best practice is to ask the cardiac physiologist to formally check and reprogramme the device in the anaesthetic room and again in the recovery room.

Defibrillators

In Switzerland in 1899, physiologists Prevost and Battelli discovered that small electric shocks induced ventricular fibrillation in dogs, with larger shocks reversing the arrhythmia. The defibrillator was subsequently invented in 1932 by Dr William Bennett Kouwenhoven. It was not until 1956, however, that external defibrillators were developed. Kouwenhoven and co-workers also published the first description of modern, closed chest-compression CPR in 1961 [3].

A defibrillator is a device that monitors the heart rhythm and delivers electrical energy to the myocardium. The energy causes simultaneous depolarization of myocardial cells, extending their refractory period, with the aim of restoring normal electrical activity. Defibrillators can be manual internal and external devices, automated, implantable and even wearable.

Defibrillation is the application of a direct current (DC) to treat VF or pulseless VT. The energy delivery is immediate, irrespective of the cardiac electrical cycle: it is asynchronous. Some defibrillators have the ability to perform cardioversion, where the administration of a DC shock is synchronized with the upstroke of the QRS complex. The aim is to convert pulsed tachyarrhythmias to normal sinus rhythm. If the energy is supplied at the wrong point in the cardiac cycle, cardioversion may fail. If the energy is delivered during the relative refractory period (corresponding to the T wave on the ECG), VT, VF or Torsade de Pointes may result; this is an example of R-on-T phenomenon (the R wave in this case is referring to the cardioversion energy).

Types of Defibrillators

Defibrillators can be classified according to their electrical systems as follows:

- Energy-based
  - The vast majority of defibrillators are energy-based, charging a capacitor by high-voltage DC (HV DC) and subsequently delivering the chosen amount of energy
- Impedance-based
  - Transthoracic impedance is assessed by means of a test pulse; the current is then selected based upon the transthoracic impedance
- Current-based
  - This delivers a fixed amount of current, independent of transthoracic impedance

Components of a Defibrillator

The key electrical components of a defibrillator are seen in Figure 13.4. These essentially consist of a power supply, capacitor, inductor and patient interface. These can be functionally divided into two principal circuits: the charging circuit (connecting a power source to a capacitor) and the patient circuit (connecting the patient to the same capacitor) (Figure 13.5).

The power to the charging circuit can be supplied as either mains power or by using an internal battery. Whichever power source is used, the patient will receive DC, as it causes less myocardial cell damage and is less arrhythmogenic than alternating current (AC). Converting voltage to DC also allows charge to be stored by a capacitor and energy to be discharged in a controlled manner.

For a 240-V AC mains supply, a step-up transformer must first be used to increase the voltage. Variable-voltage step-up transformers (producing voltages usually between 200 V and 5,000 V) can be used to allow the clinician to select different energy settings. A transformer relies on a constantly changing magnetic flux to induce a current in the secondary coil, so a DC current will not work. For this reason, if the internal battery is used (DC supply), the current must first be converted to AC before it can be transformed to provide the selected energy level. An inverter is a device or circuit that converts DC to AC (Figure 13.4). There are many different designs of inverter, such as mechanical, transistor-based and semi-conductor switches, which all rapidly alter the direction of electron flow in a circuit.

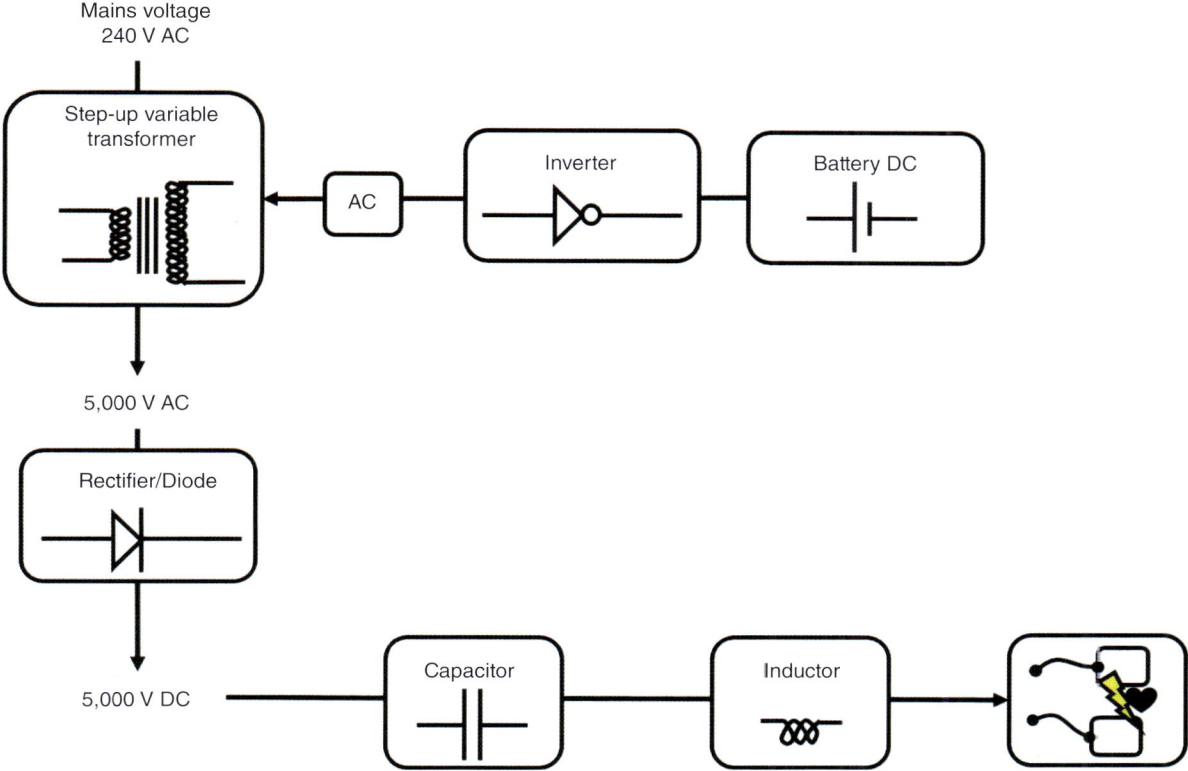

Fig 13.4 A schematic of the electronic components of a defibrillator

After the step-up transformer, the HV AC must now be converted back to DC by a rectifier. A rectifier describes a variety of different semiconductor devices, which essentially act as diodes, allowing current to flow only in one direction.

A capacitor is a device that stores electrical charge. It is usually formed by two conducting surfaces, separated by an insulator known as a dielectric. Once the 'charge' button is pressed, electrons flow from the negative terminal of the power source to one plate of the capacitor, rendering this plate negatively charged. Electrons flow from the other plate of the capacitor to the positive terminal of the power source, leaving that plate positively charged. This charge separation results in an electric field across the plates, which acts as a store of electrical potential energy.

The capacitance (C) refers to how much charge can be stored by the capacitor. It is the ratio of the charge (Q) on each conducting plate to the voltage (V) of the circuit. Its SI unit is the farad (F), defined as one coulomb of charge per volt of potential difference between the conducting plates

$$C = \frac{Q}{V}$$

The potential energy stored by the capacitor is the area under a graph of the charge accumulated on the conducting surface against the potential difference between the capacitor plates (Figure 13.6). It can be expressed as:

$$E = \frac{1}{2}QV$$
$$= \frac{1}{2}\frac{Q^2}{C}$$
$$= \frac{1}{2}CV^2$$

As a capacitor plate becomes more negatively charged it becomes less attractive to electrons. This causes

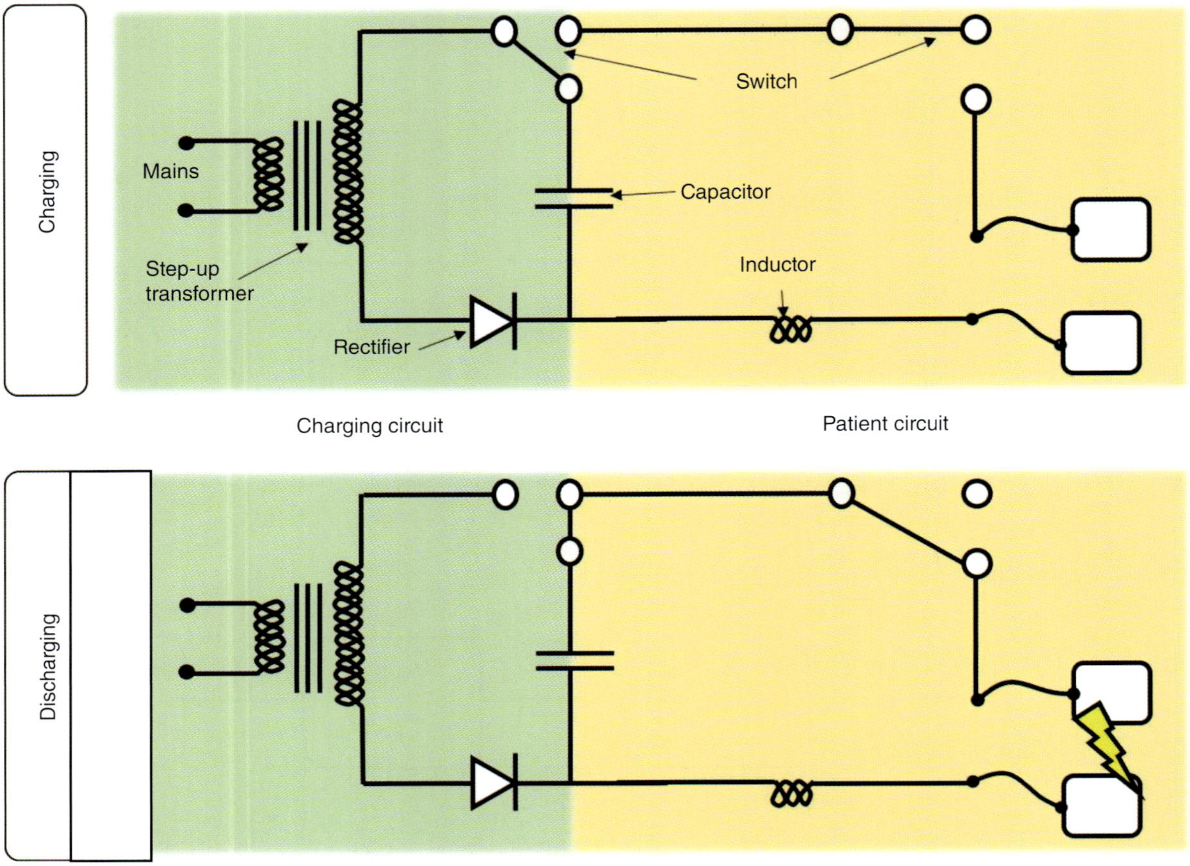

Chapter 13: Cardiac Support Equipment

Figure 13.5 A charging and discharging defibrillator

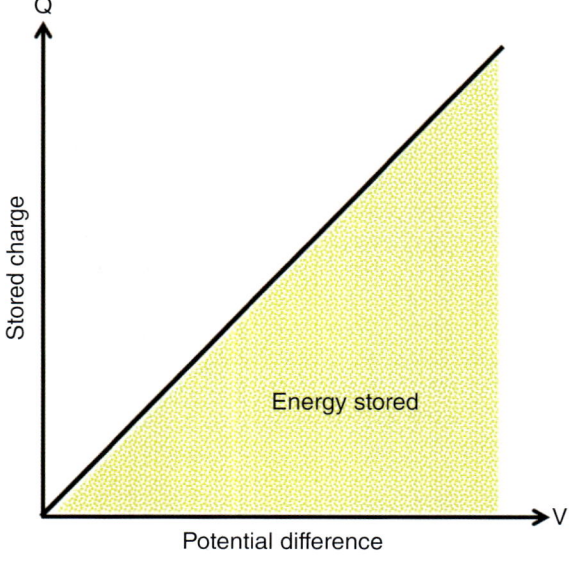

Fig 13.6 Relationship between voltage and stored charge for a capacitor

current around the circuit to reduce in an exponential manner, with a reduction in the rate of change of charge and voltage, expressed as a negative exponential build-up curve (Figure 13.7).

When the electrodes are connected to the patient, the circuit is completed when the 'Shock' button is pressed. Electrons stored on the negative side of the plate flow via one electrode, through the patient and back to the positive terminal of the power source. The potential difference falls to zero, discharging the capacitor exponentially, for the same reasons that charge accumulated in an exponential fashion initially. For successful defibrillation, the current flow must be maintained for several milliseconds. An inductor is therefore used to further prolong the duration of the current flow by modifying the waveform from the basic exponential function. Energy is absorbed by the inductor. The energy selected on the defibrillator refers to the amount of energy that is delivered; more is stored in the capacitor so as to account for such losses (Figure 13.8).

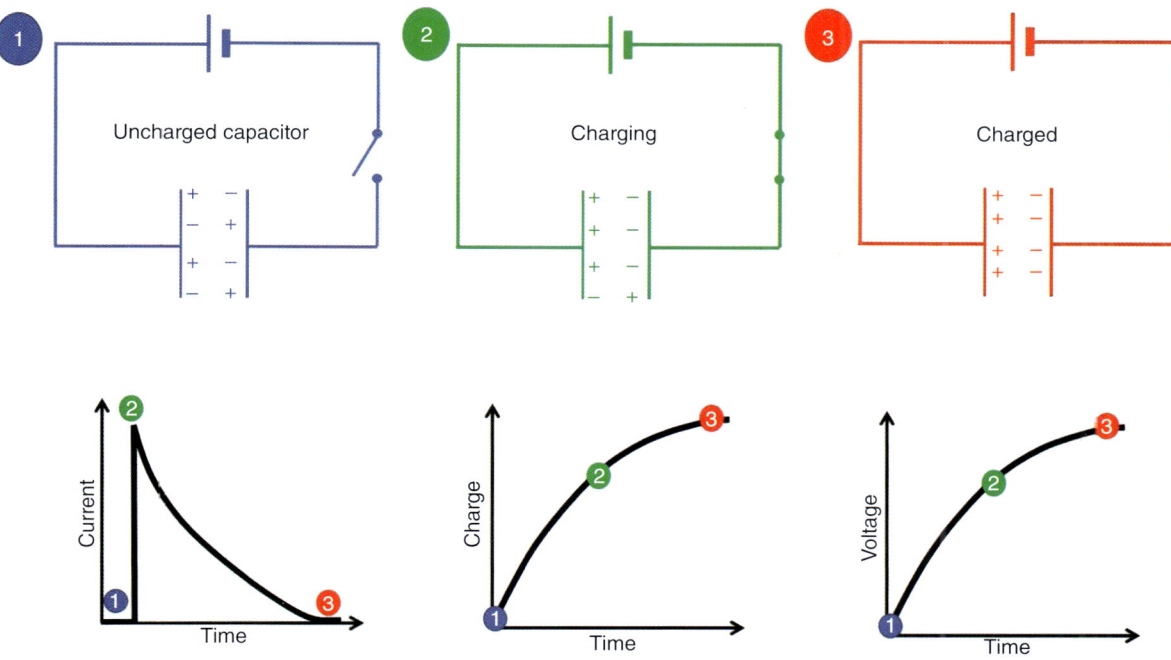

Fig 13.7 Relationship between current, charge and voltage for a capacitor with time

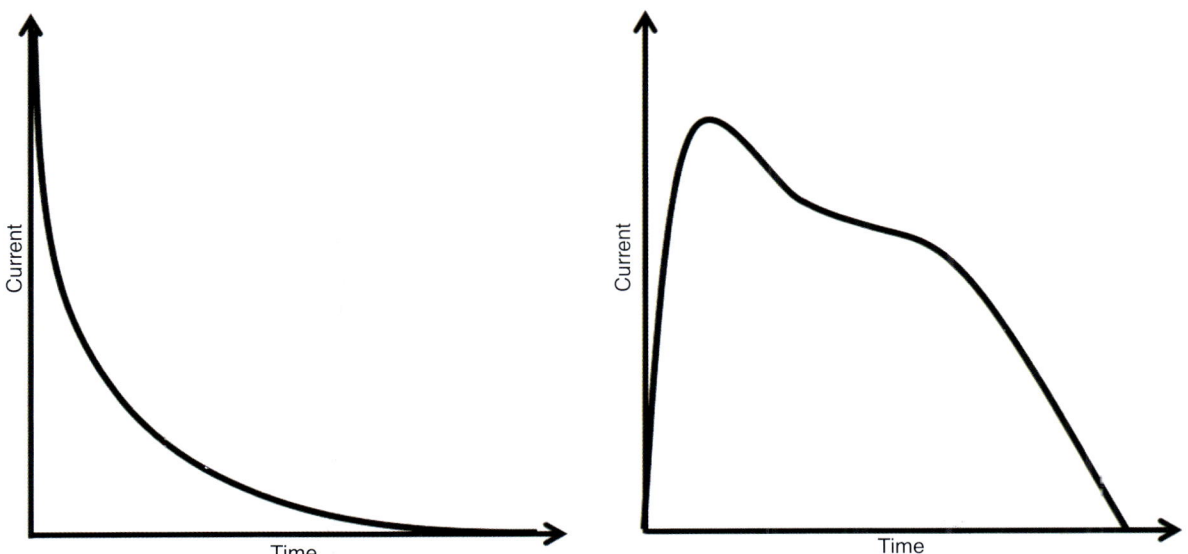

Figure 13.8 Current against time plots for standard capacitor discharge (left) compared with discharge modified by an inductor (right)

Depending on the waveform of discharge, the pad size used, the size of the patient and other factors, successful defibrillation requires a current of around 35 A to be passed through the chest to allow sufficient energy to reach the heart. Most of this is dissipated in the skin and chest wall tissues, and crossing the air/tissue gap of the lungs. This loss is quantified by the transthoracic impedance (which is at its lowest at end-expiration when the lungs are minimally aerated). The transthoracic impedance is between 50 Ω and

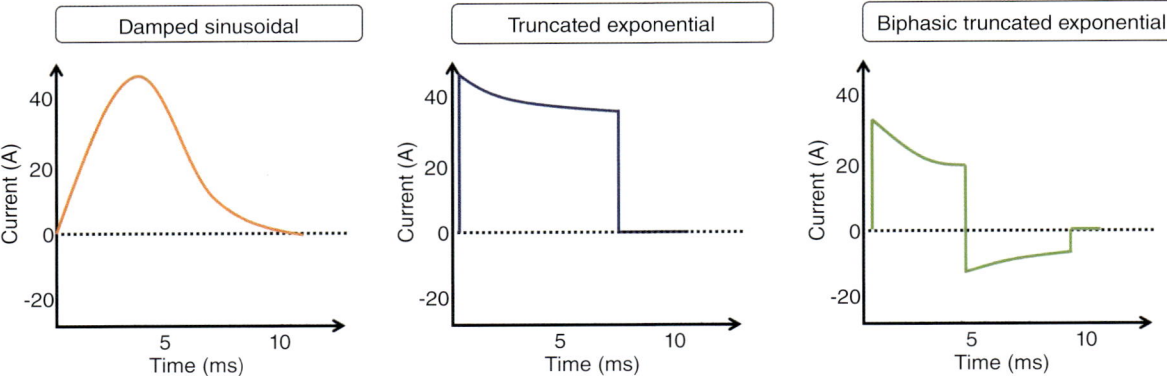

Figure 13.9 Typical defibrillator waveforms: damped sinusoidal (left), truncated exponential (centre) and biphasic truncated exponential (right)

150 Ω. By contrast, internal or implanted defibrillators only have the impedance of cardiac tissue to contend with (about 20 Ω). Internal defibrillation can be achieved with 1–2 A, delivered with a voltage of around 30 V (equating to a 30–40 J shock). Modern biphasic defibrillators measure the thoracic impedance and adjust the energy delivery during the shock accordingly; this is called impedance compensation.

Electrodes

Electrodes are connected to the patient and allow both sensing of the electrocardiogram signal and also delivery of the energy to the patient. Modern electrodes fall into two groups: internal paddles and self-adhesive, disposable external pads.

Standard adult disposable electrodes are around 8 cm × 13 cm in diameter. The larger the pad, the lower the resistance. The electrodes need to be in good contact with the skin to reduce transthoracic impedance and maximize the current flow. Disposable self-adhesive electrodes have superseded handheld external paddles. They conform to the chest better and deliver the current more efficiently as well as increasing safety for the operator. Pads degrade with repeated shocks and should generally be replaced after 10 successive shocks (sooner if they have become dislodged by chest compressions).

Four different positions are acceptable:

- Antero-lateral (default position)
- Antero-posterior
- Postero-lateral
- Bi-axillary

Waveforms

Energy delivery can be represented on a graph as current versus time. Inductors can modify these waveforms in a variety of sophisticated ways. The waveforms produced can be either monophasic or, now more typically, biphasic (Figure 13.9).

Monophasic defibrillators were developed first but are no longer manufactured. Current is delivered in one direction through the patient. If the current pulse decreases to zero gradually, as is the case for the majority of monophasic waveforms, this is known as damped sinusoidal. If the waveform initially follows an exponential decay and then falls instantaneously it is known as truncated exponential (Figure 13.9, left and centre).

Modern defibrillators produce a biphasic waveform, which is two truncated exponential waveforms, travelling sequentially across the myocardium (Figure 13.9, right). The current delivered flows in one direction between the electrodes and then reverses and flows in the opposite direction. Biphasic waveforms have a lower defibrillation threshold, which allows a reduction in the amount of energy required for successful defibrillation and therefore results in less myocardial damage. First-shock efficacy is also greater with biphasic devices.

Cardiopulmonary Bypass

Cardiopulmonary bypass (CPB) is a process whereby the function of the heart and lungs is taken over by a machine, maintaining circulation and oxygen delivery. This is mainly utilized in cardiothoracic surgery

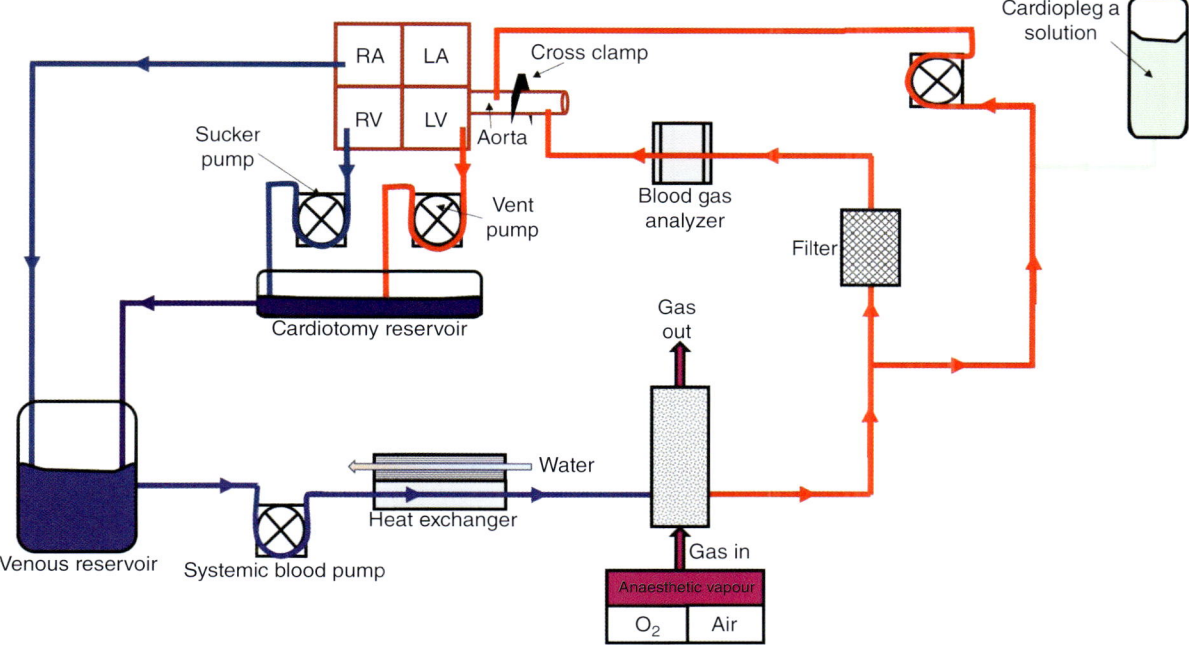

Figure 13.10 Schematic of a CPB circuit

to provide a bloodless, motionless field. The first successful open-heart procedure using CPB was performed by John Gibbon in 1953 in Philadelphia, repairing an atrial septal defect in an 18-year-old. A variation on the principle, extra-corporeal membrane oxygenation (ECMO), is used for advanced respiratory support and this can also be utilized to provide extended-duration support in cardiac arrest, for example, in cases of profound hypothermia. This is referred to as ECLS – extra-corporeal life support.

Principles

Prior to use, the circuit (Figure 13.10) is primed, usually with crystalloid. Blood can also be used as the priming fluid. This is typical in paediatric practice, where a large volume of crystalloid entering the circulation at commencement of CPB would cause significant haemodilution. Other substances such as heparin, mannitol or bicarbonate can be added to the prime. The tubing is made of polyvinyl chloride (PVC) and coated with heparin to reduce activation of the clotting cascade and an inflammatory response.

Sites for the cannulae, which need to be inserted for connection of the patient to the machine, depend on the proposed operation. The arterial cannula is often placed in the ascending aorta, but axillary and femoral arteries are alternatives. One venous cannula may be placed in the right atrium, or two in the superior and inferior vena cavae. Before cannulation or commencing CPB, the patient must be anticoagulated. This is typically achieved with intravenous unfractionated heparin.

During CPB, the aorta is usually cross-clamped distal to the origin of the coronary arteries. This means that no blood can flow around the coronary circulation. Instead, cardioplegic solutions (containing mainly potassium) can be infused into the coronary circulation. This is achieved via a cannula inserted into the aortic root. Cardioplegia leads to diastolic electromechanical arrest. This provides a motionless surgical field and protects the myocardium from the effects of minimal perfusion whilst on CPB.

A perfusionist, in communication with the surgeon and anaesthetist, operates the bypass machine. Once CPB is initiated, venous blood drains via the venous cannula(e) into a venous reservoir, under the influence of gravity. Suctioned blood from the surgical field can also empty into the reservoir. Some blood will continue to drain into the left ventricle; this is

Chapter 13: Cardiac Support Equipment

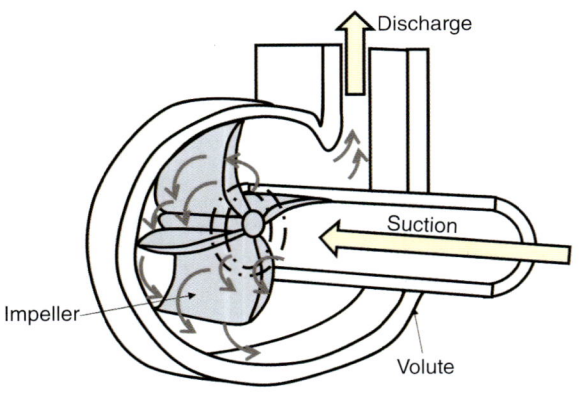

Figure 13.11 Cutaway schematic of the impeller within a centrifugal pump

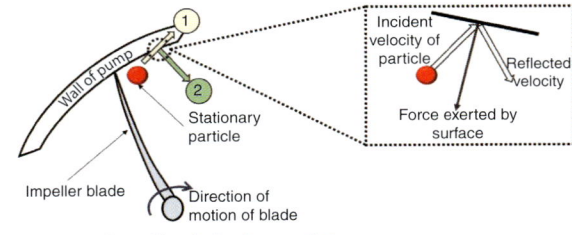

(1) Direction of travel if no further force applied
(2) Direction of force applied by collision with pump wall

Figure 13.12 Forces acting upon blood cells at the tip of the impeller blade

mainly blood and cardioplegia draining out of the myocardium from the Thebesian veins. This would continue to accumulate and so is usually collected by a 'vent' line to drain into the CPB reservoir. This venting is important as it reduces pressure within the arrested ventricle, which might otherwise reduce perfusion of the myocardium with cardioplegia.

From the reservoir, blood passes through a bubble trap into either a roller or centrifugal pump. The pump is carefully controlled by the perfusionist to produce the correct blood flow to achieve the required mean arterial pressure. A roller pump compresses the tubing, squeezing the blood along the circuit. A centrifugal pump uses a magnetically spun impeller that revolves at high speed (Figure 13.11).

The impeller blades accelerate the blood, thereby increasing the kinetic energy of the fluid. The blood will tend to move in a straight line, perpendicular to the rotation of the impeller blade (Newton's first law). When confined by the circular wall of the pump, the moving blood is acted upon by another force – centripetal force – which tends to push blood to the centre of the pump. This force is produced by the walls of the container. Centrifugal force is the equal and opposite reaction (Newton's third law) to the centripetal force and tends to push the blood out towards the sides of the container. The effect is to cause a change in momentum of the blood (Newton's second law, i.e. to change the speed and direction of the blood). In this case, the blood is accelerated around the wall of the pump (Figure 13.12). This causes a relative pressure gradient, with high pressure at the outer wall of the pump and low pressure at the centre. The in-flow port is located near the central axis of the pump where the pressure is low; this generates the suction to draw blood into the pump. The outflow port is located on the side wall of the pump where pressure is high and this allows the blood to be ejected from the pump. The pressure produced at the outer edge of the pump increases as the rate of rotation of the impeller blades increases, but is also affected by other features of the whole circuit, such as:

- Fluid viscosity
- Tube diameter
- Elevation difference between the venous reservoir and the patient
- Presence of air bubbles or blood clots in the circuit

Air bubbles are of particular concern. Air is compressible, meaning that the force required to compress or expand air bubbles is small in comparison to the force needed to overcome gravity and friction in drawing blood into the pump. In this way, the presence of elastic air bubbles will inhibit the action of the pump, as the energy of the pump is consumed in squashing the bubbles, rather than moving blood around the pump. When this happens, the negative pressure required to draw fluid into the pump is not achieved and an air lock is created.

From the pump, blood passes through a heat exchanger to regulate the temperature of the blood. Surgery is performed under hypothermic conditions to provide protection to the vital organs against the decreased blood flow they experience on CPB. The heat exchanger works by forced convection and conduction; it circulates a temperature-controlled water phase in a counter-current manner against a blood phase, separated from each other by a highly conductive surface such as stainless steel or aluminium.

Water has a specific heat capacity (SHC) of 4,181 J kg^{-1} K^{-1} and blood, 3,490 J kg^{-1} K^{-1}. The greater SHC of water means that more energy is required to change the temperature of the water than that of the blood. This means that changes in the temperature of water will have a greater effect on the temperature of the blood rather than the other way around. The rate of heat transfer depends on the SHC of different elements of the system, the temperature gradient and the surface area over which heat exchange takes place. The efficiency of the system is increased by having the water and blood flow running in opposite directions past each other – a counter-current arrangement. This maintains a temperature gradient between both fluids at all points of the exchanger so that energy is transferred from start to finish of the apparatus. There are limitations to the design of the exchanger. Firstly, as the solubility of a gas within a liquid decreases as the temperature of the liquid rises (Henry's law – see Chapter 4), rapid temperature changes, caused by a large temperature gradient across the heat exchanger, could cause gas to come out of solution and form air emboli. Secondly, the surface area is limited by the volume of crystalloid required to prime the system; large-surface-area exchangers require prohibitively large crystalloid priming volumes, which lead to problems with haemodilution at commencement of CPB.

The blood then passes to an oxygenator and gas exchanger to add oxygen and remove carbon dioxide. Bubble oxygenators, where oxygen was literally bubbled through the blood, have been superseded by membrane oxygenators, which imitate the human lung more closely. They consist of a thin membrane of polypropylene or silicone rubber, made into sheets or hollow fibres. The carrier gas – an air–oxygen mixture – passes through the layers of the membrane. Meanwhile, the blood flows in a thin film over the surface of the membrane, allowing diffusion of oxygen and carbon dioxide down their concentration gradients. The partial pressure of oxygen achieved in the blood can be adjusted by altering the partial pressure of oxygen in the carrier gas. Gas flow determines the amount of carbon dioxide that diffuses out of the blood. The greater the gas flow, the greater the amount of carbon dioxide extracted from the blood. Vaporizers can also be incorporated into this system. This allows volatile anaesthetic agents to be added to the carrier gas as a means by which to maintain anaesthesia after lung ventilation has ceased on CPB.

A haemofilter can also be included in the CPB circuit should the patient require concurrent renal support.

After the membrane oxygenator the blood then passes through another bubble trap and filter (typically 150 to 300 μm) to remove clots and bubbles before returning to the patient via the arterial cannula.

Intra-aortic Balloon Pumps

Since the introduction of the intra-aortic balloon pump (IABP) into clinical practice in the 1960s, it has remained the most effective and widely used temporary device for mechanically supporting a failing heart.

Principles

An IABP is placed in the descending aorta and is rapidly inflated and deflated, displacing the column of blood in the aorta, both distally and proximally, on inflation. The timing of inflation with the start of diastole and deflation with systole is described as counter-pulsation. This improves cardiac function by altering both preload and afterload, with the net effect of rebalancing the oxygen supply–demand relationship for the heart (Figure 13.13).

An IABP incorporates an 8–10-French-gauge double-lumen catheter with a 25–50-ml balloon at the distal end, connected to a computer-controlled pump, which drives the gas to inflate and deflate the balloon. Helium is the gas of choice. It has a low density and relatively high viscosity, ensuring a low Reynold's number and so a predisposition to laminar flow. The low density also favours high flow rates (as per the Hagen–Poiseuille equation). These two aspects together facilitate rapid inflation and deflation of the balloon. In the rare event of balloon rupture, helium is also easily absorbed into the blood with minimal risk of embolic complications.

The device is inserted via the femoral artery using a Seldinger technique and fluoroscopic guidance. The balloon should lie in the descending thoracic aorta, about 2 cm distal to the left subclavian artery (level with the tracheal carina on an anteroposterior chest radiograph) and above the renal arteries. The patient's height determines the size of balloon used which, when fully inflated, should maximally occupy 80–90% of the cross-section of the aorta. The inner lumen of the catheter monitors the arterial blood pressure in the proximal aorta, whilst the outer lumen transports the gas to and from the balloon.

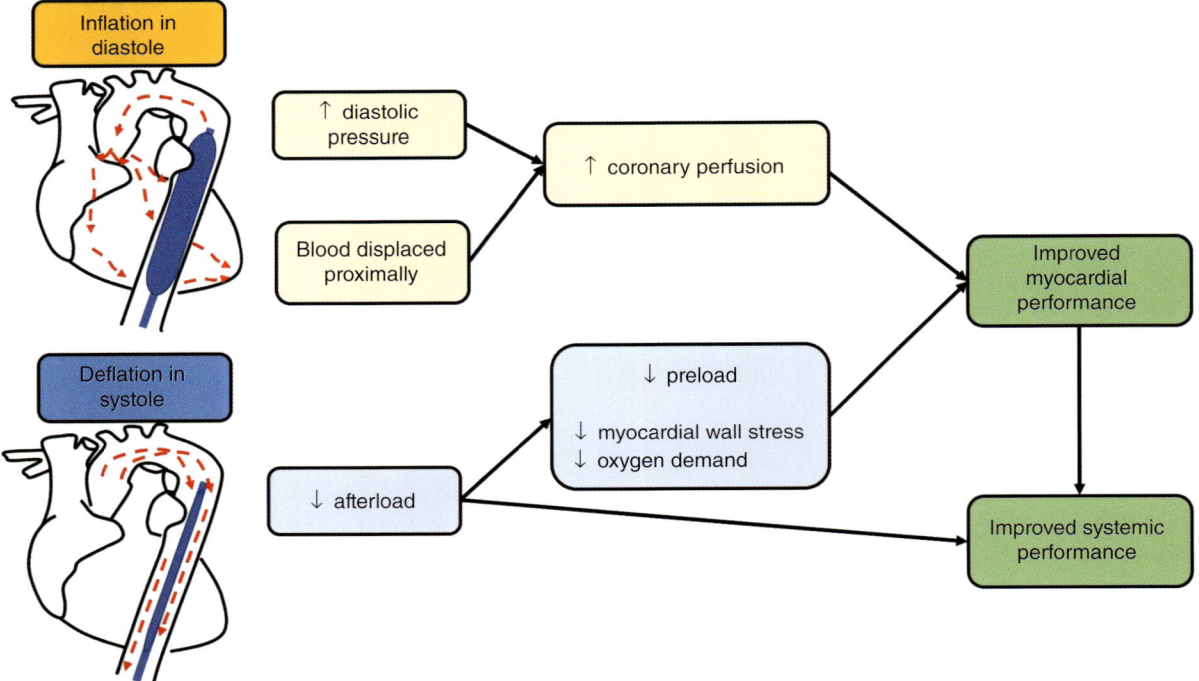

Fig 13.13 The effects of counter-pulsation therapy on cardiac performance

The machine usually uses either the aortic pressure waveform or the ECG to trigger the balloon inflation and deflation. A pressure-triggering IABP will still inflate and deflate with CPR in the event of a cardiac arrest. Inflation should occur at the beginning of diastole, when the aortic valve closes. This corresponds to the middle of the T wave on the ECG or the dicrotic notch on the arterial trace. The balloon should remain inflated for the duration of diastole, with deflation occurring just prior to left-ventricular systole and the opening of the aortic valve. This corresponds to the peak of the R wave on the ECG, or just before the upstroke on the arterial trace.

Inflation of the balloon during diastole causes a higher early diastolic pressure, creating a second peak in the arterial pressure waveform. This is known as diastolic augmentation and provides a modest improvement in downstream end-organ perfusion. This effect is most relevant to upstream perfusion, however; coronary perfusion is significantly improved with a direct benefit to cardiac performance. Deflation of the balloon results in a lower end-diastolic aortic pressure, reducing the afterload and hence the subsequent left-ventricular wall tension and myocardial oxygen demand during the next contraction. This is known as assisted systole and will be a lower pressure than native, unassisted systole. Figure 13.14 demonstrates these changes. It is important to understand that the IABP supports and optimizes cardiac function but, aside from the modest distal runoff with diastolic augmentation, it does not directly generate an increase in blood flow (see the section on ventricular assist devices below, by contrast).

The IABP can be programmed to inflate with every heartbeat, resulting in a 1:1 ratio, or in a 1:2 or 1:3 ratio. These lower ratios are generally reserved for weaning from the support at the end of therapy.

The effectiveness and efficiency of the IABP depends on several factors, including the diameter of the inflated balloon compared to that of the aorta, the heart rate and rhythm, and the compliance of the vessels. Timing, however, is perhaps the most crucial factor. Early inflation or late deflation increases ventricular afterload and may lead to regurgitation across the aortic valve. Late inflation or early deflation leads to suboptimal augmentation (Figure 13.15).

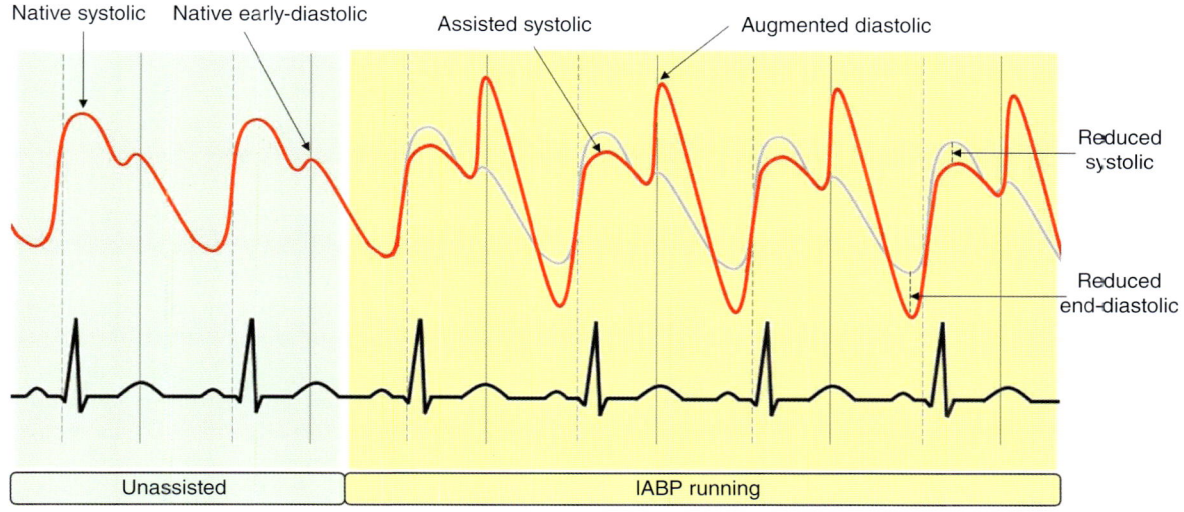

Figure 13.14 The changes seen in the aortic pressure waveform as a result of well-timed augmentation

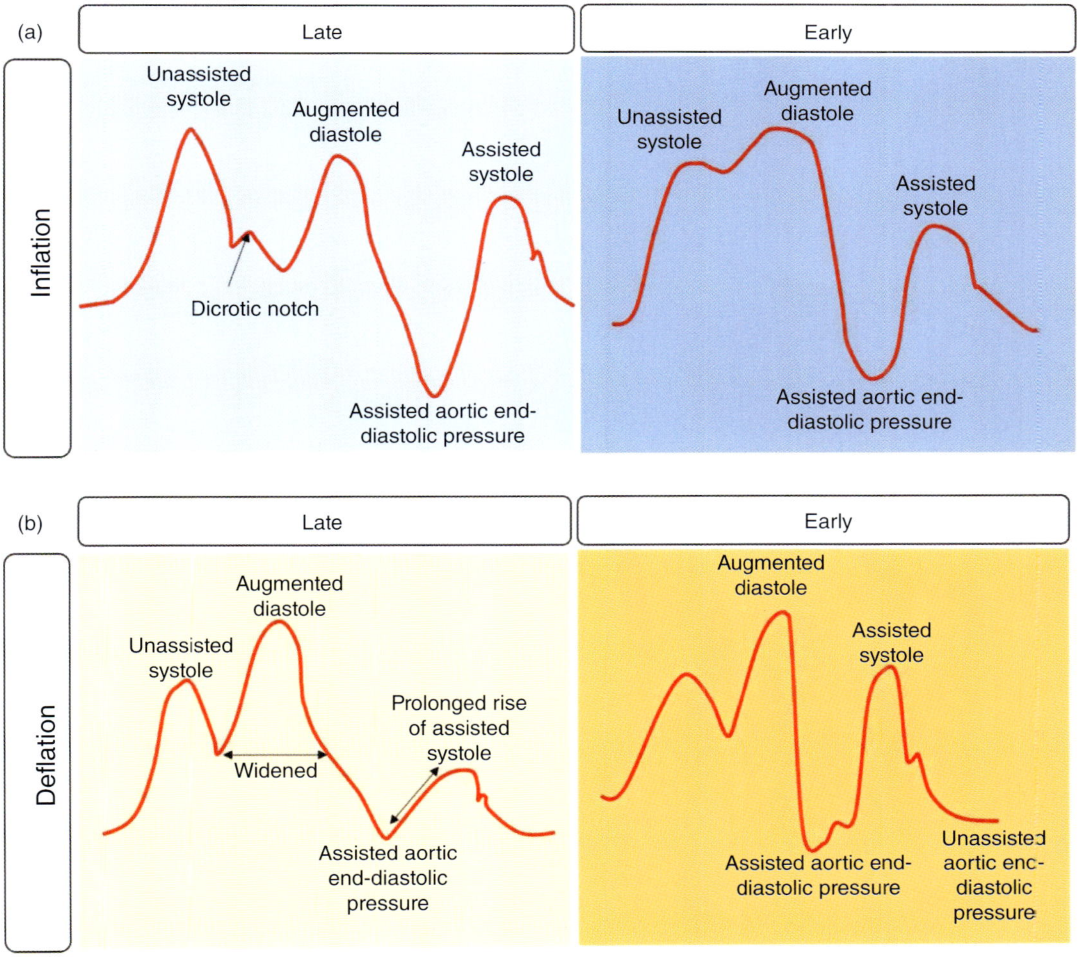

Figure 13.15 Appearance of poorly timed inflation (a) and deflation (b), showing the effects, in each case, where these are early or late in the native cardiac cycle

Chapter 13: Cardiac Support Equipment

Cardiac Assist Devices

A ventricular assist device (VAD) is a mechanical pump, used to partially or completely take over the function of the failing ventricle(s). This allows the ventricle to rest, reducing cardiac work and improving systemic and/or pulmonary circulation. LVADs are used to support the left ventricle, RVADs for the right and BiVADs, for both ventricles.

There are three main components to a VAD. An inflow cannula, an outflow cannula and a pump (Figure 13.16). The inflow cannula is inserted through the ventricle wall or atrium to drain the blood from the heart to the pump. The outflow cannula returns the blood from the pump to either the ascending aorta if an LVAD, pulmonary artery for an RVAD, or both for a BiVAD.

VADs are either *transcutaneous* (extra-corporeal), with the pump and power source located externally, or *implantable*, with an internal pump but external power source. The VAD connects to a control unit that displays information such as blood flow and provides a system status monitor with relevant alarms. Transcutaneous VADs are mainly for short-term use, whilst implantable VADs are used as a bridge to transplantation or long-term use.

These devices are typically implanted by cardio-thoracic surgeons via a median sternotomy, under general anaesthesia with CPB. However, percutaneous VADs can be inserted in the catheterization laboratory or operating theatre by passing a catheter from the femoral vein to the left atrium via an interatrial puncture. Oxygenated blood is drawn by the pump from the left atrium down the femoral venous cannula and returned to the adjacent femoral artery. The pump itself is extra-corporeal in this case.

Older VADs had a pulsatile, pumping action, mimicking the action of the heart. These were positive-displacement pumps, for example pneumatic pumps, which use compressed air as the driving force. Newer devices use continuous, non-pulsatile pumps. They have fewer moving parts, and are smaller, more durable and more reliable. Most utilize

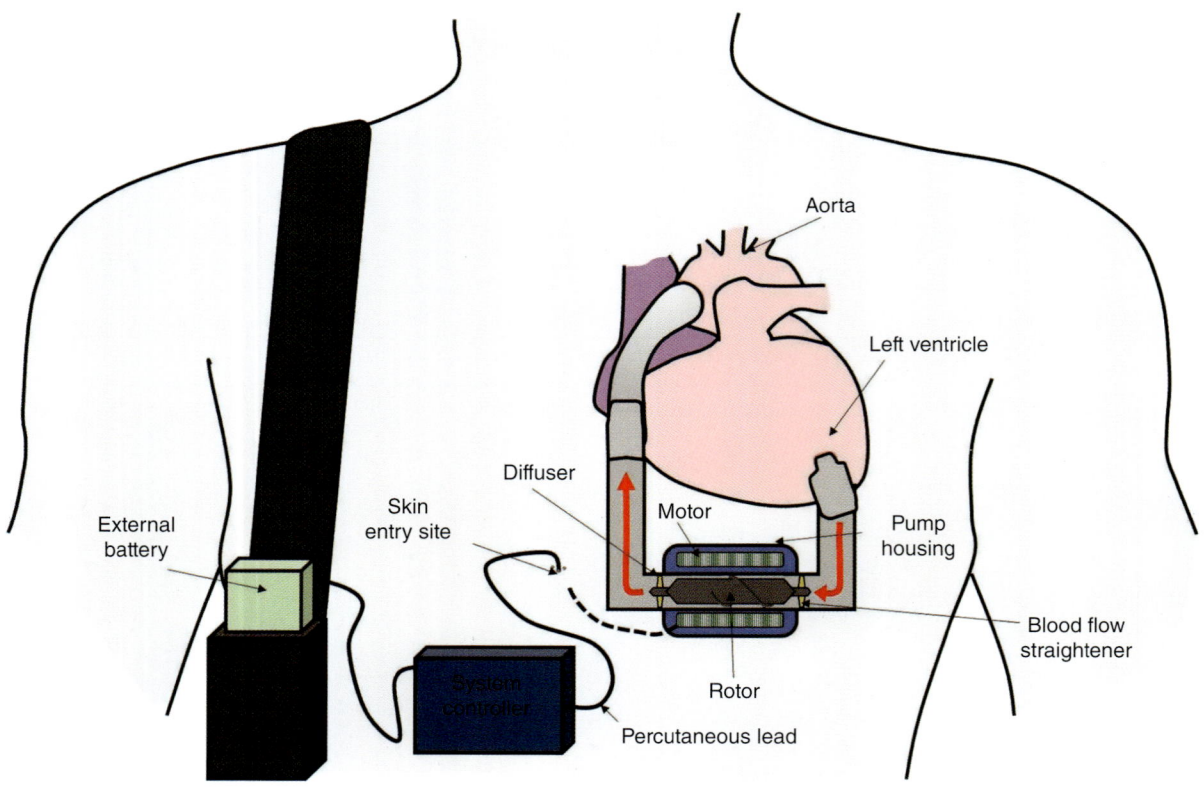

Figure 13.16 Schematic of an LVAD

either a centrifugal or axial-flow pump design. In an axial-flow pump, a helical impeller rotates within a column of blood, pushing it along the tube. With a centrifugal pump, direction of travel of the blood is perpendicular to the axis around which the impeller rotates.

The early continuous pumps contained solid bearings, which had issues with wear and eccentricity. The newer versions of these pumps instead use either magnetic levitation or hydrodynamic suspension to support the moving parts. This makes these later devices even more durable.

Patients rarely have a pulse with continuous-flow pumps. Native ventricular contraction is so weak as to be impalpable in patients who require these devices. Mean arterial pressure is used as a guide to haemodynamic adequacy of the system.

Summary

Cardiac support technologies may, superficially at least, seem to be a topic for a tertiary centre with cardiac surgical services. Whilst this is true of CPB and VADs, the vast majority of the technologies described in this chapter are regularly encountered in general anaesthetic and critical care practice in all secondary care settings.

More and more patients are undergoing pacemaker and ICD insertion, particularly as a treatment modality for cardiac failure. This, combined with increasing sophistication of the devices, demands a good understanding of the technology by all of us. In particular, it should be realized that the underlying reason for insertion may not be as straightforward as a tendency to complete heart block and that the role of magnets in the anaesthetic room to influence these devices is probably a thing of the past.

Defibrillators and cell-salvage technology are ubiquitous in anaesthetic practice and a good understanding of these devices is crucial. The balloon pump is perhaps less common than in the past but it still has a role and, in particular, will be seen in those patients with left coronary territory infarcts. The device relies on some interesting physiological and technological principles, which make it a recurrent exam favourite!

Questions

MCQs – select true or false for each response

1. The following haemodynamic effects are seen with an intra-aortic balloon pump (IABP):
   (a) A decrease in the end-diastolic pressure
   (b) A reduction in preload
   (c) Increased afterload
   (d) An increase in the left-ventricular wall stress
   (e) A reduction in the left-ventricular ejection fraction
2. Regarding defibrillation:
   (a) Transthoracic impedance increases with successive shocks
   (b) An inverter converts AC to DC
   (c) The voltage required for the shock is around 5,000 V
   (d) All shocks are synchronized
   (e) Most defibrillators are energy-based
3. Cell salvage:
   (a) May be accepted when allogenic blood is refused on religious grounds
   (b) Has a maximum final haematocrit of 50%
   (c) Typically uses axial-flow pumps
   (d) Contains platelets and clotting factors
   (e) Must be transfused within 4 hours

SBAs – select the single *best* answer

4. The following is correct regarding cell salvage:
   (a) A 7–10-μm filter is used within the machine to remove white blood cells
   (b) A 7–10-μm filter can be used to remove white blood cells on administration
   (c) A standard blood giving set has a 200-μm filter, which will remove white cells and debris
   (d) A leucodepletion filter cannot be used as the blood must be reinfused relatively quickly
   (e) The machine includes a 40–150-μm filter to separate the red cells from plasma
5. Regarding pacemakers:
   (a) A unipolar pacemaker has a cathode within the heart and an anode within the great veins

(b) Bipolar diathermy should be used as it avoids the interference issues caused by unipolar diathermy
(c) A bipolar pacemaker has the anode and cathode within the heart, allowing both ventricles to be paced
(d) Bipolar pacemakers generate smaller pacing 'spikes' on the ECG as the electrodes are embedded directly into the endocardial surface
(e) Bipolar pacemakers generate smaller pacing 'spikes' on the ECG as a smaller volume of myocardium is depolarized in completing the electrical circuit

Answers

1. TTFFF

The IABP reduces end-diastolic pressure and preload. In turn this leads to a reduction in afterload and so left-ventricular wall stress. This should result in an increase in left-ventricular ejection fraction.

2. FFTFT

Transthoracic impedance reduces with successive shocks, improving the chances of successful defibrillation. A rectifier converts AC to DC, an inverter converts DC to AC. Not all defibrillators are capable of delivering synchronized shocks (used for cardioverting perfusing dysrhythmias). All provide asynchronous shocks by default as these are required for cardiac arrest management.

3. TFFFT

Some people who reject transfusion on religious grounds may indeed accept salvaged blood although this cannot be assumed. The final haematocrit is at least 50%; somewhere between 50% and 70%. Most of these machines use roller pumps to move the blood around the machine. They also use a centrifuge but this is for separation of cells from wash and plasma, rather than pumping. The final product from the machine is devoid of clotting factors and platelets.

4. (b)

This size describes a leucodepletion filter and, whilst the blood must be transfused promptly after salvage, flow rates through such filters are more than sufficient. The machine does have a 40–150-μm filter but this is to remove debris from the salvage, not separate red cells from plasma (this is achieved by the centrifuge). A 200-μm filter is too large to remove white cells.

5. (e)

The anode of a unipolar pacemaker is the casing of the pulse generator whereas bipolar pacemakers have both the anode and cathode within the heart – although this does not allow biventricular pacing in itself. Unipolar and bipolar leads can both feature active attachment to the endocardium or simply rest within the chamber but this is not what influences the size of the pacing spike on the ECG. Bipolar diathermy is less hazardous than unipolar but it still does not avoid the risks altogether.

References

1. K. B. Absolon. Theodor Billroth and cardiac surgery. *The Journal of Thoracic and Cardiovascular Surgery*, 86(3), 1983; 451–452.
2. A. D. Bernstein, J. C. Daubert, R. D. Fletcher, D. L. Hayes, B. Lüderitz, D. W. Reynolds, M. H. Schoenfeld, R. Sutton. The revised NASPE/BPEG generic code for antibradycardia, adaptive-rate, and multisite pacing. North American Society of Pacing and Electrophysiology/British Pacing and Electrophysiology Group. *Pacing and Clinical Electrophysiology*, 25(2), 2002; 260–264.
3. J. Jude, W. Kouwenhoven, G. Knickerbocker. A new approach to cardiac resuscitation. *Annals of Surgery*, 154(3), 1961; 311–317.

Chapter 14

Ultrasound and Doppler

David Ashton-Cleary

Learning Objectives

- To understand the range of applications of ultrasound energy in clinical practice
- To appreciate the underlying physical principles of ultrasound generation and image acquisition
- To be aware of clinical limitations to image interpretation, which are a consequence of the physics principles

Chapter Content

- History of ultrasound
- Fundamentals of ultrasound energy and imaging
- Probe construction and behaviour
- Piezoelectric effect
- Basic image generation
- Image processing
- Doppler imaging
- 3D and 4D ultrasound
- Other applications of ultrasound

Scenario

A 54-year-old man is admitted to critical care following extensive debridement of the left lower limb for necrotizing fasciitis. He has established ARDS but there is also concern about a pulmonary aspiration event on induction of anaesthesia. He is on a noradrenaline infusion but remains hypotensive and oliguric. You wonder how ultrasound might be applied in this case to help guide fluid administration, respiratory management and vasoactive therapy. There is also concern about perfusion to the operative limb. Could you also use ultrasound to help here?

Introduction

Ultrasound has a vast array of applications and these are almost as varied within medicine as they are outside of clinical practice. This chapter will discuss the physical basis of ultrasound, the core clinical applications as well as some of those less commonly encountered. In general terms, the focus will be on diagnostic ultrasonography although therapeutic applications will be briefly discussed. Consideration of non-medical applications from industry, aerospace, metallurgy and communications is also relevant to understand the breadth of use of the technology.

History of Ultrasound

The appreciation of sound as an entity which can be studied and harnessed is variously accredited to the Greek philosopher and mathematician, Pythagoras, in around 6 BCE. It is believed that he noticed that the sounds emanating from a blacksmith's workshop were related to the size and heft of the tools in use. In 1794, Italian Catholic priest and naturalist, Lazarro Spallanzani, was the first to describe an application of ultrasound in the natural world. Through a series of detailed experiments, he was able to demonstrate that bats were interpreting sound, rather than light, as a means of navigation in flight. Although it would be nearly 150 years until the term 'echolocation' was coined, it is Spallanzani who is credited with its first observation. Sir Francis Galton FRS is believed to be the first to generate and use ultrasonic frequencies in a practical sense. Galton was a remarkable polymath who contributed to our fundamental understanding of basic statistical methods as well as expounding the scientific basis for forensic finger-print analysis. He was similarly fascinated with the natural world, citing Charles Darwin, his half-cousin, as a great influence in his work. In his thesis, 'Inquiries into Human Faculty and Its Development', published in 1883, Galton recounts experiments he made some years previously to evaluate the extent of human hearing with what has become known as the Galton whistle or, perhaps more commonly, the dog whistle [1]. The device, constructed from a tuneable brass tube and rubber bladder, allowed him to adjust the frequency of the sound produced. What he referred to as 'shrill notes' we now know to be ultrasound in the frequency range of 23–54 kHz. He used the apparatus attached to a modified walking cane to carefully approach animals in London Zoo in order to determine if they were aware of the sound. It was, in fact, domestic cats on the city streets that he found to have the best perception of those animals he tested.

Brothers Jacques and Pierre Curie discovered the piezoelectric effect (see below) in 1880. Building on a theoretical prediction of its existence by Gabrielle Lippman, the brothers demonstrated the reverse effect the following year. This allowed accurate and reproducible generation of ultrasound waves but, in addition, opened the door to detection of the sounds. A Canadian, Reginald Fessenden, developed the first sonar hydrophone in 1912, following the sinking of the *Titanic*, and Paul Langevin, a former PhD student of Pierre Curie's, subsequently filed patents with Constantin Chilowsky for a practical application of the technology for submarine detection in 1916 and 1917. Interestingly, Langevin also noted during his work that fish were killed by ultrasound and pain was experienced if a hand was placed in a water bath through which ultrasound waves were transmitted. These were the first observations of the effects of ultrasound on living tissue. The next significant advance was with the work of a Russian physicist, Sergei Sokolov, who developed quartz detectors operating in the 3-GHz range for revealing flaws in metal machine parts. This particular field was further advanced by Raimar Pohlman, who also later made the link to the clinical arena describing, in 1938, the use of ultrasonic waves as an adjunct to physiotherapy.

Clinical application of ultrasound as an imaging medium only really began to take off around the middle of the twentieth century. In the late 1930s, Karl Dussik, an Austrian neurologist and psychiatrist, pioneered imaging of the brain using what he referred to as 'supersonic waves' in the science of 'hyperphonography'. The veracity of these images was subsequently questioned but they spurred interest in the field, and Dussik is generally regarded as the father of diagnostic ultrasonography. In 1949, Wolf Dieter-Keidel produced the first ultrasound imagery of the heart while George Ludwig and John Wild each independently proposed the pulse-echo principle; American radiologist, Douglas Howry, coupled this technique with 35-mm film to capture the image, a concept he further improved on, 3 years later, with the first B-mode array. Much of the equipment was improvised from spare parts from World War 2 radar and radio arrays. Howry's 'pan-scanner' incorporated the ring-gear from the gun turret of a B-29 bomber, which allowed the scanning element to rotate fully around the subject.

A string of developments further developed echocardiography in particular, during the 1950s. A physician–engineer team in Sweden, Inge Edler and Carl Hellmuth Hertz (great-nephew of Heinrich Hertz, whose name is given to the unit of frequency), pioneered M-mode in 1954 and Shigeo Satomura, of Japan, developed Doppler ultrasonography in 1955. Ian Donald, an obstetrician and inventor, born in Cornwall, pioneered obstetric ultrasound in 1958 with a publication in *The Lancet*. Various incremental improvements through the early 1960s led to more portable machines until, in 1965, Walter Krause and Richard Soldner produced the first real-time scanning machine, the Siemens Vidoscan. In 1966, Don Baker, John Reid and Dennis Watkins introduced pulsed Doppler to demonstrate blood flow through the heart. A year later, Gene Strandness also applied the Doppler effect in diagnosis of peripheral vascular disease.

The next leap came in 1973, from James Griffith and Walter Henry, with the introduction of 30-frames-per-second, sectoral real-time scanning, which transformed imaging quality in a stroke. In 1974 came the advent of duplex scanning, with further advances from Baker and Reid. Then, in 1975, Marco Brandestini developed 128-point, multi-gated, pulsed-Doppler imaging, which allowed flow information to be colour-encoded over a 2D image. In 1987, Olaf von Ramm, at Duke University, added the third dimension but it was nearly a decade later before Thomas Nelson published work on 4D: real-time 3D fetal echocardiography in 1996.

Fundamentals of Ultrasound

Ultrasound, like any other acoustic phenomenon, is a mechanical wave and transmits energy through the sequential compression and rarefaction of particles within a medium, e.g. oxygen and nitrogen molecules in the case of air. Mechanical waves therefore cannot travel through a vacuum, unlike electromagnetic waves of which light is an example. Whilst light waves possess all the properties of mechanical waves, mechanical waves do not obey all the laws of electromagnetic waves. Light exhibits properties, some of which can only be explained by particle physics, hence the concept of a photon, a particle of light. Light is thus described as demonstrating wave–particle duality.

The peaks of a sound wave represent maximal compression of the medium and the troughs, maximal rarefaction. One complete progression from rest to peak compression, through rest to peak rarefaction and back to rest, comprises a cycle. Each cycle takes a defined time to complete – the period of the wave (seconds). The frequency of the wave is thus the number of cycles in 1 s (Hertz, Hz).

Any point of the cycle can also be described by its phase, measured in degrees. As demonstrated in Figure 14.1, one complete cycle sees the phase move through 360 degrees. Phase also provides a frame of reference when defining the wavelength of a wave; this is the longitudinal distance between points of equal phase on consecutive oscillations of a wave.

The maximal displacement from rest is defined as the amplitude of the wave: the force per unit area to produce the displacement of molecules (N m^{-2}). The defined minimum threshold for human hearing, under laboratory conditions, is 0.00002 N m^{-2} for a 1 kHz tone. By contrast, the threshold for pain is around 60 N m^{-2}; and 85 N m^{-2} is generally accepted as causing noise-induced hearing loss. The square of the amplitude is proportional to the energy carried by the wave. In turn, the power of the wave is defined as the energy transferred per unit time. This has the units of watts (J s^{-1}). The intensity of the wave describes the power passing through a given area (A), considering an area perpendicular to the direction of wave propagation through which the sound is travelling (Figure 14.2a). This has the units of W m^{-2}. Sound intensity level (SIL) reduces predictably with distance from the source. In the case of a point source, sound waves emanate spherically in all directions. Therefore, as the radius (r) from the source increases, the surface area of a hypothetical sphere at that distance also increases and the energy is distributed equally across the whole surface (Figure 14.2b). Therefore, the SIL reduces according to the inverse-square of distance from the source in accordance with the geometric definition of the surface area of a sphere. The SIL is conventionally quoted as a decibel (dB), which expresses the logarithm of the ratio of

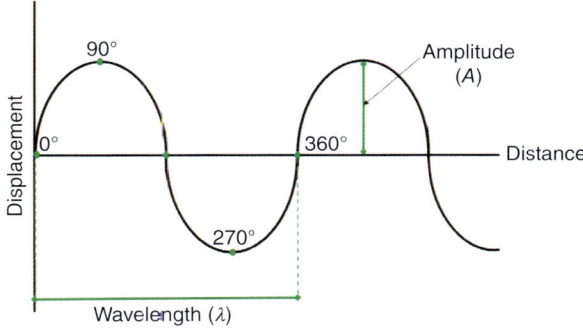

Figure 14.1 A wave can be fundamentally described by a number of key properties such as amplitude and wavelength

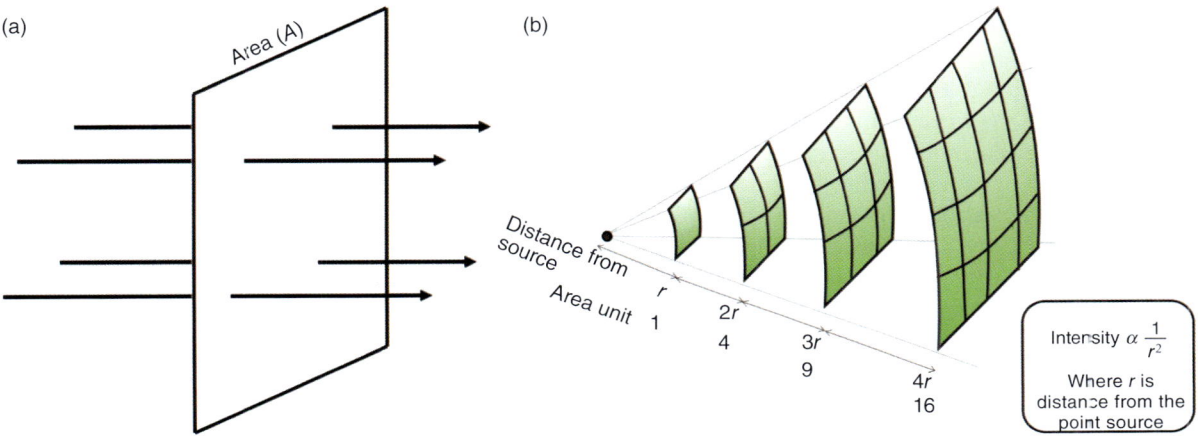

Figure 14.2 The power per unit area is the intensity of the wave (a) and this varies with distance from the source according to the inverse-square law (b)

Chapter 14: Ultrasound and Doppler

intensity at two points, e.g. measured point (I) vs. source (I_0).

$$\text{SIL (in dB)} = 10 \times \log_{10}\left(\frac{\text{Intensity}}{\text{Intensity}_0}\right)$$

Sound pressure level (SPL) is the conventional means of comparing pressure levels in the context of audible acoustics. Unlike SIL, it is affected by the acoustic properties of the environment and thus SPL and SIL are only equivalent in an anechoic chamber, which removes all reverberation and reflective effects. The reference pressure level is taken to be the threshold of human hearing (0.00002 N m^{-2} for a 1 kHz tone). Thus, as SPL is a ratio, it stands that the human hearing threshold is, for an 'average' human, 0 dB SPL by definition. Similarly, a human with exceptional hearing may have a threshold of hearing measured at –10 dB to –15 dB.

The speed of propagation of a wave depends on the medium through which it is transmitted but is a constant for that medium. This allows wavelength and frequency to be related:

$$\text{Velocity} = \text{Frequency} \times \text{Wavelength}$$

$$\text{Wavelength} \propto \frac{1}{\text{Frequency}}$$

Interpretation of reflected ultrasound waves by an ultrasound machine depends fundamentally on the speed at which the wave travelled through the tissues. However, since many tissue types may have been encountered along the path of the wave, each with differing propagation velocities (dictated by density and bulk modulus), the ultrasound machine must make the assumption that only a single tissue type is encountered by the beam. This is assumed to be a tissue with a conduction velocity of 1,540 m s^{-1} but Table 14.1 demonstrates the range of actual velocities.

Acoustic impedance of the tissues is a further property which determines the ultrasound propagation. Electrical impedance is analogous. For direct current (DC) circuits, only ohmic resistance effects apply and resistance and impedance are equivalent. In this setting, Ohm's law applies ($V = IR$). For alternating current (AC), however, electromagnetic effects due to the oscillation of the current result in reactance within the circuit; this is a frequency-dependent phenomenon. The electrical impedance is a combination

Table 14.1 Propagation velocities and acoustic impedance values for human tissues

Tissue	Speed (m s^{-1})	Impedance (kg s^{-1} m^{-2} × 10^6)
Air	333	0.0004
Lung	500	0.18
Water	1,480	1.5
Fat	1,446	1.3
Blood	1,566	1.7
Muscle	1,542–1,626	1.7
Bone	4,080	7.8

of the Ohmic resistance and reactance. Ohm's law, therefore, does not completely describe the relationship between potential difference and current in an AC circuit. To understand acoustic impedance, a simple analogy of air blown through a tube is helpful. In crude terms, the impedance represents the opposition to flow through the tube as a result of a pressure differential from end to end (see the Hagen–Poiseuille equation). More accurately, impedance reflects that the flow through the tube is not related simply to static properties of the system but also varies with oscillatory effects set up within the tube as the air pressure increases at the opening of the tube (therefore comparable to AC circuits). As the frequency of these oscillations varies, so does the flow through the duct as predicted by the impedance. The impedance (Z) mathematically is the product of the density and the velocity.

$$\text{Impedance} = \text{Density} \times \text{Velocity}$$

Human tissues all have varying impedance values (Table 14.1) and this is of key importance when considering reflection (see below).

As with any wave travelling through a medium, ultrasound is susceptible to attenuation – the reduction in energy along the path of transmission. This occurs as a result of absorption of the energy, i.e. conversion to other forms of energy, principally heat. Different tissues absorb the energy to differing extents (Table 14.2). Higher frequencies are absorbed to a greater extent so the attenuation coefficient must always be reported at a reference frequency, usually 1 MHz.

There is also a reduction in energy which results from geometric expansion of the wave front as it

Table 14.2 Attenuation coefficients of various tissue types

Tissue	Attenuation coefficient (at 1 MHz)
Blood	0.18
Fat	0.6
Liver	0.9
Muscle	1.2–3.3
Bone	20
Lung	40

Table 14.3 Reflection at various tissue type interfaces (Reproduced from J. Aldrich. Basic physics of ultrasound imaging. *Critical Care Medicine*, 35, 2007; S131–7 [1])

Boundary	Percentage reflected
Fat–muscle	1.08
Fat–kidney	0.6
Soft tissue–water	0.2
Bone–fat	49
Soft tissue–air	99

radiates from the source (see earlier). Additionally, reflection of the energy reduces that which can reach deeper tissues and may interfere with energy returning to source. Reflection occurs at the interface of any two tissue types of differing impedance. Table 14.3 demonstrates the proportion of energy reflected by some typical tissue interfaces.

Whilst attenuation therefore reduces the available energy to interrogate deeper tissues, if reflection did not occur, there would be no energy returned to the probe from which to generate an image. Attenuation, at a wave level, is represented by a reduction in amplitude of the wave. In a uniform material, the effect of attenuation can be predicted by a negative exponential relationship:

$$Amplitude = A_0 \times e^{-\alpha d}$$

where A_0 is the initial amplitude, α is the attenuation coefficient for the material and d is the distance travelled in the direction of the outgoing wave. This relationship, whilst only describing absorptive effects, forms the basis of timed gain compensation (TGC), an image-processing technique which optimizes the image to adjust for predictable reductions in energy with depth of penetration. It is important to appreciate that this function amplifies the returning signal rather than increasing the power of the transmitted waves leaving the probe. TGC is applied by all modern machines and compensates for loss of amplitude of reflections from deeper structures. By assuming the propagation velocity to be 1,540 m s^{-1}, the machine times echo-returns for each structure and uses this information to determine its depth within the subject. This is the basis of building the image but TGC then predicts the reduction in amplitude at any given tissue depth (d) and applies a correction by means of progressively increasing gain down the image.

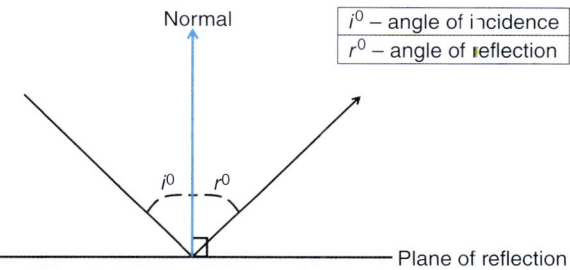

Figure 14.3 The laws of reflection

To come back to reflection, this occurs in two principal forms; specular (mirror-like) and diffuse reflection. Reflection is a very familiar concept with respect to visible light and this provides a useful analogy through which to discuss the principles. The underlying physics applies equally to acoustic and light waves. For specular reflection, the laws of reflection (derived from the Fresnel equations) apply (Figure 14.3):

1. The incident wave, reflected wave and 'normal' (a line perpendicular to the reflecting surface from the point of reflection) are in the same plane
2. The angle of incidence to the normal is equal to the angle of reflectance to the normal
3. The incident and reflected wave are on opposite sides of the normal.

A good understanding of these laws will make you a master of snooker because you'll be able to expertly judge deflections of balls off the cushions! A specular reflector has a surface dimension greatly in excess of the wavelength of the reflected wave. The reflected waves thus maintain their spatial relationship to one another and an 'image' is produced of the emitting source. This is the underlying principle of a mirror and, in ultrasonography, needles, the diaphragm,

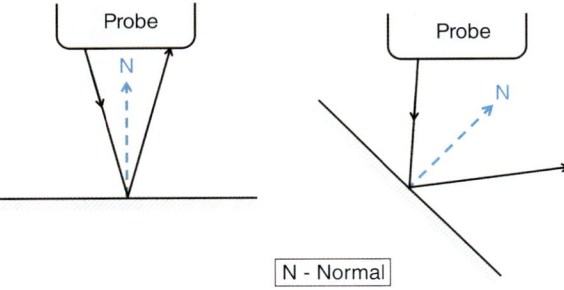

Figure 14.4 Specular reflection

bone cortex and blood vessel walls all provide specular reflections. Whilst these are very strong reflections, generating a high-intensity return and a bright image, they are highly dependent on the angle of incidence; if the incident wave strikes the surface tangentially, no reflected energy reaches the transducer and there is no image (Figure 14.4).

Diffuse reflection, on the other hand, is the basis of how our eyes work to perceive the world around us and also how the vast majority of ultrasound energy is returned to a probe. Here, the reflecting surface is of a dimension similar to, or smaller than, the wavelength of the incident wave. This results in wide scattering of the energy in multiple directions but not with the focus to produce a mirror-like image (Figure 14.5).

Surfaces generally exhibit a combination of specular and diffuse reflection. A highly polished stone surface, for example, will provide some mirror-like properties but will always retain the appearance of surface texture and colour. Similarly, a blood vessel wall provides a strong, specular return but, due to co-existent diffuse reflection, visualization by ultrasound is not very angle-dependent. An in-plane visualization of a non-ultrasound-specialized needle, however, provides a challenging target with ultrasound; visualizing it depends on surface imperfections in the metal or adherent tissue fluids.

The final form of reflection is Rayleigh scattering, which is sometimes incorrectly regarded as a sub-type of diffuse scattering (it does share the attribute that scatter is from small targets). Diffuse scattering results from multiple reflections in differing directions, generated by small surface irregularities, usually where the reflecting surfaces are arranged at any number of angles relative to the incoming beam. Rayleigh scattering, meanwhile, is a specific interaction seen when the target is very much smaller than the wavelength of

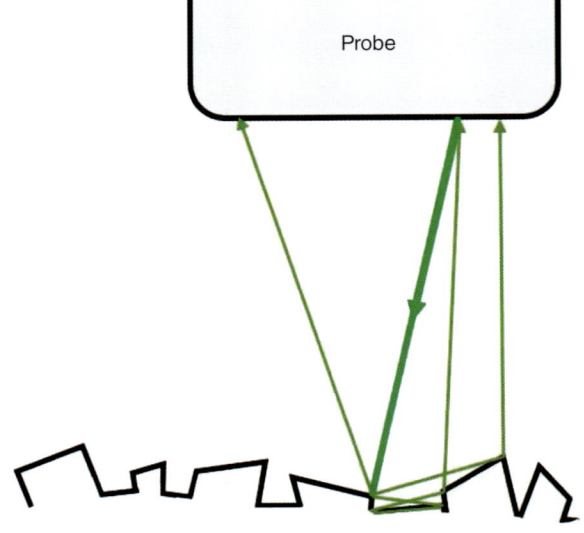

Figure 14.5 Diffusion reflection from a fine, irregular surface

the incident beam, and occurs even when the beam arrives perpendicularly to the target. A 5-MHz probe will produce energy with a wavelength of 300 μm. The archetypal, biological Rayleigh scatterer is a red blood cell, with an average diameter of 7 μm, much smaller than the wavelength of the beam. In basic terms, Rayleigh scattering results in scattering in all directions except back towards the source. This is the conventional explanation as to why the interior of blood vessels appears anechoic on B-mode – the red cells scatter the signal in all directions except back to the probe. The reality is that there is indeed some small return which is, in fact, the basis of Doppler ultrasonography of blood flow (see later). Rayleigh scattering is highly dependent on the properties of the incident wave; the intensity of scattered energy is proportional to the fourth power of the frequency (therefore, also wavelength to the power of -4). This explains the most widely known example of Rayleigh scattering: the blue sky caused by scatter of solar radiation by atmospheric constituents. Long wavelengths of solar radiation (red and infrared) are scattered least and that is why the heat of the Sun is felt as a point source from the direction of the Sun in the sky. Meanwhile, short wavelengths (blue) are scattered maximally so any blue light incident on the solar-facing hemisphere can be scattered in the direction of the observer's eye (Figure 14.6a). At sunset, light reaching the observer travels almost parallel to

Table 14.4 Comparison of common probes

	Linear	Curvilinear	Phased-array
Application	Superficial, vascular	Lung, abdomen	Echocardiography
Frequency (MHz)	6–18	2–5	3–7
Depth (cm)	1.5–6	5–20	5–16
Axial resolution (mm)	0.5	2	2
Lateral resolution (mm)	1	3	3

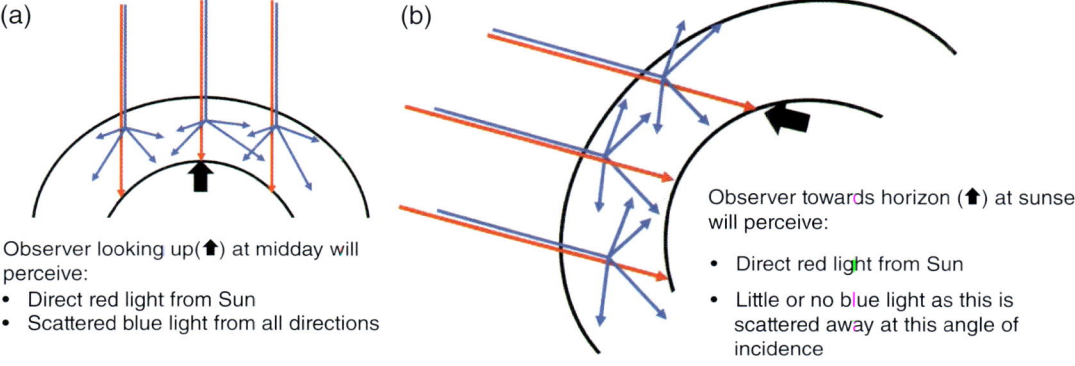

Figure 14.6 Rayleigh scattering of sunlight at (a) midday – blue sky; and at sunset – red sky

the Earth's surface with a longer course to reach the observer's eye. This gives more opportunity for the blue wavelengths to be scattered away and only the red-end wavelengths reach the eye (Figure 14.6b).

Probe Construction and Behaviour

Probes are varied in their configuration but are designed for a defined purpose, with properties to suit. The common probes in clinical diagnostics are the linear, curvilinear and phased-array probes. These are compared in the table above (Table 14.4).

Each probe consists of the same constituent parts (Figure 14.7). In modern probes, ultrasound is generated by an array of transducer crystals. Behind the array is a backing material which absorbs energy, ensuring emission only occurs from the front face of the crystals. In turn, this minimizes vibration within the probe, maintaining a narrow pulse width, a crucial requirement for good axial resolution (see below). The front face of the probe – a rubber layer, often grey or black in colour – is in fact an acoustic lens.

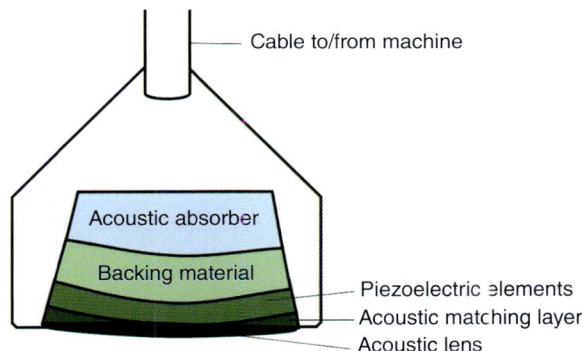

Figure 14.7 Basic probe construction

This seals the probe for infection control considerations but is also vital in focusing the beam to improve the image quality and lateral resolution (see below). Lenses produce their effects by refracting waves (Figure 14.8). In order to do this, they must simply be made of a material in which the speed of the

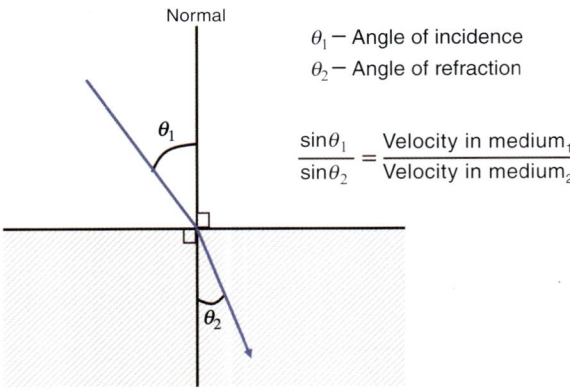

Figure 14.8 Snell's law, relating the angle of incidence and refraction to speed of the wave within the media

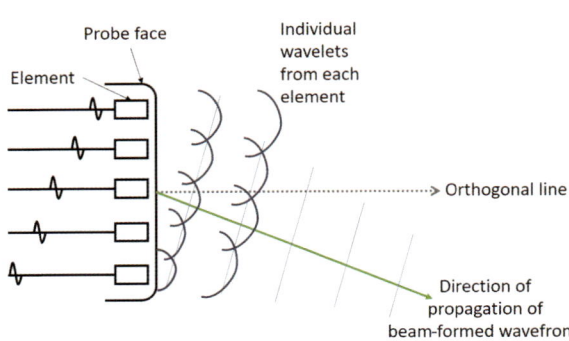

Figure 14.9 Staggered activation of individual piezoelectric elements to steer or 'beam-form' a wave

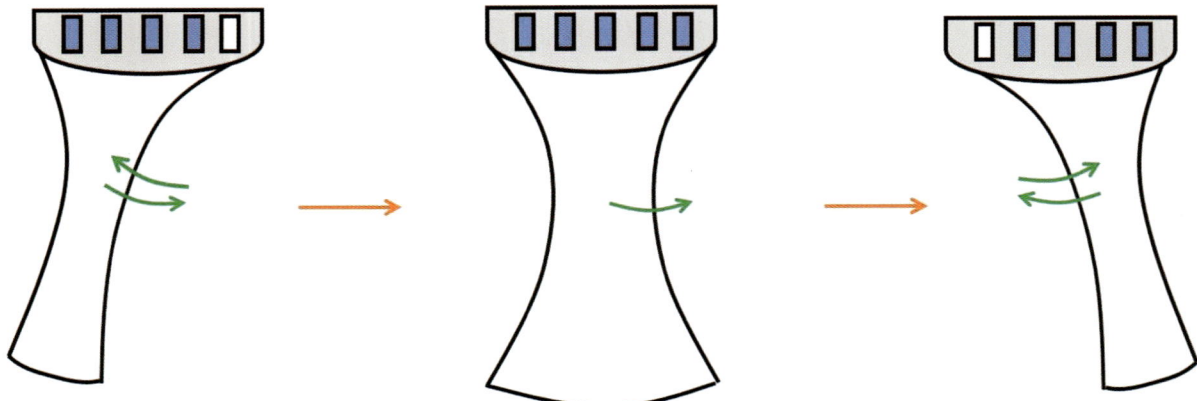

Figure 14.10 Cluster-activation of the elements to construct numerous slices in the sector, to build up a single image frame

wave changes on entry to the lens. In fact, an optical lens will also be an acoustic lens, just not necessarily a very good one. The angle of refraction of a lens is predicted by Snell's law.

The beam is also focused electronically in a process known as beam-forming. This process relies on staggering the pulse from each element of the transducer to manipulate the wavefront interference and hence steer the beam relative to the probe face (Figure 14.9). At the high frequencies used in ultrasound, the staggering interval is so minute that the pulses trail one another by only a few degrees of phase. This is the origin of the term 'phased array'.

It is important to realize that the moving image is not a live recording of all elements, continually activated and receiving information about the tissue directly beneath them. Instead, the image is composed of numerous slices, rapidly assembled as a narrow, focused beam, originating from a small fraction of the probe surface, sweeps across the transducer. Each one of these beams is generated by beam-forming the output of many or nearly all crystals in clusters. The image is then constructed by rapidly forming similar beams, in quick succession across the probe face (Figure 14.10). The speed at which this can be achieved determines the temporal resolution of the probe (see below). Beam-forming is also part of the processing of the received information as the image is reconstructed by essentially reversing the beam-forming process. It is also used to gather diffuse scatter from a target on multiple crystals, to form a better image of the structure.

Anywhere along the course of the ultrasound beam where attenuation or refraction could degrade performance, it is necessary to introduce a medium to minimize these effects. Between skin and probe,

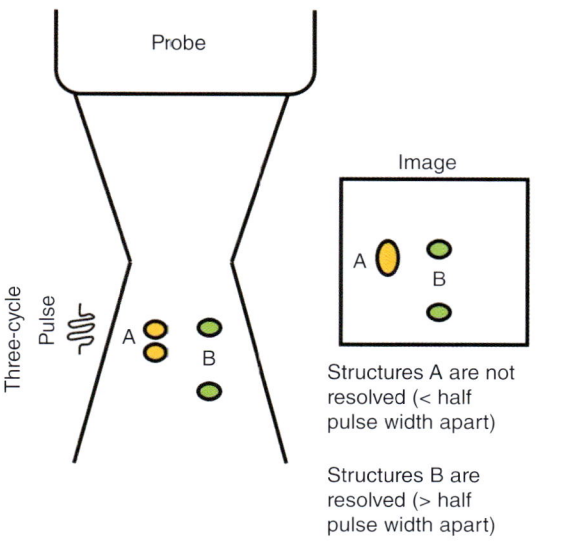

Figure 14.11 Axial resolution

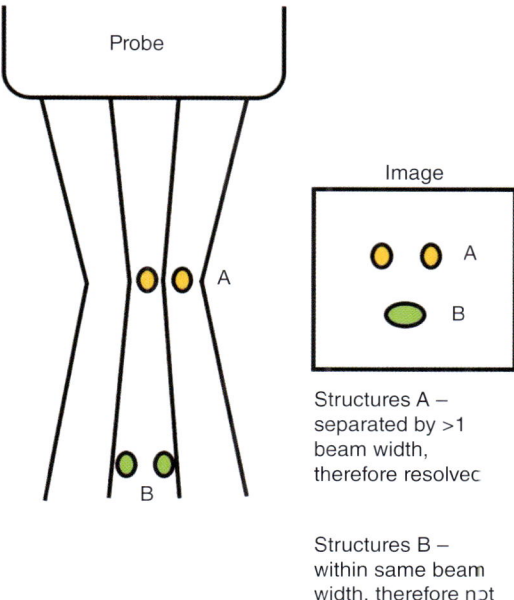

Figure 14.12 Lateral resolution

water-based gel is used to ablate the air gap. A similar effect would be found between the transducer elements and the acoustic lens within the probe and this problem is dealt with by the acoustic matching layer.

Frequency is a crucial determinant of probe functionality. Most modern probes can be described as being wide-band, i.e. they operate over a number of frequencies rather than at one specific frequency. This allows them to be tuned and optimized during use. The two key reasons for selecting the correct frequency probe are penetration and resolution. Penetration cannot be achieved at higher frequencies due to the frequency-dependent increase in attenuation effects. However, higher-frequency probes deliver significantly higher resolution and this trade-off must be considered when selecting the probe for the task at hand.

Resolution is the ability to distinguish features or effects separated in time or space. It has three principal facets: axial and lateral (together comprising spatial) resolution; and temporal resolution. Frequency is a key determinant of spatial resolution. Axial resolution concerns the ability to separate structures along the beam (Figure 14.11). In order to be distinguished, the features must be located with a separation no less than half the pulse length of the beam. A typical probe will produce a pulse consisting of two to three cycles. The length of that pulse is therefore dictated by wavelength and frequency. Higher-frequency ultrasound will result in a shorter pulse length. This leads to greater axial resolution but progressive problems of attenuation with depth, as discussed. So, whilst a high-frequency probe delivers excellent axial resolution it can only do so for superficial targets. Alternatively, the probe can be constructed to reduce the number of cycles in a pulse and this is achieved by the damping material behind the crystals. The trade-off here is a reduction in amplitude and so penetration again becomes problematic.

Lateral resolution is determined by beam width; structures close enough laterally to be within the same beam width will not be resolved (Figure 14.12). Beam width varies with depth from the probe according to focusing and divergence of the beams. At the probe face, the beam is almost the full width of the probe head. The width then reduces until it is maximally narrow at the focus zone (see Figure 14.13). The converging zone between these two points is referred to as the near field or Fresnel field. From the focus zone, the beam again diverges through the far field or Fraunhofer field. This is important: any two structures existing with lateral separation less than one beam width will not be resolved. Therefore, understanding the shape of the beam demonstrates that lateral resolution is best at the focus point (which can, and should, be actively set for this reason), next best in the near field and worst in the far field. A high-frequency, narrow-face probe will have the best lateral resolution on account of a short near-zone length and narrow beam width at the focal point.

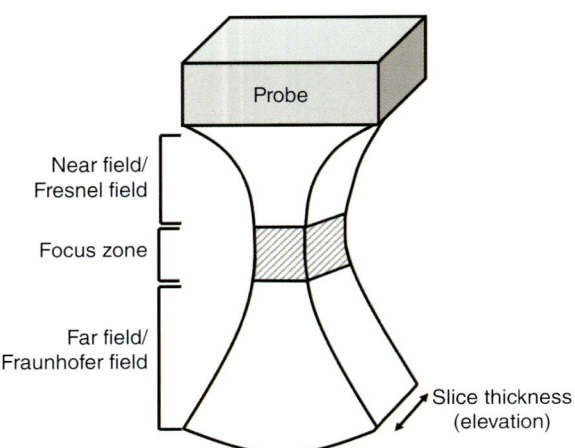

Figure 14.13 Near field and far field and the focus zone of an ultrasound probe

Temporal resolution relates to the frame rate that is achievable by the machine and whether this can keep pace with rapidly moving subjects, e.g. can the fine motion of the mitral valve leaflets be accurately depicted? This depends principally on the computational power of the machine and the mode in which it is being used. Shallower imaging means a shorter round trip for the ultrasound pulse so inherently this improves the speed at which information can be collated about the moving target. Therefore, deeper structures cannot be visualized with the same temporal resolution as superficial targets, irrespective of the capabilities of the machine. Reducing the sector width does help, however, as fewer slices are required to construct each frame. Taken to the extreme, M-mode (see later) is a single slice and no scanning is required to construct an entire frame. This mode therefore delivers the maximal temporal resolution possible for any given machine.

Piezoelectric Effect

The transducer elements themselves are made, conventionally, of lead zirconate titanate (PZT). This is used due to its high efficiency in converting between electrical and mechanical energy; however, crystalline DNA, quartz and even bone (in fact the collagen, rather than the hydroxyapatite) will exhibit some piezoelectric activity in the correct circumstances. Piezoelectricity has a very wide range of everyday applications. In any circumstance where a micro-actuator or electromechanical transducer is required, the piezoelectric effect often has a role. Another ubiquitous clinical application is in bubble detectors for extra-corporeal circuits such as cardio-pulmonary bypass and haemodialysis systems.

> Piezoelectric crystals have an enormous range of everyday applications: a bit like the saying regarding rats in London, you are probably never more than 6 feet from a piezoelectric crystal! Consider cigarette lighters, gas barbecue starters, quartz watches, microphones, guitar pick-ups, flat-panel loudspeakers, inkjet printers and fuel injectors for internal combustion engines: all rely on the piezoelectric effect.

The effect results from application of pressure to a substance and, in fact, thinking about the word 'piezoelectricity' can help in remembering the difference between the direct and reverse effect. The word 'piezo' derives from the Greek for pressure and so the direct piezoelectric effect describes pressure generating electrical charge. The reverse effect (think of the word, 'piezoelectricity' backwards now) is electrical charge creating pressure by distorting the crystal. This aide-memoire is useful as, perhaps a little confusingly, the work of an ultrasound probe starts with the reverse effect, to generate the ultrasound, and then detects reflections with the direct effect.

In order to demonstrate piezoelectricity, a crystal must exhibit sufficient structural asymmetry to result in an electrostatic dipole. So, whilst the ions within a single unit of the crystal result in a net charge of zero, the spatial arrangement of positive ions relative to the negative ions results in a polar axis (Figure 14.14). If mechanical stress distorts the crystal along this axis, moving the negative and positive elements further apart, a charge is produced.

The polar axes of adjacent crystal units are randomly arranged throughout the material and so applying pressure in any given direction will result in very little net change in polarity. This explains the weak piezoelectrical properties of some natural substances. Engineered piezoelectric materials undergo a process known as 'poling' during manufacture whereby a high-intensity electromagnetic field is used to align all the polar axes. When the field is removed, the crystal lattice structure tends to resist return of the individual axes to their original state. As all poles

Chapter 14: Ultrasound and Doppler

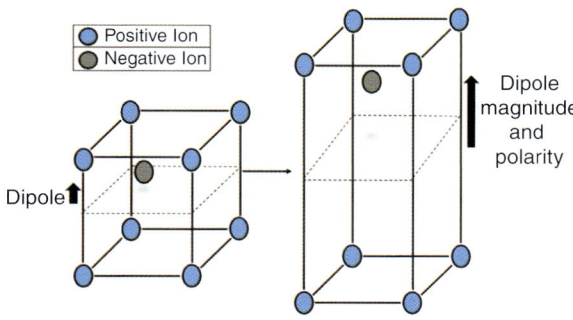

Figure 14.14 Electrostatic dipole within a crystal which is augmented by mechanically stressing the crystal

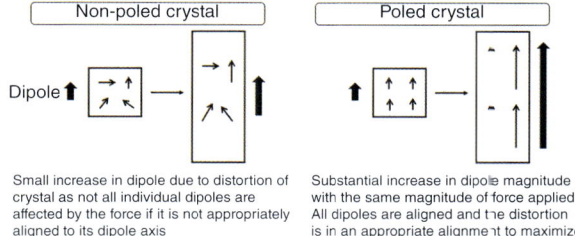

Figure 14.15 The result of poling an engineered piezoelectric crystal

are now virtually aligned, the piezoelectric effect for any given mechanical stress is very much stronger (Figure 14.15).

Interestingly, and of particular relevance for industrial applications, temperature is a relevant design consideration when selecting a piezoelectric material. Above a particular temperature for each material, the Curie temperature, any degree of poling is lost and the alignment of dipoles becomes random again. Magnetic materials also lose their inherent magnetism at this temperature for the same reasons. Consequently, the operational temperatures for the proposed crystal dictate the material type because the Curie temperature should be about twice the operating temperature. The particular species of PZT used in medical diagnostic ultrasound has a Curie temperature of around 185 °C.

Basic Image Generation

Ultrasound imaging has a number of recognized modes which will be discussed further throughout the chapter. To start with, however, basic A- and B-mode imaging will be discussed.

A-mode (amplitude mode) describes the very first form of ultrasound imaging. It still has a use in industry, particularly for non-destructive testing (NDT) to assess for cracks and other defects within welds or materials, e.g. gas cylinders and metal components of aircraft such as turbine blades or wing components. The information produced is a graphical plot of depth from the probe against strength of the return (Figure 14.16).

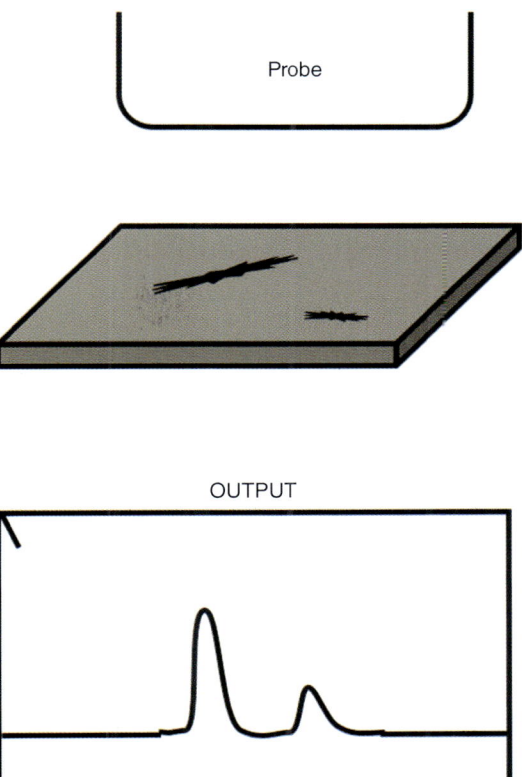

Figure 14.16 A-mode imaging

B-mode (brightness mode) is the mainstay of conventional imaging. Amplitude values of an A-mode scan are converted into a grey-scale value to form an image. The sector image was initially produced by

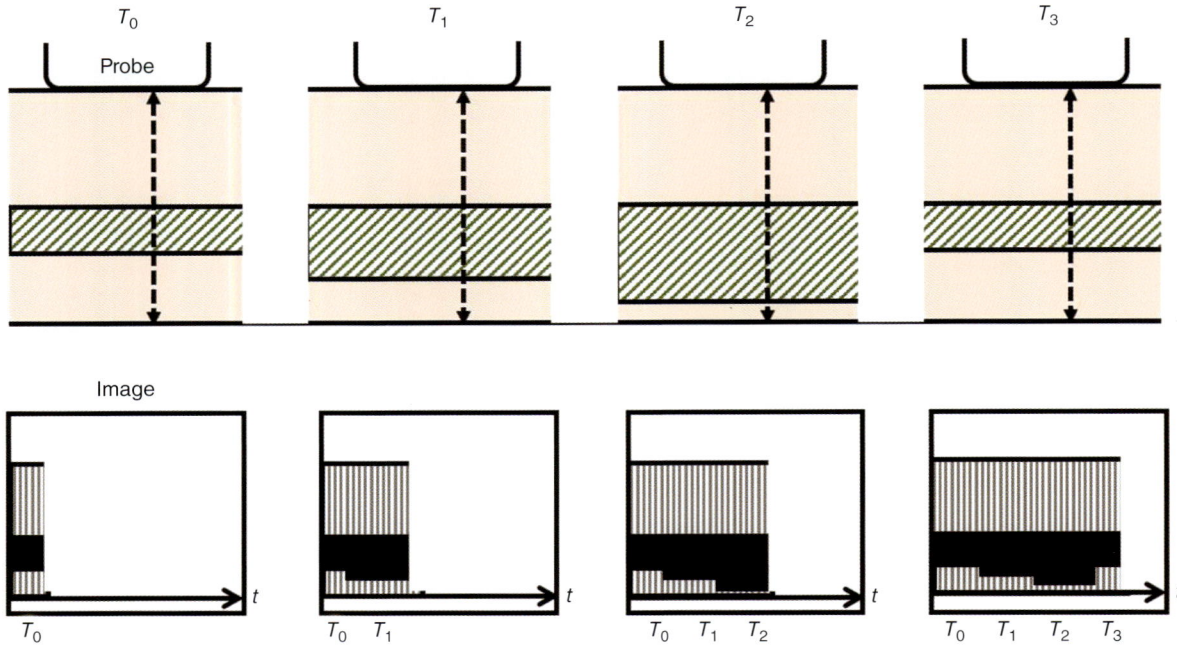

Frame-by-frame assembly of an M-mode image of the change in size of structure 's'. The width of the frames on the time axis (*t*) is grossly exaggerated for diagrammatic purposes

Figure 14.17 M-mode imaging

moving the transducer element around the patient (who had to sit very still for minutes at a time). Later, it became possible to mechanically scan the transducer element through an arc within the probe head. Modern scanners use multiple transducer elements and beam-forming, as discussed earlier, and this dramatically improves the resolution of the images.

M-mode (motion mode) utilizes the principles of B-mode but along a single scan line, which is selected by the user. The image generated is of brightness values against time on the *x*-axis. As there is no scanning to form a complete sector, the frame rate is very high and temporal resolution is thus maximized (Figure 14.17).

The heart of any ultrasound is a phenomenally accurate clock. With the exception of continuous-wave Doppler (see later), the probe operates on the pulse-echo principle. Around 99.9% of the work-cycle of the probe is concerned with receiving echoes of pulses sent out in the remaining 0.1%. The timing of when these echoes return in relation to the time when the pulse left is the basis for determining the depth from which the echo has returned within the patient. This also underpins some artefacts produced on the image – interfaces between tissue and gas, e.g. lung and bowel, will produce an echo artefact of that interface. The returning energy is part-absorbed, part-reflected at the probe. The re-reflected energy travels to the same interface and reflects again but will return to the probe for a second time, with twice the delay of the first return; the machine portrays this as an echo twice as far down the image. These artefacts are collectively referred to as reverberation artefacts – the ultrasound energy passes repeatedly between the probe and a structure (Figure 14.18).

There are other artefacts of particular relevance. A strong reflection or attenuation by one structure, for example, will lead to an acoustic shadow deep to that structure. This renders any deeper structures impossible to image without adjusting the probe to view from another angle. Meanwhile, low attenuation structures or poor reflectors, e.g. fluid, tend to result in enhancement of deeper structures as the

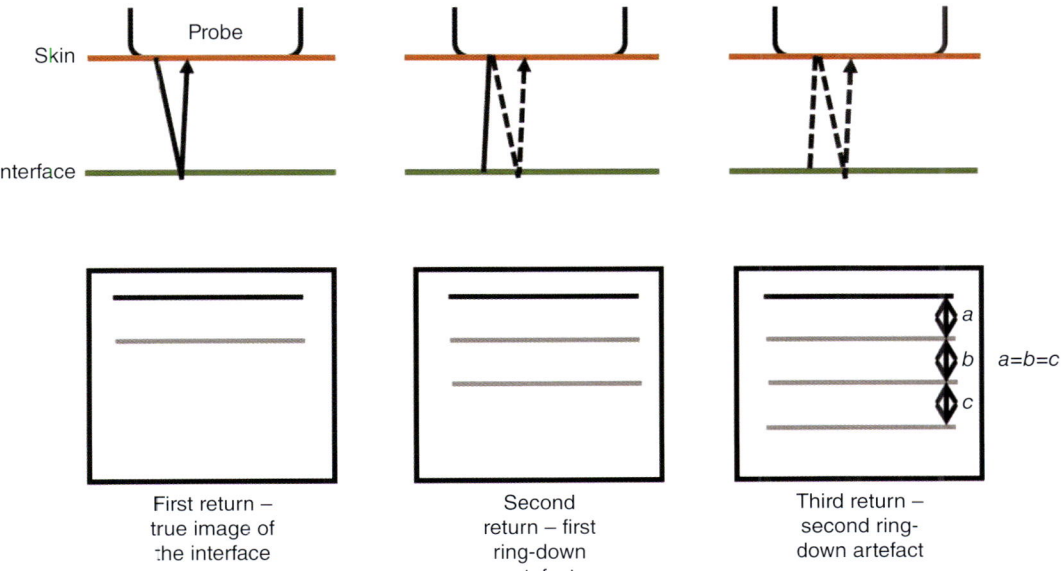

Figure 14.18 Reverberation artefact

ultrasound freely travels to and from the deeper tissues. The classic example of both of these effects in one place is the gallbladder. A gallbladder filled with bile will lead to post-cystic enhancement of the structures beneath whereas a stone in the gallbladder will provide a bright image due to strong reflection by the surface of the stone and strong attenuation of the remaining energy by the substance of the stone. The result is an acoustic shadow down the image below this point (Figure 14.19).

The effects of refraction and reflection can lead to misplaced or duplicated structures or even mirror images of some structures about the plane of a specular reflector. The machine can only assume energy has left and returned to the probe along a straight line. If the energy encounters a refracting or reflecting interface, the machine portrays the return along the assumed trajectory of the outbound energy (Figure 14.20).

A final phenomenon which introduces artefacts is that of anisotropy. The term refers to any mechanical or physical property of a system which changes with direction. A very simple example is that of wood grain, which results in differing properties for cutting and working the wood depending on the direction of the cutting strokes relative to the grain. In ultrasonography, this artefact applies principally in the fields of nerve and musculoskeletal imaging.

Parallel bundles of fibres in tendons, muscles and, to some degree, nerves will return a strong echo when the incoming beam is perpendicular. This renders the interior of the structure as a hyperechoic space. If there is a slight change in the angle, the reflection from the fibres becomes much weaker and the structure may now appear hypoechoic. This can lead to misinterpretation: nerves mistaken for blood vessels, intact tendons mistaken for those which are torn. Experience and careful angulation of the probe help to truly reveal the characteristics of the structure.

Image Processing

The raw data from the probe undergo a significant degree of processing to generate the image. This involves amplifiers, various filters and analogue-to-digital conversion. In addition, TGC is applied (see earlier) to compensate for depth-related attenuation. Numerous image enhancements can be applied but these are beyond the scope of this chapter.

Doppler Imaging

The Doppler effect was first observed and studied by Christian Doppler, an Austrian physicist, in 1842. It describes the effect on observed frequency of a wave

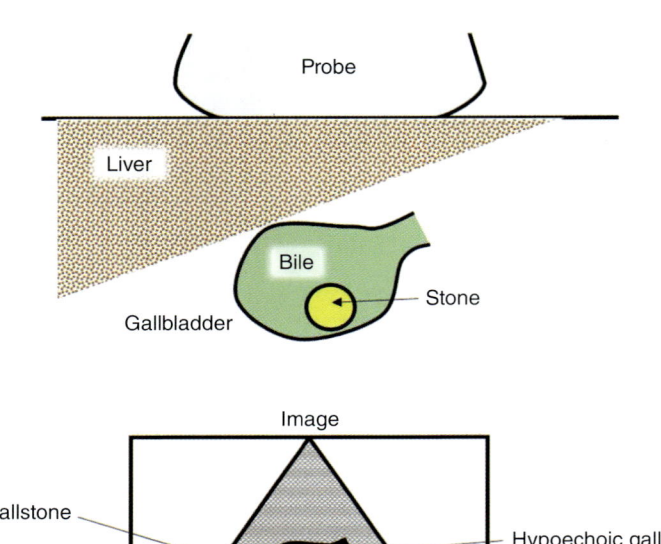

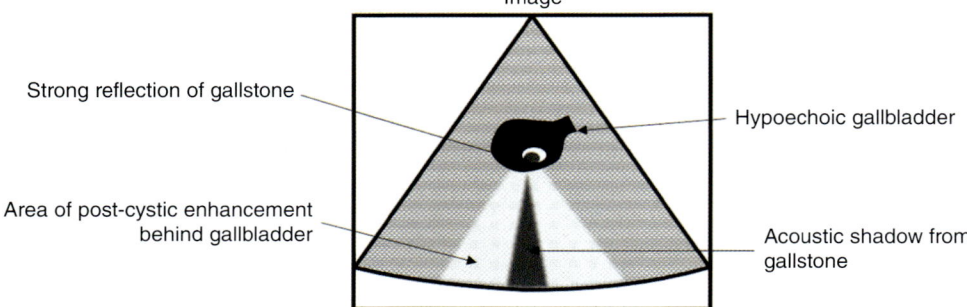

Figure 14.19 The range of artefacts resulting from fluid and gallstones in the gallbladder

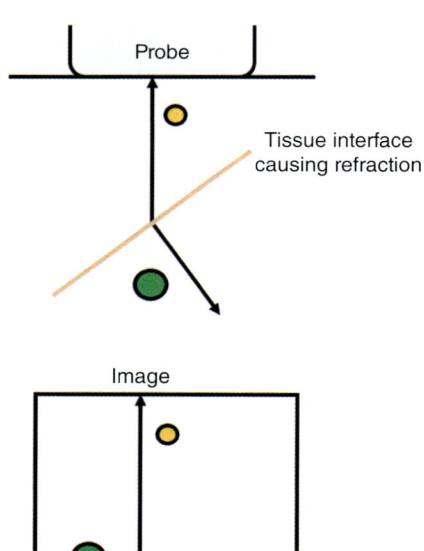

Figure 14.20 The spatial misrepresentation of structures due to a refraction artefact

produced by relative movement of the source to the observer. The conventional example is the siren tone of an ambulance. As the siren approaches, each successive wave front of the sound is closer to the observer than the previously emitted one. This has the effect of spatially compressing wave fronts and so the perceived frequency (hence tone) increases on the approach. As the ambulance passes the observer, the reverse effect leads to a reduction in frequency. The effect is also exaggerated by relative movement of the medium through which a mechanical wave moves (i.e. including sound). So, if the ambulance is approaching from upwind, the effect of the wind will contribute to the effect.

The Doppler effect in a given system can be described mathematically by the Doppler equation:

$$\text{Observed frequency} = \frac{(c + v_r)}{(c + v_s)} \times f_0$$

where f_0 = emitted frequency, c = speed of wave in the medium, v_r = velocity of receiver relative to medium (positive for receiver moving towards source) and v_s = velocity of source relative to medium (positive for source moving away from source). The application

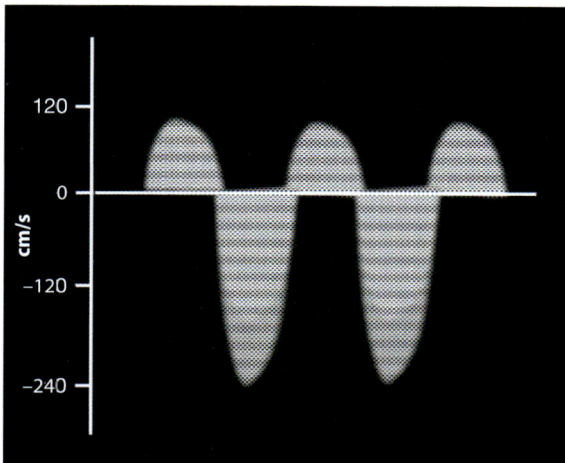

Figure 14.21 Velocity–time profile of CWD

of the Doppler effect in ultrasound is therefore in quantifying velocity, be this of tissue structures, e.g. valve leaflets in the heart, or of fluids, particularly blood. Conceptually, the Doppler effect in medical imaging is more akin to a radar speed gun than the classic ambulance siren example. The source of the signal is co-located with the receiver and both are stationary relative to the medium through which the energy moves. The moving element is the reflecting surface (be that red blood cell or speeding car). In this setting, the Doppler shift (f_s, which equals $f - f_0$) is more relevant than simply the observed frequency, f, as this can be used to determine velocity of the reflecting surface. In a system where v_r and v_s are small compared to c, the Doppler shift is approximately calculated by:

$$f_s = \frac{v}{c} \times f_0$$

where v = velocity of the reflector. This is then solved for v:

$$v = \frac{f_s \times c}{f_0}$$

In a reflective system such as this, the Doppler effect occurs twice; once as the beam arrives at the moving surface and once as it is reflected. This requires adaptation of the relationship by multiplying the term f_0 by 2. Furthermore, the ability to accurately quantify the velocity of the surface in question is highly dependent on the direction of motion being parallel to that of the beam. The cosine of the angle between beam path and the path of the moving target (θ) must also be incorporated. It is for this reason that the sample box superimposed on the B-mode image is not, in fact, a square but a sector or parallelogram; whilst the B-mode beam may be perpendicular to the blood vessel in question, the Doppler beam is ensured not to be. The final relationship to determine velocity is given by:

$$v = \frac{f_s \times c}{2f_0 \times \cos\theta}$$

The applications of the Doppler effect fall into two principal types: continuous-wave Doppler (CWD) and pulsed-wave Doppler (PWD). In CWD, as the name implies, one region of the transducer continuously transmits whilst another receives. The result is a velocity–time profile (Figure 14.21). This technique lacks spatial resolution as the peak in velocity could result from a phenomenon at any depth along the beam. The technique does, however, have excellent velocity resolution (see below).

PWD utilizes one element to send repeated pulses. After a set delay (determined by the user-set depth on a 2D image, according to the area of interest), the element listens for the return. The result is a spectral profile of velocity versus time (Figure 14.22). This profile, when displayed alongside a B-mode image of the anatomy, constitutes Duplex ultrasonography.

Because a defined sample volume is interrogated, PWD is superior to CWD in resolving the depth from which a flow phenomenon originates. The restricted size of the sample also allows characterization between turbulent and laminar flow when interrogating, for example, blood within a vessel. For laminar flow, most red blood cells have the same velocity and the profile will be represented as a thick outline (multiple returns all with a very similar velocity). Turbulent flow is thus denoted as a filling-in of this profile as there are now a wide-range of velocities within the sample. This is referred to as spectral broadening.

A common critical care application of the Doppler effect is the oesophageal Doppler monitor (ODM). This acquires a velocity profile of the descending aorta from an ultrasound probe placed adjacently in the oesophagus. An estimation of the geometry of the aorta is made from details of the patient (age, weight, gender, height) in comparison to reference tables. This allows computation of flow from velocity data. Similar data can be acquired via echocardiography

Chapter 14: Ultrasound and Doppler

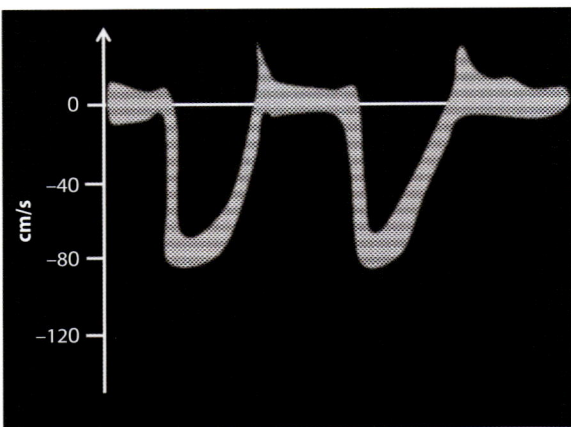

Figure 14.22 Spectral profile of PWD

with the left-ventricular outflow tract velocity–time integral (LVOT VTI). The theoretical advantage of this over the ODM is that the patient's aortic dimensions are measured rather than estimated.

The finite speed of the ultrasound beam and the depth of interest (i.e. the distance of the round-trip for the beam) contribute to the pulse repetition frequency (PRF). This underpins the key disadvantage of PWD over CWD. The maximum velocity which can be measured is dictated by the magnitude of the resulting Doppler shift. For a velocity to be measurable, its resulting Doppler shift must be below the Nyquist limit (defined as half the PRF). As the PRF is infinite for CWD (because the pulses are continuously emitted), there is no theoretical upper limit on the velocity which can be measured. For PWD, however, there is a limit. Referring back to the Doppler equations above, it can be seen there are some work-arounds. A lower frequency can be used as this will reduce the Doppler shift for any given velocity, bringing it within the Nyquist limit. This has a cost in terms of spatial resolution, however. Increasing the angle between the beam and the motion path will have a similar effect but at the expense of underestimating the true velocity. Fundamentally, the PRF itself can be increased by reducing the depth or increasing the speed. Neither of these is practical in real terms; the speed of sound is assumed to be a constant by the machine and an anatomical structure of interest is generally scanned from the most superficial location by default, for reasons of practicality.

A natural extension of PWD is colour Doppler (also variously referred to as colour flow imaging, colour flow Doppler or, simply, Doppler). This consists of the familiar colour overlay on a conventional 2D B-mode image. It is generated by performing PWD on a very large number of sample points rather than a single point, as described earlier. Conventionally, flow away from the probe is depicted as blue, towards as red ('BART' – blue away, red towards). Colour Doppler suffers all the flaws of PWD as would be expected. It is also computationally intensive and this, and the limits of PRF, influences frame rate. Reducing sector width, depth and Doppler box size to the minimum necessary can all compensate for these limitations. The other consideration common to all applications of Doppler imaging of blood flow is the effects of Rayleigh scattering, the principal interaction between blood cells and ultrasound. This necessitates very sensitive equipment as the returns are very low in amplitude compared to surrounding tissue – Rayleigh scattering returns little or no energy in the direction of the source. This again limits the technique to more expensive equipment and, until relatively recently, it was not available on hand-portable scanners.

3D and 4D Ultrasound

Three-dimensional ultrasound is perhaps most colloquially associated with obstetric 'keepsake' scanning, allowing expectant parents to see their unborn baby in a more visually intuitive manner. 4D scanning refers simply to real-time 3D imaging (the fourth dimension being time). It does fundamentally assist in appreciating the true nature of structures. We scan the human body which is a 3D structure but conventionally we have to mentally interpolate a number of 2D images to reconstruct the true nature of the target. This is labour-intensive, training-dependent and prone to error, which 3D and 4D scanning help to alleviate. 3D imaging has specific roles in precise volumetric measurements, such as trans-rectal scanning of prostate tumours.

As with CT scanning, one of the principal limitations is the computational power available. Having acquired information from a block of tissue, this must then be assembled with 3D coordination. This allows 2D images to be reconstructed in any plane from the sampled volume and rendered into a 3D image on the screen.

Other Applications of Ultrasound

Ultrasound has a range of other applications outside of clinical imaging. A wide range of these are within other aspects of medical therapy. Energy between 1 MHz and 2 MHz is used in ultrasonic nebulizers. These have the advantage over conventional gas-driven nebulizers in that they do not require a source of compressed gas. This cuts down on noise and weight. Additionally, the droplet size is much more homogeneous and generally smaller than with conventional systems. This allows deeper and more uniform penetration of the lungs, which is particularly important for humidification and delivery of some drugs.

Lower-frequency energy is employed in technologies which produce tissue lysis. Ultrasonic scalpels have the ability to simultaneously cut and coagulate vessels with minimal collateral damage to surrounding tissue. In this respect they are perhaps superior to electrocautery and also do not produce smoke. Other devices rely on cavitation to selectively disrupt dense tissue (e.g. tumour) whilst sparing softer tissues (e.g. healthy brain, liver, nerves or blood vessels). Cavitation is the creation of small gas bubbles within the medium, which then collapse with the generation of a highly destructive shock wave. All these forms of devices operate in the low-ultrasound, kilohertz band, usually between 20 kHz and 80 kHz.

A relatively new application in therapeutics is high-intensity focused ultrasound (HIFU). Using a similar philosophy to stereotactic radiosurgery, HIFU focuses multiple low-frequency beams at the target point in such a way as to achieve summative interference. This delivers point-focused energy only within the target tissue, with minimal damage to other tissue. It is often guided by real-time magnetic resonance imagery; this is known as MRgFUS (magnetic-resonance-guided focused ultrasound). This technique has been used in treatment of uterine fibroids and is gathering pace in ablation of a range of tumours including prostate, pancreas, breast and others. It also has potential applications in Parkinson's disease and essential tremor, depression and OCD. The frequency band used is around 250 kHz to 2 MHz; although this is close to the band used in imaging, the energy is significantly higher.

Perhaps the most established applications in therapeutics are lithotripsy and those in physiotherapy and musculoskeletal tissue healing. The latter was in fact the very first therapeutic use of ultrasound. Lithotripsy is as longstanding as it is ubiquitous, being the most common treatment for renal stones in the UK. It uses a heterogeneous 3–4-microsecond pulse of waves with frequencies ranging from 100 kHz to 1 MHz. This generates a shock wave within the stone, fragmenting it into pieces, which can usually be passed in the urine without further issue. Unfortunately, the technique can result in damage to the surrounding renal parenchyma, predisposing to infection, parenchymal haemorrhage, acute kidney injury and hypertension. Lithotripsy can be used elsewhere in the body to treat pancreatic, biliary and salivary stones but this is less common.

Outside medicine, ultrasound has a wide range of applications. For example, SONAR (sound navigation and ranging) is used to detect topographical features underwater as well as locate objects within the water, e.g. boats and submarines, shoals of fish, shipwrecks, etc. Generally speaking, it utilizes a comprehensive spectrum of acoustic energy, particularly from the infrasound and audible sound bands but it also involves ultrasound from 100 kHz to 600 kHz in some applications.

Other industrial applications are principally of ultrasonic cavitation effects. This can be used to mix industrial slurries and constituents. It also has a role in imparting energy to chemical reactants or assisting in their mixing – an application referred to as sonochemistry. It can be used to weld plastics. Ultrasonic cleaning can be experienced in the home with off-the-shelf toothbrushes but there are also industrial applications; disinfection can be achieved by disrupting biological cells on surfaces. It can also be used to separate other non-biological contaminants from surfaces for cleaning equipment and components.

Summary

Ultrasound has a wide range of clinical applications and, in anaesthesia and critical care, is most frequently used as a diagnostic tool. Our necrotizing fasciitis patient is a prime candidate for multimodal ultrasound deployment: lung ultrasonography to track the progress of his aspiration pneumonia, cardiac echo and oesophageal Doppler to guide haemodynamic support, Doppler studies of the perfusion to the affected leg and B-mode imaging to assist with placement of intravenous lines. Ultrasound has limitations but, without us perhaps realizing it, it has become ubiquitous in our practice over the last decade.

Questions

MCQs – select true or false for each response

1. Increasing frequency of ultrasound:
   (a) Reduces attenuation
   (b) Increases lateral resolution
   (c) Increases axial resolution
   (d) Increases velocity for a fixed wavelength
   (e) Reduces the effects of Rayleigh scatter
2. Regarding the piezoelectric effect:
   (a) The effect is only demonstrated by materials which are also magnetic
   (b) The reverse piezoelectric effect describes the process by which echoes are received
   (c) The Curie temperature is the maximum temperature at which a piezoelectric probe can perform
   (d) All elements in the probe must receive the same trigger voltage but the timing of activation can be staggered
   (e) Collagen is a piezoelectric substance
3. The Doppler shift of sound in air is dependent on:
   (a) The velocity of the observer within the medium
   (b) The velocity of the source within the medium
   (c) The atmospheric pressure
   (d) The humidity
   (e) The frequency of the original source

SBAs – select the single *best* answer

4. In a patient with cardiogenic shock, the best method to easily assess cardiac function using bedside ultrasound is:
   (a) Oesophageal Doppler monitoring
   (b) Assessment for evidence of pulmonary oedema with lung ultrasound
   (c) Measurement of LVOT VTI on echocardiography
   (d) Trans-oesophageal echocardiography (TOE)
   (e) Visual estimation of left-ventricle function and filling on transthoracic echocardiography
5. A high-velocity flow phenomenon can best be characterized using which form of Doppler imaging?
   (a) Continuous wave Doppler (CWD)
   (b) Pulsed wave Doppler (PWD)
   (c) Tissue Doppler imaging
   (d) Colour Doppler
   (e) Duplex imaging

Answers

1. FTTTF

   As with all forms of resolution, attenuation is a frequency-dependent phenomenon. Similarly, Rayleigh scattering is proportional to frequency to the fourth power. Velocity is directly proportional to frequency.
2. FFFFT

   Piezoelectric properties do not depend on a substance being magnetic. The reverse effect generates ultrasound energy, the direct effect allows it to be received by a transducer. The Curie temperature is that at which a substance loses its piezoelectric properties and probes should generally use a material whose Curie temperature is around twice the anticipated operational temperature for the device. Both timing and voltage can be differentially applied to the crystals in a probe to control beam generation.
3. TTTTT

   These are all statements of fact.
4. (e)

   Of the choices given, basic bedside echo is the best evaluation of cardiac function which is easy to achieve. LVOT VTI or TOE may be technically superior but they require specific skill so are not easy to do. Oesophageal Doppler monitoring relies on assumptions and estimations to generate the numbers so may be unreliable. Lung ultrasound is a useful complement to cardiac assessment but will only yield useful findings where pulmonary oedema exists as a result of any cardiac dysfunction.
5. (a)

   Duplex and colour Doppler involve PWD; PWD is poor at quantifying high-velocity flow by comparison to CWD. Tissue Doppler imaging is, as the name suggests, for tissue motion not flow. That means it is attuned to low-frequency phenomena like the movement of myocardium or valves, rather than high-frequency phenomena such as blood flow.

References

1. F. Galton. *Inquiries into Human Faculty and Its Development* (London, McMillan, 1883).
2. J. Aldrich. Basic physics of ultrasound imaging. *Critical Care Medicine*, 35, 2007; S131–137.

Chapter 15

Atomic Structure, Radiation, Imaging and Lasers

David Ashton-Cleary and Jumana Hussain

Learning Objectives

- To understand the fundamental structure of the atom and how this relates to other important disciplines of science
- To be able to explain exponential processes using radioactive decay as an example
- To understand the principles of X-ray, gamma and magnetic imaging techniques
- To be able to describe the difference between spontaneous and stimulated emission of light and the laser principle in terms of population inversion and lasing threshold
- To be able to explain the principles of fibre-optic transmission and total internal reflection

Chapter Content

- Atomic structure
- Radiation and decay
- Radiation safety
- Computed tomography
- Gamma scintigraphy, PET and SPECT
- Magnetic resonance imaging
- Lasers and fibre optics

Scenario

You are asked to anaesthetize a 56-year-old man for laser-debulking of a glottic tumour. He has already undergone various imaging processes and some of these are of direct relevance to you.

What role does PET scanning have in these cases and how are the images obtained? The patient has had a CT scan of the head and neck; what is the particular relevance in this case? Having undergone radiotherapy, what are the anaesthetic challenges to you as the anaesthetist? Does he pose any health hazard to you and the team, having received such therapy?

Introduction

The nature of matter is of fundamental importance to many of the other principles discussed in this book. Bond structure underpins many of the gas-analysis techniques. Electrons and their shell arrangements form the basis of chemistry, electricity, electronics and light emission. The properties of crystals are central to ultrasound and other applications of piezo-electricity. The topics in this particular chapter are key examples of areas where it is necessary to understand the physics at this atomic level. The next few pages deal almost exclusively with protons, electrons, neutrons, photons and various combinations of the above. For some, it will be a welcome review of a fascinating corner of the A-level physics syllabus. For many, there may be a little trepidation but the aim of the chapter is to focus only on the relevant detail which informs your anaesthetic practice.

Atomic Structure

Although the ancient Greeks coined the term 'atom', much of their understanding was plainly incorrect. It was James Dalton who first explained the atomic basis of chemistry in the nineteenth century. The model was then gradually refined over the next 150 years to that which we recognize today. However, so small are these particles that their behaviour does not obey classical mechanics, and the focus of research in the last 80–100 years has been on producing a model which accurately predicts the behaviour of subatomic particles. This model is quantum mechanics.

It is useful to have a brief understanding of the standard subatomic particles so that we can understand the building blocks of the atom. The nucleus of an atom is composed of nucleons: neutrons (uncharged) and protons (positively charged) (Figure 15.1). The protons are able to exist in close proximity due to the very short-range nuclear force;

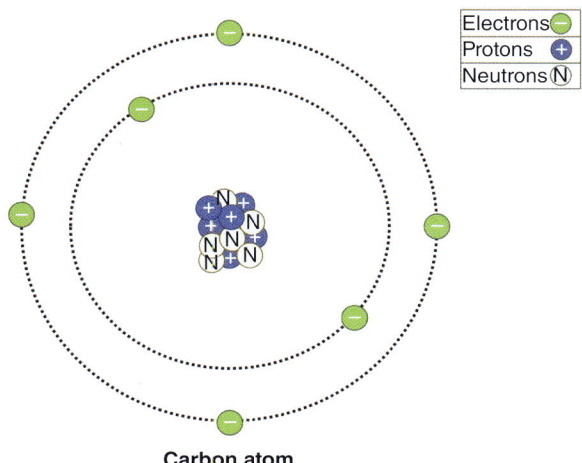

Figure 15.1 Subatomic structure of a carbon atom

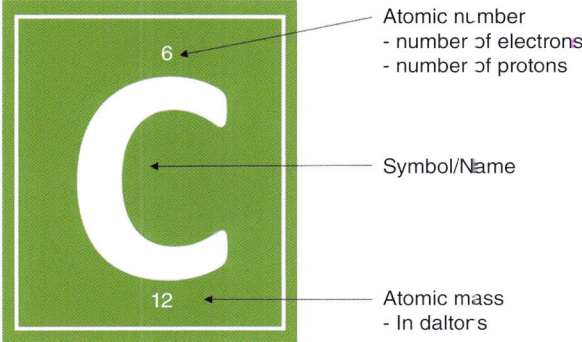

Figure 15.2 Understanding the periodic table

this overcomes the electrostatic force otherwise repelling them from one another. The number of protons in the nucleus (the atomic number) determines the chemical element while the combined total of nucleons determines the atomic mass number. For example, a nucleus containing six protons defines it as that of an atom of carbon. That carbon atom may have six neutrons (an atom of carbon-12) or eight neutrons (an atom of carbon-14). These two represent two different isotopes – species which share an atomic number but differ in mass number. Mass number is the count of nucleons but the weight of a single nucleon (one dalton) is so small as to be impractical in most settings. The mole is a more useful construct and the SI definition of this relies on Avogadro's constant, which defines the number of particles present in a mole; 6.02×10^{23} mol^{-1}. One mole of a substance will weigh the mass number in grams, e.g. 1 mol of lead atoms weighs 208 g. The mass number and atomic number often appear with the symbol in the relevant square on the periodic table of elements (Figure 15.2).

The term 'nuclide' may also crop up and, although it's often used synonymously with 'isotope', they are different terms. As discussed earlier, isotopes are identical in respect of the same number of protons in the nucleus (but differ in neutron count). This is a little like the term 'ion', which refers to differences in electron count but with the same nucleus. For example, iron can exist as Fe^{2+} or Fe^{3+} – both different ionic species of iron. A 'nuclide' is specified in terms of not just proton count but also neutron count and energy state. Also, don't confuse the nuclear physics term, nuclide, with the genetics term, 'nucleotide' – these are very different!

Surrounding the nucleus are the electrons. Classical models consider these as particles and, for ease of description, that construct will be used here. In reality, they are better described as clouds, the shape of which is dictated by a standing wave that models the probability of the electron existing in any one location relative to the nucleus. The electrostatic attraction between electrons and protons means that electrons are most stable closest to the nucleus, in the so-called ground-state, having lowest energy. As additional electrons are added, however, the electrostatic interaction with their neighbours dictates that they must exist further away from one another. Quantum mechanics describes how electrons have discrete energy levels at which they can exist and, in turn, this gives rise to the shell model of electrons, as taught in school chemistry lessons (Figure 15.1). This is relevant in two particular ways.

Firstly, electrons can change energy level by absorbing energy from photons and climb up an energy state – or emit energy as a photon and drop an energy state. It was Niels Bohr who postulated the concept of a series of stable energy states for electrons. This deals with the paradox which would otherwise see all electrons immediately emit photons to allow them all to reach the ground state (which they do not do). This gives us the basis for understanding the production and absorption of light by elements according to their electron configuration (see later).

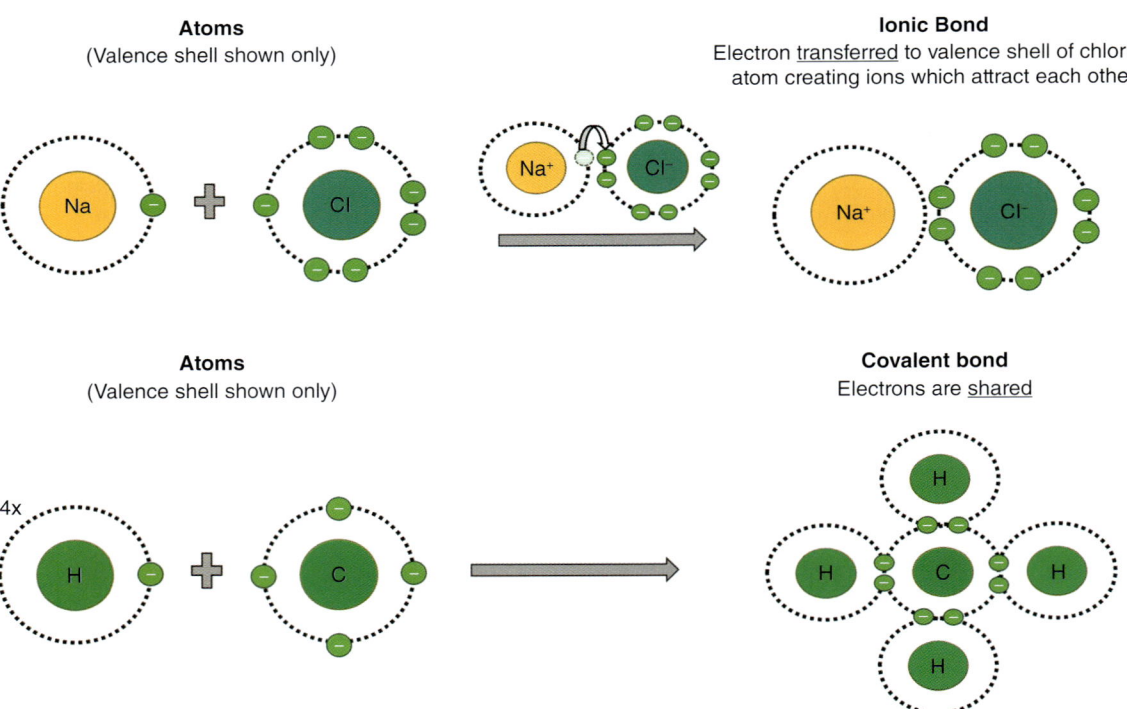

Figure 15.3 Ionic and covalent bonds

 The energy change of an electron moving between two states can be related to the frequency of the photon involved in the transaction by Plank's constant (h). $E = hf$ predicts the frequency and hence wavelength (colour) of light absorbed from a beam of white light. Since the energy transitions possible are unique to each element, this produces a characteristic pattern of black absorption bands in the spectrum of light when shone through a substance. This is the basis of spectroscopy, used to identify atoms. It is also how sunscreen works – the ingredients are selected to produce an absorption band in the ultraviolet range.

Secondly, the physical chemistry of an element is principally determined by the completeness, or otherwise, of its outermost electron shell. This is known as its valence shell. An element will react with others in a mutually convenient manner to fill their respective valence shells. A number of prototype bonds exist (Figure 15.3). Ionic bonds, e.g. metal salts such as sodium chloride, involve electrons localized, but not exclusive, to an adjacent sodium and chloride ion within the crystal. Covalent bonds involve the sharing of pairs of electrons, usually one, two or three but sometimes four: single, double, triple bonds etc. Covalent bonds are particularly prevalent in organic chemistry. Metallic bonding is similar to ionic except that the electrons are entirely free to roam the crystal lattice; hence the properties of metals, particularly thermal and electrical conductivity. The completeness of the valence shell also determines the position in the periodic table, with each row of the table corresponding to a shell progressively filled from left to right across the table. The right-most element has its shell filled and is unreactive as a result – the inert gases. Elements in the same column of the table share the same number of electrons in their valence shell.

Radiation and Decay

So far, we have alluded principally to stable elements and described their nucleus as an equal mix of neutrons and protons. In fact, once you pass calcium (atomic number 20) on the periodic table, that model begins to change; stable isotopes of the elements tend to have more neutrons than protons. Once the nucleus of an element is too large to be contained by the radius of the nuclear force (about 1 femtometre, 10^{-15} m, a

Table 15.1 Comparison of the key forms of radiation

Radiation type	Nature	Change to nucleus	Energy	Shielding
Alpha	Helium nucleus, 2^+ charge	$A-4$ and $Z-2$	4–9 MeV	Paper or a few centimetres of air
Beta	High-energy electron or positron	$Z \pm 1$, A unchanged	Variable	Aluminium or thick clothing
Gamma	Photon, $>10^{19}$ Hz	Lower energy state	>41 KeV	Lead
X-ray	Photon, 3×10^{17} Hz	No change	0.1–100 KeV	Lead

Z – atomic number (proton count), A – mass number (nucleon count)

quadrillionth of a metre), the electrostatic repulsion between the protons can prevail, leading to break-up of the nucleus. This is radioactivity. All isotopes of all elements heavier than bismuth-83 are radioactive. Of course, there are radioactive isotopes of lighter elements too, but there are also stable isotopes of those elements. Radioactive emission takes a number of key forms. The most relevant are the forms of ionizing radiation which, by definition, is any emitted energy or particle with sufficient energy (>10 electron-volts, eV) to liberate electrons from atoms or molecules, converting them to ions (see Table 15.1).

Alpha Radiation

Alpha radiation is the emission of a helium nucleus (two neutrons and two protons). This particle is highly energized but also relatively high in mass, compared to other forms of radiation, and it is positively charged. As a result, even though it is ejected from the nucleus at close to 5% of the speed of light, it is absorbed by a sheet of paper or a few centimetres of air. The clinical corollary to this is that alpha particles cannot penetrate skin. Alpha sources can, however, have fatal effects if ingested.

Americium-241 is used in smoke detectors. The alpha particles that are produced ionize the air in the sample chamber, allowing an electrical current to pass through. Smoke particles do not ionize and the conducted current through the chamber reduces, triggering the alarm.

Beta Radiation

Beta decay results from the transformation of a neutron to a proton, releasing a high-energy electron (the beta particle) and an anti-neutrino. Alternatively, conversion of a proton to a neutron can produce a positron and a neutrino (this is the basis of PET scanning, as discussed later). Beta emission is driven by the tendency of the nucleus to reach the lower-energy state inherent of a more stable proton–neutron ratio. The energy of the beta electron depends on the proportion of the total energy release which is taken by the anti-neutrino and this can vary over a wide range. The emission is less ionizing than an alpha particle but penetrates matter much more readily (lower mass and charge) so requires more shielding; an aluminium plate will suffice. Interaction with heavier elements, e.g. lead, can actually worsen matters by triggering secondary gamma emission, in a process known as *bremsstrahlung* (German for 'braking radiation' – rapid slowing of the particle results in electromagnetic emission).

Release of alpha or beta particles causes a predictable transmutation to another nuclide, e.g. alpha decay of uranium-235 yields thorium-241. Decay continues until a stable species results; ^{235}U decays to ^{207}Pb via thirteen intermediary radionuclides. Decay of all radionuclides proceeds according to an exponential relationship over time, i.e. the rate of decrease depends on the current amount present. This can be represented mathematically as:

$$N_t = N_0 \times e^{-kt}$$

where N_t is the number of particles at time t, N_0 is the number of particles initially, k is the decay constant and t is the time elapsed. From this, the time taken for the amount of the parent nuclide to halve (half-life – $t_{1/2}$) can be determined:

$$t_{1/2} = \frac{\ln(2)}{k}$$

Note that the half-life does not determine when radioactivity will diminish to safe levels. Seven half-lives will reduce the parent nuclide to 0.78% of the original amount, but if this is still a large quantity in absolute terms, it is a very radioactive species or has decayed to other radionuclides, a hazard to life will persist.

Gamma Emission

Most alpha and beta decay is accompanied by gamma emission. This is defined as any electromagnetic energy release as a result of radioactive nuclear decay. These high-energy photons have no mass (a defining property of anything which moves at the speed of light) or charge but are highly ionizing through indirect interactions on account of their very high energy. The most powerful gamma source is interstellar radiation but the vast majority is absorbed by the atmosphere. That said, secondary gamma emission from interaction between cosmic rays and the atmosphere does occur. Despite its biological hazard, gamma radiation has a wide range of medical applications, including gamma-knife surgery, gamma camera, PET and SPECT diagnostics, and in the sterilization of equipment and instruments. Shielding from gamma emission relies on the total mass within the path of the beam. Lead is the prototype shielding material because high-atomic-number elements and those in a dense form (both properties of solid lead) ensure a large mass in the beam path. A denser material allows for a thinner shield with obvious practical benefits: a 0.5-mm lead foil is much easier to wear as a radiation protection apron than 1.3 cm of steel plate!

You may be thinking, 'if $E = mc^2$, surely photons have a mass as a consequence of their energy and velocity?' Actually, $E = mc^2$ only applies to stationary objects. $E = mc^2$ is the end-derivation of energy relating to the square root of $(m^2 \times c^4) + (p^2 \times c^2)$. For a stationary object, momentum (p) is zero (because velocity is zero), and so the rest of that equation resolves to the familiar $E = mc^2$. For a massless photon (objects moving at the speed of light have to be massless), it instead becomes $E = pc$ which equates to $E = hf$. Special relativity defines momentum differently to classical physics and the end result is that the momentum of a photon is equal to 0/0 – this is 'indeterminate', which is not mathematically equal to zero. All of which means a photon doesn't have to have mass to make the maths work. In fact, if a photon is assigned mass by application of Newtonian physics, a number of other important aspects of physics fall apart, for example, electrodynamics.

X-Ray Radiation

X-Radiation is a further form of electromagnetic emission. Various definitions distinguish between X- and gamma-rays, based on frequency or source; the current consensus states that gamma rays originate from nuclear decay whereas X-rays originate from orbiting-electron interactions. X-rays are generally produced by two types of interaction: *bremsstrahlung* (see above) and K-shell emission. The latter is the principal mechanism in an X-ray tube (Figure 15.4). High-energy electrons bombard a tungsten-alloy target and strip electrons from the inner shell of the atom (the inner shell is the K shell, hence the name). Electrons from higher shells fall to refill the K shell and emit the energy difference as a high-energy photon – an X-ray. A conventional X-ray tube consists of a cathode and an anode in a vacuum tube. Historically, the anode was copper or copper with a platinum film but modern tubes use a tungsten–rhenium alloy or molybdenum. A voltage of around 100 kV is applied, causing electrons to be accelerated towards the anode. They strike the target, releasing X-rays, which are directed towards the patient. The process is very inefficient – only around 1% of the energy is converted to usable X-rays; the rest causes point-heating of the target to temperatures of 1,000–2,000 °C. Increasing the voltage across the tube (or, more accurately, the peak voltage – kV_p) increases the *energy* of the predominant X-rays produced, whereas increasing the current and duration of the current pulse through the tube (milliamp seconds – mA s) increases the *number* of X-ray photons produced. In simple imaging terms, increased kV_p increases tissue penetration but at the expense of reduced image contrast (number of greyscales depicted in the whole image), and an increase in milliamp seconds increases density or 'blackness' of the image.

Table 15.1 compares and summarizes the key forms of radiation.

Radiation Safety

All forms of ionizing radiation are, by definition, biologically harmful. Ionization of DNA, RNA, proteins and other biological molecules can lead to acute radiation poisoning, burns or mutation risk, i.e. cancers and heritable defects. Dose can be described in a number of ways and the nomenclature can be a little confusing. There are a number of key factors: amount of energy absorbed; what type of emission is bringing that energy to bear; and the type of tissue irradiated and its sensitivity to irradiation.

The 'absorbed dose' describes the energy absorbed per unit mass (J kg^{-1} or gray). This is non-specific to the other factors mentioned above, however. Tissue sensitivity (see Table 15.2) and emission type are combined to consider the biological impact of a given dose in terms of risk of long-term harm: this converts the absorbed dose to the 'effective dose'. Confusingly, the derived units for this are also J kg^{-1} but it is given the special name of a sievert (Sv). One sievert equates to a 5.5% lifetime risk of cancer resulting from the exposure. For X-ray, gamma and beta radiation, all three cause similar degrees of biological harm and so this isn't factored into the conversion from absorbed dose to effective dose. The result is that, for these emissions, the absorbed dose (Gy) and effective dose (Sv) will be numerically equal. Alpha sources, however, are 20 times more hazardous and so 1 Gy of alpha exposure gives an effective dose of 20 Sv. Some effective doses of various radiological investigations and real-world exposures are given in Table 15.3.

The effective doses for medical exposures in Table 15.3 are based on a specified amount of energy which is deemed to be justifiable for that examination or intervention. This is set down for each radiology intervention by the Ionizing Radiation (Medical Exposure) Regulations (IRMER) in the UK and the hospital medical physics and radiology departments are required by law to stay within these limits. Additionally, there are legal requirements on referring clinicians to justify the exposure, with sufficient information to allow the radiologist to determine the best and most appropriate imaging modality which allows the exposure to adhere to the ALARP principle: the residual risk should be As Low As Reasonably Possible.

Safety depends on minimizing the number of people exposed to ionizing radiation and minimizing

Table 15.2 Tissue weighting (larger number = more sensitive to ionizing radiation) (Reproduced from The 2007 Recommendations of the International Commission on Radiological Protection. ICRP Publication 103 [1])

Bone marrow (red), colon, lung, stomach, breast, remainder tissue group*	0.12
Gonads	0.08
Bladder, oesophagus, liver, thyroid	0.04
Cortical bone, brain, salivary glands, skin	0.01

* Remainder tissue group includes adrenals, heart, kidneys, pancreas, small bowel, spleen and thymus

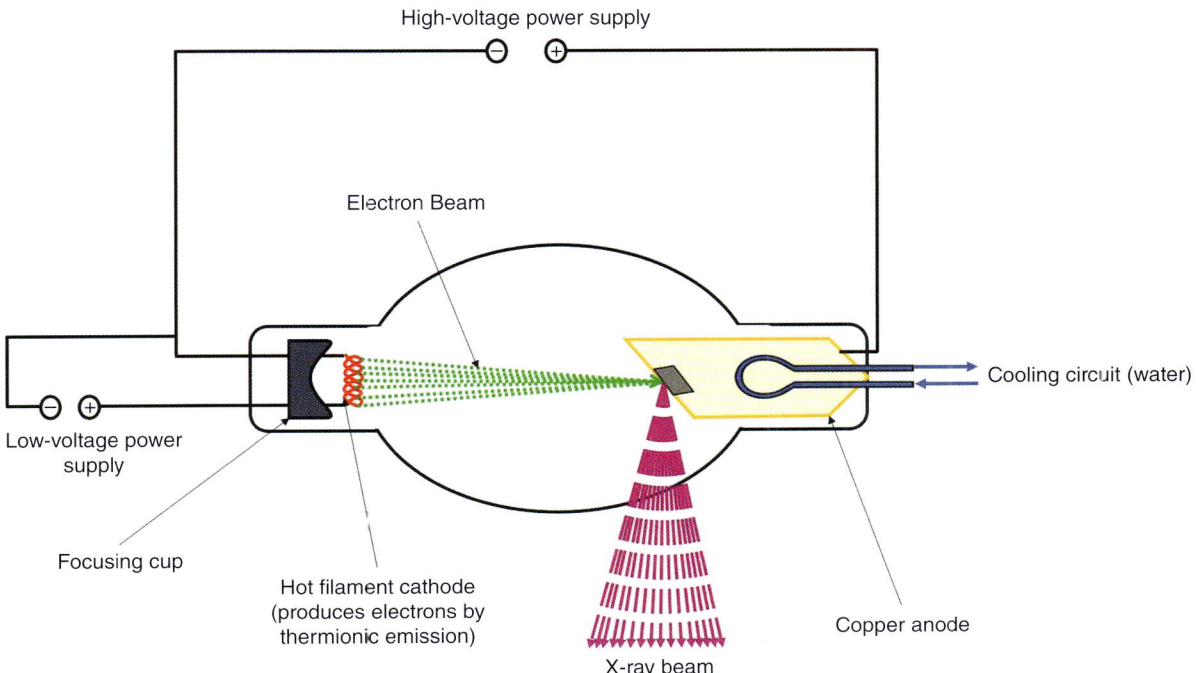

Figure 15.4 K-shell emission X-ray tube

Table 15.3 Example effective doses (medical examples in bold)

Eating a banana	0.1 μSv
Dental X-ray	5 μSv
CXR	20 μSv
Living in a stone, brick or concrete house for 1 year	70 μSv
CT head	1.4–2 mSv
Annual background dose (UK average)	2.7 mSv
Spending 1 hour at Chernobyl plant	6 mSv
Chest CT	7 mSv
CT pulmonary angiogram	11 mSv
Myocardial perfusion scan	18 mSv
Annual maximum dose for radiation workers	20 mSv
Full-body CT	30 mSv
Short exposure, causing poisoning	400 mSv
Short exposure, causing severe poisoning or death	2 Sv
Dose causing death within 30 days	4–8 Sv
10 minutes next to recently exploded Chernobyl reactor	50 Sv

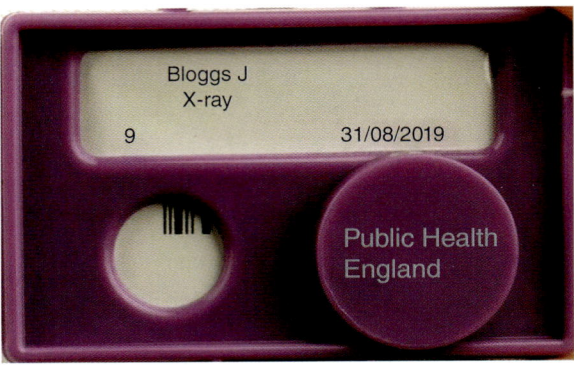

Figure 15.5 Thermoluminescent dosimeter (Photograph reproduced with kind permission of Public Health England Personal Dosimetry Service, Didcot, UK)

the dose they receive. For patients, this largely means ensuring that exposures are clinically justifiable and that, for any given intervention, the dose is minimized. For personnel, there needs to be adequate shielding to contain the particular type of emission being utilized. This includes shielding of rooms, e.g. X-ray suites, storerooms where radionuclides are kept, as well as personal protection, e.g. lead aprons, thyroid shields, bismuth pads for interventional radiology, etc. Those working continuously with ionizing radiation, e.g. radiology and interventional cardiology staff, should also have their personal exposure monitored. In its simplest form, this is achieved by wearing a cassette, containing a piece of photographic film. There is a portion of the film fully exposed (to quantify beta exposure), and a series of metal filters allow the energy and exposure of gamma/X-ray exposure to be determined. These devices are simple and cheap but lack accuracy and cannot be used for finger doses for interventionalists. They are being superseded by thermoluminescent and electronic dosimeters (Figure 15.5). Thermoluminescence usually employs magnesium- or manganese-doped crystals of calcium fluoride or lithium fluoride. Incident gamma/X-radiation boosts electrons in the crystal to a higher energy state, where they are trapped (due to the influence of the dope). When the detector is heated, the electrons are released and fall to ground state, emitting the energy difference as a photon of visible light. The intensity of luminescence correlates to exposure.

Computed Tomography

Computed tomography (CT) is ubiquitous in modern practice. In fact, with the exception of plain chest radiography, CT is by far the commonest modality that anaesthetists and critical care clinicians now encounter. It has the clear advantage of being able to demonstrate the location of structures in three dimensions. Even a combination of a lateral and postero-anterior plain chest radiograph still leaves some mental interpolation to be done to determine where a lesion lies within the thorax, for example. In addition, the contrast resolution of CT is vastly superior to plain radiography. For a plain film, two adjacent tissue types need to differ in radiopacity by at least 10% to be distinguishable on the image. For CT, the necessary difference is only around 0.3%. This is in addition to the greater spatial resolution (see later) which allows CT to distinguish structures that are much less widely separated in physical space. The idea of CT only really took off in the 1960s with the advent of the necessary computer power to undertake the massive data processing and storage required. At this stage, a single slice took up to 5 minutes to acquire

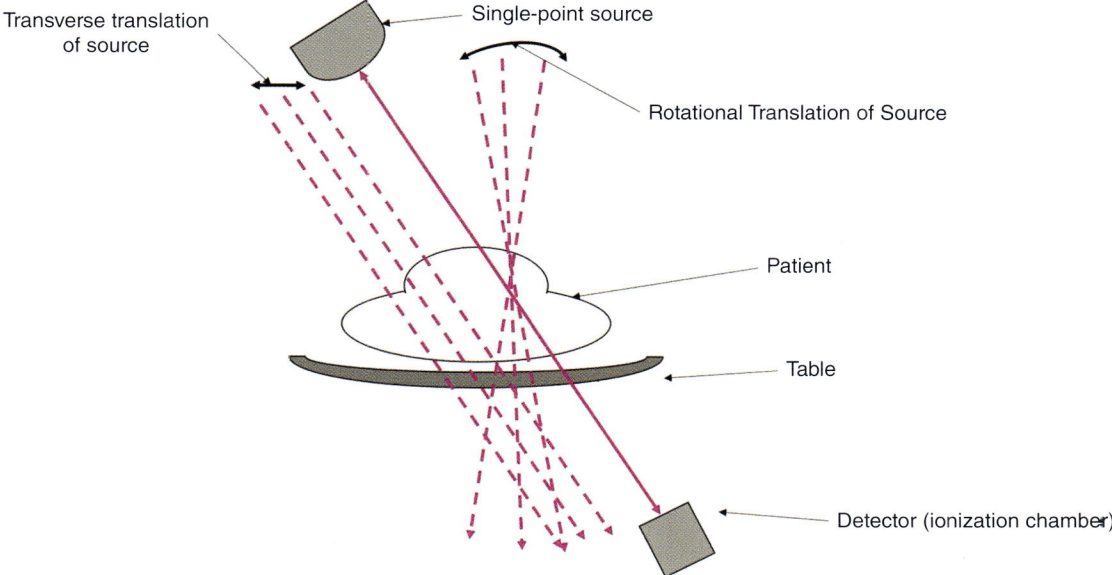

Figure 15.6 Basic layout of an axial CT array

and a further 90 seconds to process. Consequently, brain imaging alone could take up to an hour to acquire.

In its earliest and simple form, CT consisted of a single pencil-point beam of X-ray energy directed through the patient to an ionization chamber, acting as the detector on the opposite side of the apparatus. The entire emitter–detector assembly would rotate around the patient and also traverse across the patient, making a number of exposures (Figure 15.6). Then the patient was moved through the scanner in a small increment and the whole process started again. Although we have moved a long way since this, it is a relatively simple way to understand how the process of tomography works. We need to think about a single slice (i.e. with no movement of the patient through the scanner along the z-axis). Each slice of the image is assembled from multiple beams passed through the tissue from multiple angles. The data are assembled into a grid and, ultimately, the value of each cell of the grid is translated into a greyscale value, displayed as a pixel (short for 'picture element') on the image. Each cell of the grid has a dimension in the x-plane and y-plane (a width and height in the patient) but it also has a z-plane dimension, dictated by the thickness of the beam. So, in fact, this 'slice' of the patient is actually a 3D volume and each cell in the grid is also a volume referred to as a voxel

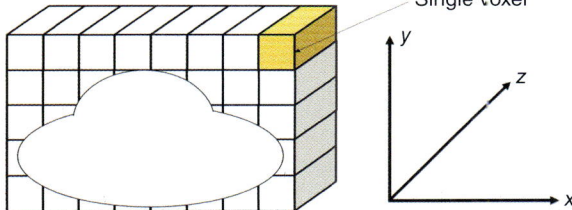

Figure 15.7 An axial image constructed of an array of voxels

(a 'volume element') (Figure 15.7). This concept becomes particularly important when talking about reconstructions later.

Each individual beam passes through numerous voxels on its way through the patient. The extent to which tissue absorbs X-rays can be quantified by the X-ray attenuation, and each voxel will have a different X-ray attenuation coefficient, depending on the tissue type present. So how can we determine the attenuation of the tissue for each single voxel when we can only image a whole beamful of voxels at once? By interrogating the whole slice from numerous angles, it is possible to mathematically combine the data from multiple beams. The data from all the beams which intersect a single voxel can be used to determine the attenuation of that volume of tissue and discard the data from the other voxels in the contributing

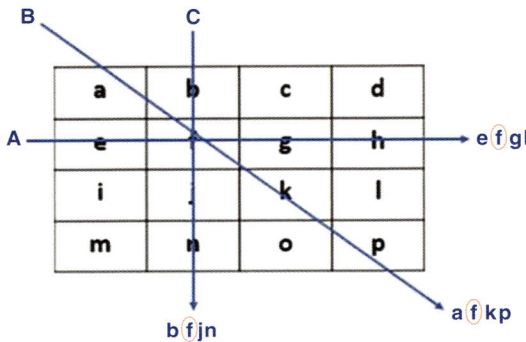

Figure 15.8 Intersection of multiple beams allows information to be determined about an individual voxel: beams A, B and C all have only one voxel in common (f)

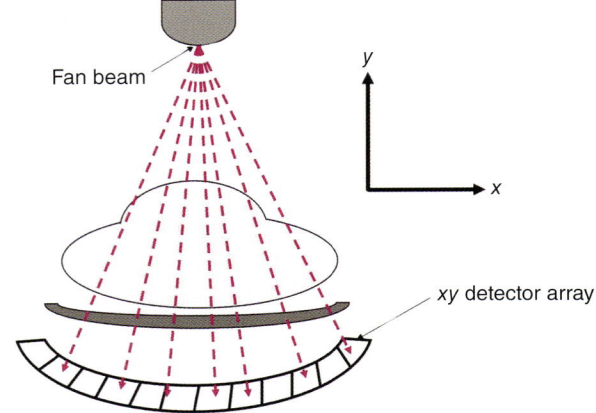

Figure 15.9 Detector array in the x–y-planes

beams (Figure 15.8). This is actually surprisingly simple mathematics but must occur on a huge scale as it must be repeated for every voxel of every slice, just to create one axial image of the patient.

There may be a significant variation in attenuation within a single voxel, e.g. a small clot within a blood vessel. The best the machine can manage is to provide an average value for all the attenuation occurring in a voxel. This can lead to poor contrast resolution of very small targets. This is known as the partial volume effect.

What we have described so far is a single beam and a single detector. While this avoided the problems of X-ray scatter and the associated artefact, it was very slow. The next step is to use an X-ray source which produces a fan of beams radiating out towards an array of detectors in the x–y-plane (x–y because the detectors wrap around the circular aperture of the scanner so they cross behind the patient plinth and rise up around the sides as in Figure 15.9). This advance produces a dramatic improvement in speed and spatial resolution but there are compromises with scatter from one beam onto an adjacent detector. This is managed with collimators between the patient and the detectors, to absorb the incoming scatter-photons and ensure that, as far as possible, the scanner behaves more like an array of individual beams. Rather than ionization chambers, modern scanners use solid-state photodetectors. Typically made from cadmium tungstate, these fluoresce visible light when exposed to

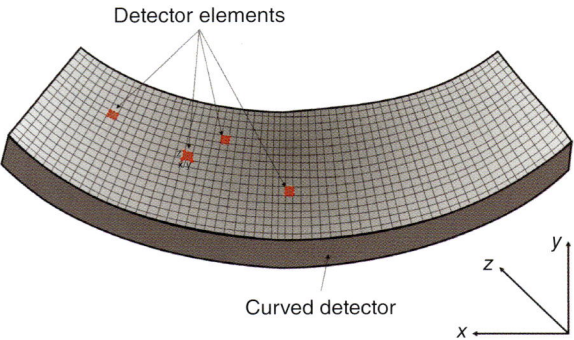

Figure 15.10 Detector array in the x-, y- and z-planes

X-ray energy. A photodetector then captures this visible light and converts it into an electric current. Crucially, these detectors can be made much smaller than an ionization chamber, allowing for arrays of detectors and for smaller detectors; this improves spatial resolution (for a more complete discussion of spatial resolution see Chapter 14).

Single-slice detector arrays, as described above, were a huge advance but they remained quite slow. With the miniaturization of detectors, it next became possible to have detectors in the z-plane. This allows so-called multi-slice scanning. The thickness of the slice in these arrays is not solely dependent on the beam width but also the thickness of the detectors in the z-plane and, in fact, on whether or not multiple detectors are grouped together; 0.625-mm detectors could be grouped together to give slices of 1.25 mm or 2.5 mm for example (Figure 15.10). Thin slices have the clear advantage of increasing spatial resolution although they are more susceptible to noise issues.

It is common to acquire data in thin slices and utilize filters and algorithms for reconstruction of this data in order to reduce the noise in the reformatted images.

Historically, CT has gone by the term 'CAT' scanning, the 'A' standing for 'axial'. In axial imaging, a slice was acquired, the patient was advanced along the z-axis by a pre-determined increment, a further slice was acquired and so on. The distinct disadvantage to this is that any reconstruction of images into other planes or thicknesses had to be planned before acquiring the required imaging data. Helical scanning has changed that. With helical scanning, the emitter–detector array spins continuously and the patient moves through the scanner continuously. Let's say we want to make some sandwiches, so we go to the baker and buy just enough slices of bread. If we realize we need to make more sandwiches or someone prefers thicker bread slices, we don't have the option once we've bought the bread in this way. That's a little like classic axial imaging. If, however, you bring home the whole loaf, you can slice it however you want and that's the difference with helical imaging; you have data for a complete volume of tissue, not pre-selected slices from it. This allows for multiplanar reconstruction. The final hurdle was getting detectors small enough in the z-plane. An x–y resolution of 0.5 mm has been possible for some time. Now that a similar resolution is possible in the z-plane it means the voxels are cuboid rather than a rectangular prism. That means that it is possible to reformat the data in any direction; it is even possible to follow curving blood vessels and reconstruct them into a linear representation. This allows accurate measurements to be made to plan endovascular procedures or assess for coronary vessel patency, for example.

Display of the data presents a different problem. X-ray attenuation coefficients for various tissue types are known (see Table 15.4) but these need to be converted into a more useful system. The Hounsfield scale mathematically references all attenuation coefficients to a scale where water has a value of zero. The data acquired from the scanner are 12-bit data, in other words, the greyscale data contains a range of up to 4,096 shades (2^{12}). Most computer displays can only display 8-bit greyscale (256 shades, 2^{8}) but the real problem is the human eye, which is a 6-bit device! That means we can only perceive around 60–90 shades of grey. This gives rise to the concept of 'windowing' the image. This means selecting the

Table 15.4 X-ray attenuation coefficients (for 70 keV) and Hounsfield scale for several matter types

Matter or tissue	X-ray attenuation coefficient (cm^{-1})	Hounsfield units
Distilled water at STP	0.19	0
Air at STP	0	−1,000
Fat	0.171	−100
Grey matter	0.197	38
Cortical bone	0.38	3,000

range of raw data values we are interested in (depending on the body region we are investigating) and representing them across the 256 shades the display can depict. We set the lowest value we are interested in as the black point and the highest value as the white point and then we 'level' the window to ensure the mid-grey value corresponds to the value of the tissue we are particularly focused on.

X-Ray Contrast Agents

Both plain and CT imaging can be enhanced by the administration of contrast agents. Typically, intravenous agents contain iodine and oral agents for gastrointestinal imaging contain barium. In the setting of diagnostic X-ray imaging, attenuation of the beam occurs through two principal mechanisms: Compton scattering and the photoelectric effect (there are three other X-ray-matter interactions but they only occur at energy levels well outside the band used for diagnostic imaging). The photoelectric effect involves absorption of a photon by an electron, which is then ejected from the atom due to the energy it absorbs. This effect dominates at lower energy levels. The Compton effect, or Compton scatter, dominates at the higher energy levels and involves partial absorption of the photon energy by an electron (which, as with the photoelectric effect, is ejected from the atom). With Compton scattering, the X-ray photon is not fully absorbed by interacting with the electron but it does change its frequency as a result of transferring part of its energy to the ejected electron. This frequency change causes refraction (direction change), with scatter possible in any direction, including back towards the source. Compton scatter is the principal cause of occupational risk to clinicians (through backscatter) and also introduces noise and contrast reduction in the image. High-density substances increase Compton interactions. High atomic number (irrespective of density) increases photoelectric absorption. Both of these result in the radiopaque properties of iodine and barium. Note that both of these interactions strip an electron from an atom. In other words, these are ionizing interactions and this is the mechanism by which radiation produces cellular damage in sufficient dose.

> The photoelectric effect is the basis for night-vision technology. Photons of light strike a metal plate, causing ejection of electrons. These pass through a photomultiplier that accelerates them and increases their numbers. Finally, the photoelectrons strike a fluorescent substance causing it to glow, with an image derived from the original few incoming photons.

Gamma Scintigraphy, PET and SPECT

The discipline of nuclear medicine is largely concerned with detection of gamma radiation from radionuclide tracer agents injected into the patient. The agents are selected for the preferential way in which they bind to the tissue of interest. The gamma photons are photographed by a gamma camera. This consists of a sodium iodide crystal which fluoresces in response to an incident gamma photon. A photomultiplier behind the crystal detects the fluorescence and converts it to an electrical signal for conversion into a digital image. In scintigraphy, the radionuclide produces gamma photons directly. In PET (positron emission tomography), an administered tracer substance produces a positron which annihilates a nearby electron, producing two gamma photons that are subsequently detected in a similar way with a form of the gamma camera. Having two photons released per event, as in the case of PET, produces significantly better spatial resolution but it is a much more expensive modality (mostly due to the cost of tracer production). It is typically combined with conventional CT or MRI to allow overlay of the PET signal on anatomical imaging; strictly speaking, this is PET-CT or PET-MRI. Currently, the commonest PET tracer is ^{18}F-fluorodeoxyglucose (FDG), which acts as a glucose analogue. This means it is concentrated by highly metabolically active tissues such as tumours or seizure foci.

Single-photon emission computed tomography (SPECT) is a combination of gamma scintigraphy with CT to provide a 3D scintigram. As with PET-CT, this can also be combined with conventional X-ray CT. Perhaps a little confusingly, this provides a SPECT-CT image. The key point here is to realize that the term 'computed tomography' is not specific to X-ray imaging; it refers to the process of gathering data about voxels and rendering 2D or 3D images from this data. In a similar way to the X-ray array of CT, SPECT utilizes a gamma camera head (or sometimes two to three heads) which rotate around the patient gathering data in three dimensions. In a process not dissimilar to the glass lens of a photographic camera, a SPECT or standard gamma camera needs a collimating filter to focus an image. The collimator consists of a thick lead plate with a number of very small channels through which the photons can pass. This actually screens out the majority of photons and yet also, unfortunately, allows some photons to interact with the photodetectors in adjacent areas of the camera. This results in an image which is relatively blurred and lacks contrast. This is why superimposition on X-ray imaging can be very helpful. Typical applications of SPECT include cerebral perfusion scanning, location of certain tumours, particularly of the endocrine system, and white-cell scans (using infused radio-labelled white cells) to locate infection. Perhaps the most widely encountered SPECT modality in anaesthesia is myocardial perfusion scanning. This is sometimes known as MIBI scanning after one of the several radiotracers which can be used for cardiac imaging, Technitium-sesta-mibi-99m ('m' stands for metastable).

Magnetic Resonance Imaging

Magnetic resonance imaging (MRI or sometimes simply referred to as MR) also utilizes the principles of CT. The process of generating and detecting a signal to delineate the anatomy is entirely different from the modalities discussed so far.

All the protons of every nucleus of every atom have a quantum spin state (Figure 15.11, left). This is an inherent property, just like the positive charge and mass they carry. MRI exploits this characteristic. The spin of the proton results in a magnetic field and, therefore, an external magnetic field will interact with

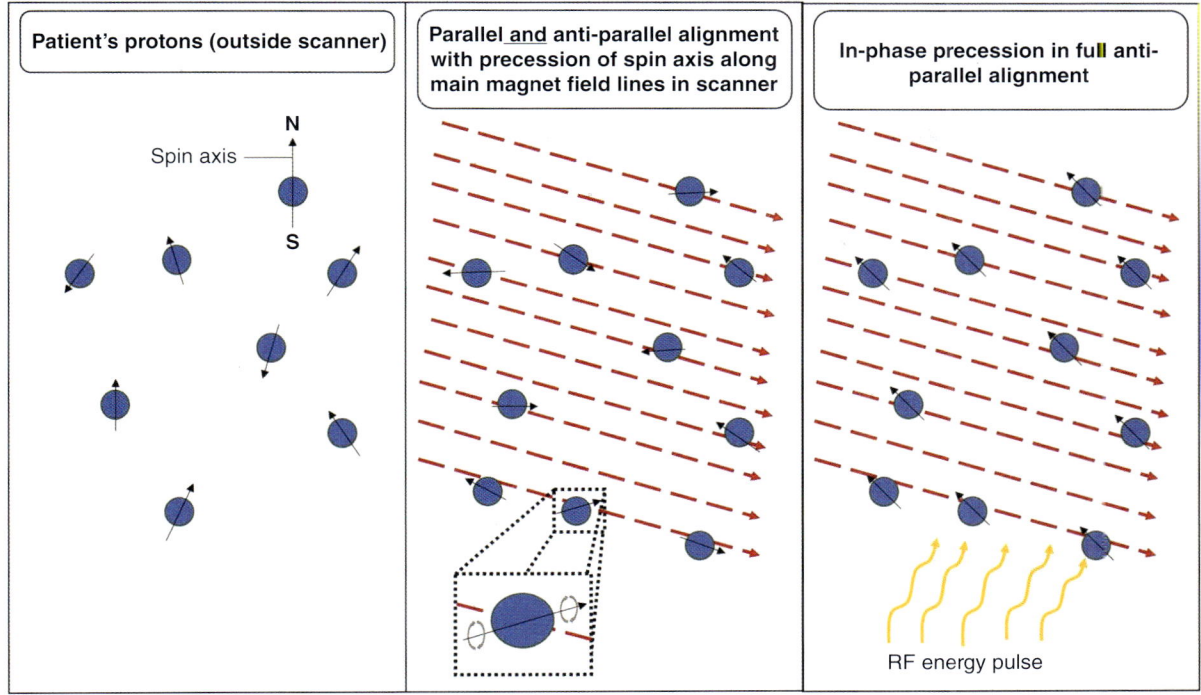

Figure 15.11 State of proton spin outside an MRI scanner (left), under the influence of the main magnetic field (centre) and resonating after application of the radio-frequency (RF) pulse (right).

the proton. In an MRI scanner, the main magnet is actually an electromagnet. It consists of a niobium–titanium coil which is cooled to around 4 K with liquid helium. At this temperature, the electrical resistance falls to zero and the coil becomes a superconductor, allowing massive currents to flow, resulting in a magnetic field of 2–3 tesla (the Earth's magnetic field is around 30–60 microtesla). This magnetic field can align the field and spin axes of the protons; some assume a low-energy, stable alignment with their field parallel to the scanner's main field, but others align parallel but in the opposite direction, i.e. anti-parallel (Figure 15.11, centre). The anti-parallel state is much less stable and is a higher energy state. The protons' spin axes are never perfectly aligned and in fact, precess around the field lines of the scanner's magnet. This is very much like a spinning top or gyroscope. A gyroscope precesses around the vertical field lines of the Earth's gravitational field. The frequency with which the protons precess is directly related to the strength of the main field. We'll come back to why that relationship is particularly important later on.

The second component of the MRI scanner is a coil. Coils are the components added around the body-region of interest when the patient gets in the machine. If electromagnetic energy is applied to the aligned photons with the exact frequency of their precession, they will resonate (hence the name of the scan). The required frequency is in the megahertz band, so this is radio-wave energy and is supplied by the coil. Proton resonance involves two effects. Firstly, the parallel-aligned protons are boosted to the higher-energy, anti-parallel alignment. Secondly, all the protons now precess in phase. Imagine people swimming chaotically in a pool. If we apply lane barriers (analogous to the scanner main field lines), we cause the swimmers to swim in lanes. However, they can still choose to swim in one of two directions within these lanes (parallel or anti-parallel). An instruction from the swimming teacher (the RF pulse) causes them all to swim in the same direction *and* to have their arm strokes all in sync. This is resonance (Figure 15.11, right).

When the RF pulse is switched off, the protons undergo a process known as relaxation in which they either flip back to parallel alignment (with emission of electromagnetic energy) or lose their phase alignment with their neighbours. Flipping from anti-parallel alignment is known as T1 relaxation (or spin–lattice relaxation) and loss of phase alignment is T2 or spin–spin relaxation. Different tissue types have characteristic curves for the rate at which they undergo both T1 and T2 relaxation and detection of this signal decay allows the scanner to determine tissue characteristics with a very high degree of precision.

The third component of the MRI scanner is the array of gradient magnets. These are responsible for the characteristic loud noises in the scan suite. They superimpose a graded field in the x-, y- and z-planes throughout the whole scanner, on top of the primary field. The result is that the field strength is very slightly different in every single voxel of the patient. As discussed earlier, field strength determines the frequency of electromagnetic energy required to induce proton resonance. By knowing the field strength in every location of its core, the scanner is able to determine that signals generated by a particular frequency of electromagnetic pulse can only have come from tissue in a very specific location in 3D space. This is how spatial encoding works in MRI and it gives spatial resolution of less than 0.5 mm in modern scanners. This method is, unfortunately, also the reason why MRI scanning is so slow; scanning must be repeated at numerous frequencies for every slice to acquire the required spatial information.

Next is the topic which probably causes most confusion to non-radiologists: imaging sequences. There are a baffling number of different sequences available but the core ones are T1-weighted, T2-weighted, STIR, FLAIR and DWI. T1-weighted means that the image is captured in a way which predominantly depicts the signal relating from T1 relaxation. T2-weighted scans similarly reflect mainly T2 relaxation signals. Since both relaxation phenomena occur simultaneously, an image never depicts just T1 or just T2 signals but, as T1 and T2 occur at different rates, it is possible to focus on one relaxation type. Table 15.5 lists the differing signal intensity (not 'density', that is an X-ray term) for different tissue types depending on the weighting. In short though, T1 weighting is considered to give the best anatomical depiction while T2 is arguably better for pathology. Since most pathological processes lead to a greater localized presence of water (oedema, vascularity or both), the lesion

Table 15.5 Comparison of tissue appearance on T1- vs. T2-weighted scans

Tissue type	T1-weighted appearance	T2-weighted appearance
Air	Black	Black
Bone cortex	Black	Black
Bone medulla	Bright	Isointense
Water, CSF	Dark	Bright
Fat	Bright	Darker
Grey matter	Darker	Brighter
White matter	Brighter	Darker
Blood (flowing)	Black	Black

appears brighter on a T2-weighted sequence; remember 'WW2' – water white on T2-weighted).

STIR (short T1 inversion recovery) and FLAIR (fluid attenuated inversion recovery) are two sides of the same coin. They are methods to reduce signal artefact from fat or water, respectively. STIR is useful for suppressing adipose artefact and for looking at bone marrow, adrenal tissue and fatty tumours (remember, 'STIR is slimming' because it removes fat!). FLAIR is particularly good for cerebral oedema or the sort of periventricular and cortical lesions seen in multiple sclerosis.

Diffusion-weighted imaging (DWI) uses two brief pulses from the gradient magnets to quantify the extent to which water moves by Brownian motion at a cellular level. Only stationary water molecules will return a signal as the molecule needs to be in the same position for both pulses in order for an overall signal to be detected. Normal diffusion of water molecules therefore results in a weaker diffusion-weighted signal.

Different tissues have different apparent diffusion coefficients (ADCs) depending on various factors such as the degree of cellularity; cell and organelle membranes physically obstruct Brownian motion and so reduce the diffusion of water. Reduction of the ADC as compared to the normal value for that tissue type shows up as a high-intensity signal on a DWI image. Diffusion may be restricted in highly cellular masses, ischaemic tissue or purulent collections.

MRI can be enhanced by injection of contrast agents. The typical agents contain gadolinium because it exhibits strong paramagnetism on account of having seven unpaired electrons in its outer shell when in the 3+ oxidation state. The result is to shorten the T1 relaxation time of adjacent protons, causing a high-intensity signal on T1-weighted images. The gadolinium ion is chelated to various ligands depending on the contrast agent. The ligand used determines the distribution and uptake of the contrast agent to various tissue types. Agents that bind preferentially to albumin are useful in magnetic resonance angiography (MRA), for example. As these agents do not cross an intact blood–brain barrier, they are useful in highlighting cerebral tumours because they cross the localized breach in the barrier associated with these tumours. Gadolinium-containing agents are available in orally administered forms to image the gastrointestinal tract, particularly for small-bowel studies. Like X-ray contrast agents, gadolinium contrast is problematic in renal failure as it can lead to a disorder known as nephrogenic systemic fibrosis.

The term 'chelation' derives from the Greek 'chele', referring to the main claw of crustaceans such as lobsters. This describes the way in which the coordinating groups of the ligand encircle and grab on to the metal ion.

Lasers and Fibre Optics

Laser light is highly versatile, with applications in microscopy, measurement, communications, surgical resection, photocoagulation, lithotripsy, welding and optical drives (CD and Blu-ray) to name just a handful. The myth is that lasers were initially an invention without an obvious use. There is actually little truth in that. The invention of the laser is mired in a 20-year battle in the US patent courts. One of the early contributors, Charles Gould, had patents granted on appeal in 1977. His original notes from the late 1950s include a wide array of potential applications, all of which have since come to fruition.

The acronym 'laser' stands for 'light amplification by stimulated emission of radiation'. This section will focus on production of laser light. Specifics of laser safety and anaesthesia equipment modifications required when using lasers will not be covered here (see Chapter 10). To understand what is special about lasers and stimulated emission, an understanding of spontaneous-emission ('normal') light sources is first required. Energy is applied to the atoms of the source of light. The electrons are excited to various

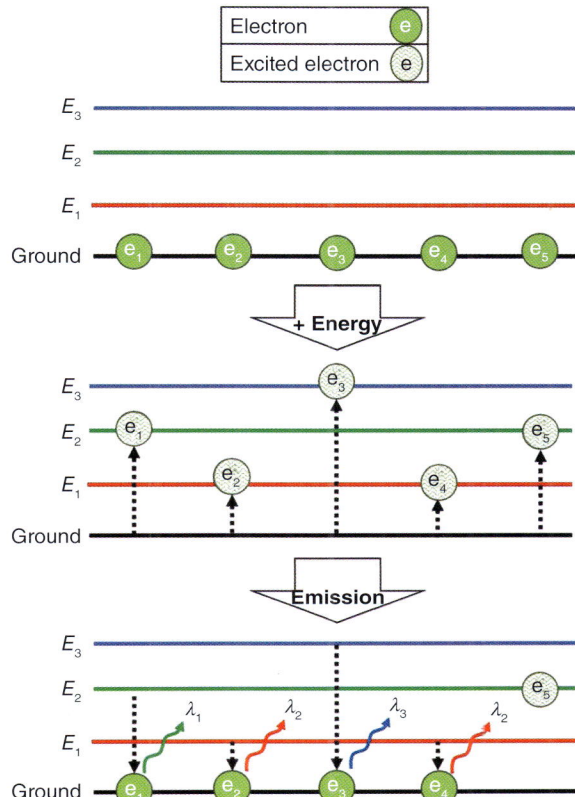

Figure 15.12 Spontaneous emission of light

higher-energy states and then randomly fall back to ground state (Figure 15.12). As the energy transitions of the various electrons are different (E_1, E_2 or E_3 in this case), the frequency of the photons released as they drop back to the ground state also differs (as related by Plank's constant). Differing frequency means different wavelengths (λ_1, λ_2 and λ_3 here) so the light emitted is polychromatic or even white (a full array of visible wavelengths). Because the decay of electrons back to ground state is a random process, the phases of the emitted photons all differ; in Figure 15.12, electron 5 (e_5) has yet to decay so, even though it will produce a photon with the same wavelength as e_1, it will not be in phase due to the temporal delay between the two emissions.

Before we go on to discuss stimulated emission, it is worth briefly considering two other forms of luminescence which are encountered in everyday life; fluorescence and electroluminescence. This is particularly relevant given that, superficially, they may appear to have features similar to stimulated

Table 15.6 Some common laser systems and their applications

Gain medium	State	Wavelength (nm)	Application
Helium–neon	Gas	633	Optics research
Carbon dioxide	Gas	10,600	Cutting, welding, medical
Helium–silver	Gas	0.0005	Raman spectroscopy
Neodymium yttrium–aluminium–garnet (Nd:YAG)	Solid	1,064	Laser-TURP, numerous ophthalmological applications
Rhodamine-6G	Liquid	635–560	Cosmetic skin lesion removal, astronomical interferometry, spectroscopy
Potassium titanyl phosphate (KTP)	Solid	532	Energized by Nd:YAG to produce light at double the frequency – port wine stain, tattoo and rosacea removal

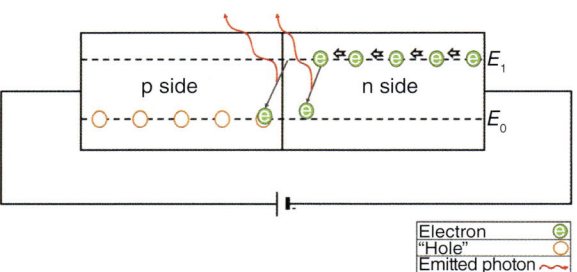

Figure 15.13 Electroluminescence at the p–n junction of an LED

emission. Fluorescence is the principle underlying 'strip lighting'. The system consists of a vacuum tube lined with a phosphor material and containing a small amount of mercury vapour. Electrical current passes through the vapour, causing spontaneous emission of light, predominantly in the ultraviolet range but also some green and orange visible light. This, in turn, excites the phosphor material, which fluoresces, i.e. produces further light (in the visible range for strip lights) by spontaneous emission. In most examples of fluorescence, the light produced by the phosphor is of lower energy than that of the exciting source. Consequently, the frequency is lower and the wavelength longer; hence ultraviolet excitation leads to visible-light fluorescence. Note, despite the term 'phosphor', phosphorescence is a different process again, the defining characteristic being that phosphorescent materials continue to luminesce after the exciting radiation is switched off. Electroluminescence, meanwhile, is the mechanism behind light-emitting diodes (LEDs). Diodes are in fact the principal format of most lasers in everyday use (laser pointers, Blu-ray players, etc.) but these laser diodes are a special case and will be discussed later. The standard LED is composed of a semiconductor 'p–n junction' (Figure 15.13). This simply means two semiconductor substances within a single crystal. The n (for negative) side has a relative excess of free and mobile electrons whilst the p (positive) side has a series of 'holes'. An electrical current drives the electrons from n to p, where the electrons fill the holes, dropping to a lower energy state (E_1 to E_0) and releasing a photon. The light emitted is not, unlike laser light, coherent (see below), and therefore not truly monochromatic (although it may not be far off to the naked eye).

Laser light has a number of distinct properties compared to other forms of luminescence. These centre around two key points: the light is produced by stimulated emission (see below) and this results in it being coherent. Coherence means that the phase difference between photons is constant and the frequency is the same. As a result, the light is monochromatic. That said, for all its ideal properties, laser light is not necessarily parallel and so most devices use collimating filters or lenses.

The process of lasing involves stimulated emission. The lasing substance, or 'gain medium', can be any state of matter and some examples are given in Table 15.6. The medium is typically enclosed by a mirror at one end and a half-silvered mirror at the other to form an optical resonator (Figure 15.14). The process starts with adding energy to the gain medium, typically in the form of light from a flash tube but alternatives include another laser, a heat source, a

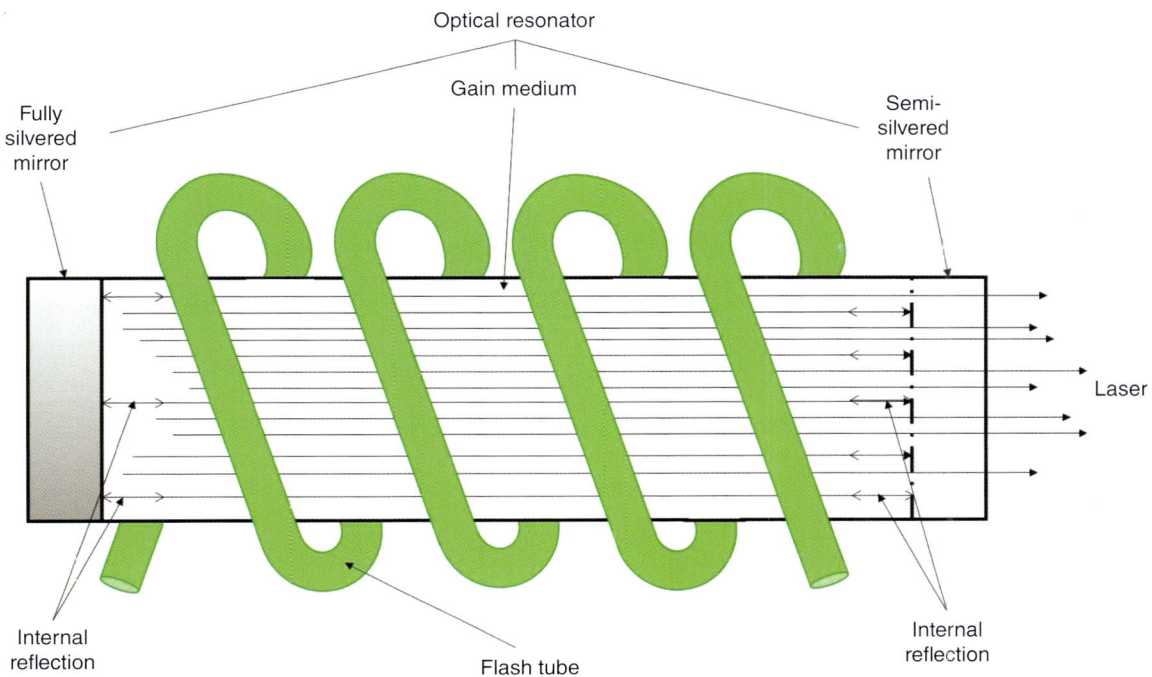

Figure 15.14 Typical optical resonator of a laser

current across the p–n junction of a laser diode or even a chemical reaction. This drives electrons up to higher energy states, a process referred to as electron pumping. Initially, this leads to what, in essence, is the same photonic emission seen in spontaneous luminescence; some electrons decay back to the ground state and emit a photon. The difference is that the photon is internally reflected within the optical resonator where it has the potential to interact with another pumped electron, triggering it to transition back to the ground state with emission of another photon. The energy transition is identical to the energy of the stimulating photon and so the frequency of the emitted photon matches that of the stimulating photon (this is stimulated emission). The original photon is not lost in this encounter (it is an electromagnetic interaction rather than an energy transfer) so the result is two photons of identical frequency, phase (coherent) and direction as the original one (this is light amplification).

There are some key terms which underpin the functioning of a laser. The first is 'population inversion'. This describes a state where more electrons in the gain medium are in an excited energy state than those in the ground state. This is crucial and was actually mathematically modelled by Einstein around 40 years ahead of the invention of the laser. He noted that the fate of incoming photons was either to be absorbed by ground-state electrons, causing them to become excited, or to trigger stimulated emission. It follows that only when a population inversion has been achieved can there be a net emission of photons. To understand this better, consider a simple system of six electrons in a lasing medium with six incoming photons. If, at the point of entry of the photons, two electrons are excited and four are at ground state, then four of the incoming photons will be absorbed and two will trigger stimulated emission, passing through the medium with an extra photon each (Figure 15.15a). This is a net absorption of two photons. If five are excited and one at ground state (a population inversion), six photons incoming leads to 10 emitted, an amplification of 66% (Figure 15.15b). At the 50:50 point, as many photons enter as leave and the medium is said to be optically transparent (Figure 15.15c).

The second term is 'lasing threshold'. This refers to the minimum energy which must be provided by

Optical discs such as the CD, DVD and Blu-ray all rely on laser diodes. Microscopic pits pressed into the disc encode the information, almost like a mechanical form of Morse code, spiralled onto the disc. When the reading laser light is reflected by a pit, it results in destructive wave interference, which is detected by a photodiode. For this phenomenon to occur, the size of the pits must be around one-quarter of the wavelength of the light being employed. As the wavelength decreases with each newer format (CDs – near-infrared, DVD – red, Blu-ray – violet blue), the pits can become more closely packed on the disc and so more data can be compressed onto the same-sized physical disc. If you look inside a Blu-ray player, you will see it actually has two lenses – one for a red laser to play DVDs and one for a blue laser to play Blu-rays.

Lasers have numerous applications but, certainly in clinical applications, generation of laser light is only part of the problem. There needs to be a method to convey the light in a controlled manner to the point of interest. Optical fibres are the answer and, of course, these have applications for transmitting conventional light as well, e.g. fibre-optic bronchoscopes, indirect laryngoscopes.

Glass or plastic optical fibres have numerous advantages, particularly in communication, when compared to copper wires: greater bandwidth, faster transmission, cheaper and less open to materials theft (copper has a high scrap-value), no susceptibility to electromagnetic interference, ground loops or lightning strike and much more secure. The way in which mechanical stress alters the light transmission properties of fibres makes them ideally suited for remote sensing, e.g. sensors within jet engines of temperature, torque, vibration, acceleration, etc. In medicine, it is their flexibility, compact form and efficiency of light transmission which makes them attractive.

It has been hypothesized that if the ocean had the clarity of an optical fibre, it would be possible to see the bottom of the Marianas Trench from the surface (over 10,000 meters).

Fibre transmission relies on total internal reflection of the light beam within the fibre and that is achieved by wrapping the core in a material of higher refractive index (Figure 15.16). Refractive index is the ratio of the

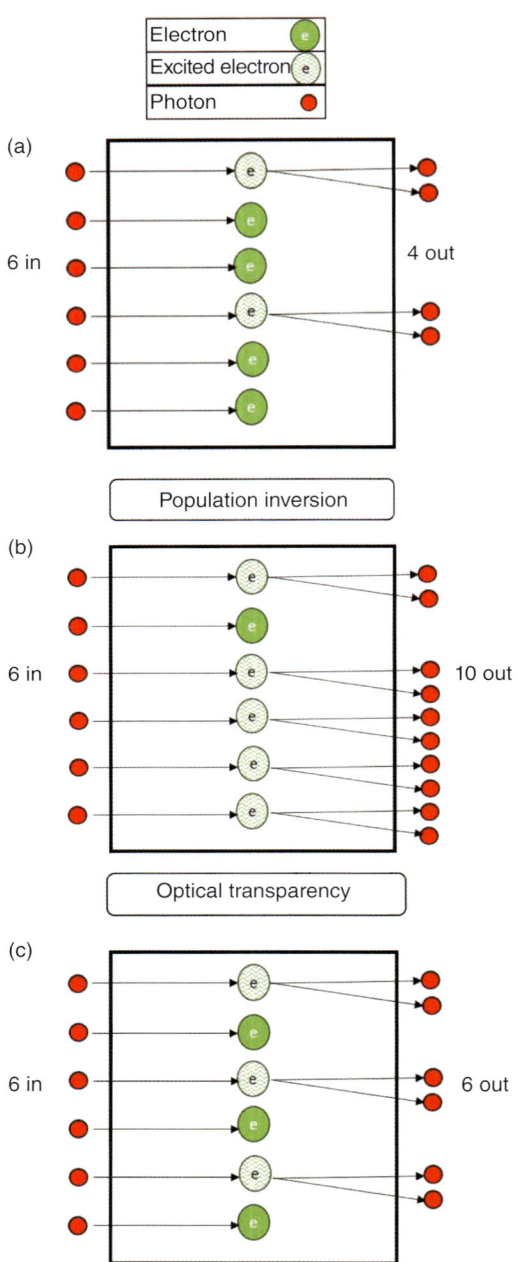

Figure 15.15 (a) Net absorption of photons as they interact with a group of electrons; (b) net gain of photons (light amplification) in a medium where a population has occurred; (c) no change in photon numbers, in versus out; defined as 'optical transparency'

pumping to ensure that photon gain from light amplification exceeds losses to absorption. Only above this threshold will a population inversion be achieved and will lasing commence.

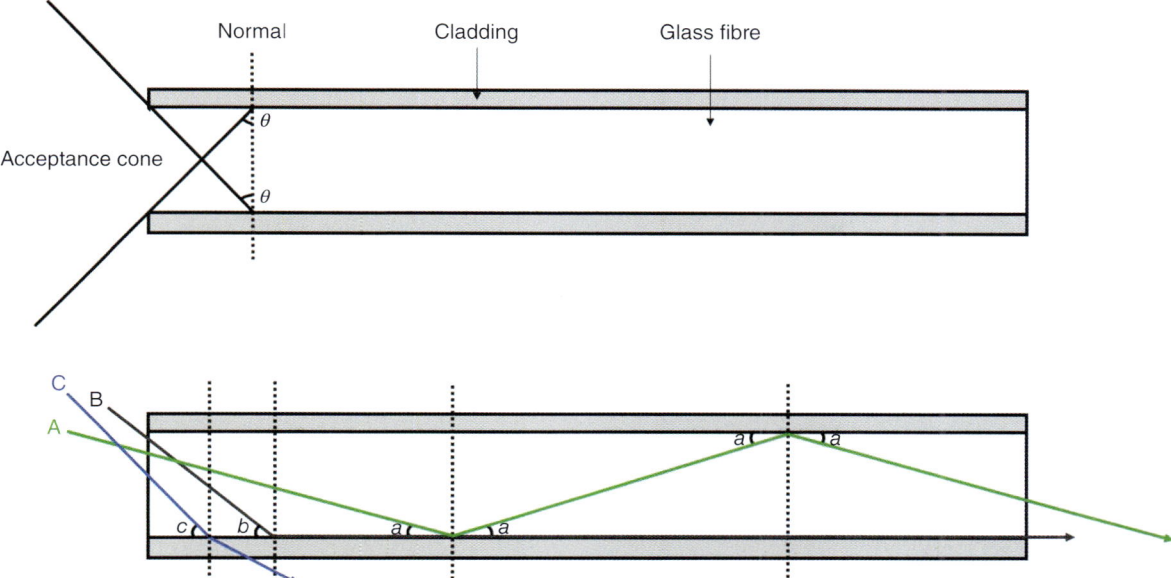

Figure 15.16 Acceptance cone for a fibre-optic (top) which describes the maximal angle of entry of a beam of light which can follow a path of total internal reflection down the fibre (bottom).

speed of light in a medium to that of its speed in a vacuum; the higher the index, the slower the speed of transmission. Figure 15.16 demonstrates that light entering the fibre must do so at an angle less than the critical angle (θ) of the fibre, otherwise it will be transmitted into the cladding (ray C, entering at angle $c > \theta$) rather than undergo total internal reflection with propagation down the fibre (ray A, entering at angle $a < \theta$). Light entering exactly at the critical angle will be propagated parallel to the fibre (ray B, entering at angle $b = \theta$). The critical angle is determined by the extent of the disparity between the refractive indices of the fibre core and its cladding. This can be derived from Snell's law, which relates the ratio of incident and refracted angles of a wave meeting a second medium to the ratio of the velocity, wavelength or refractive index of the wave within those two media (note, for refractive index it is the inverse ratio which is proportional to that of the angles):

$$\frac{\sin \text{Angle of incidence}}{\sin \text{Angle of refraction}} = \frac{\text{Refractive index}_2}{\text{Refractive index}_1}$$
$$= \frac{\text{Velocity}_1}{\text{Velocity}_2}$$
$$= \frac{\text{Wavelength}_1}{\text{Wavelength}_2}$$

From this, the critical angle (of incidence) can be calculated from knowledge of the refractive indices of the core and cladding (by definition, the critical angle is the angle of incidence giving an angle of refraction of 90°):

$$\frac{\sin \text{Angle of incidence}}{\sin \text{Angle of refraction}} = \frac{\text{Refractive index}_2}{\text{Refractive index}_1}$$
$$\frac{\sin \text{Critical angle}}{\sin 90°} = \frac{\text{Refractive index}_2}{\text{Refractive index}_1}$$

As $\sin 90° = 1$ this simplifies to

$$\text{Critical angle} = \sin^{-1} \frac{\text{Refractive index}_2}{\text{Refractive index}_1}$$

This also has a number of practical consequences for implementation of optical fibres. The critical angle can be used to map the extremes at which light can successfully enter the fibre and be transmitted by total internal reflection. This is known as the acceptance cone of the fibre (Figure 15.16). This in turn has relevance for the precision required at junctions and connections between one fibre and the next, to avoid loss, as well as the maximal field of view possible when using fibres as a fibrescope. Typically, an adequate field of view is only achievable with a lens at the end of the fibre, to increase the width of the acceptance cone. Another everyday clinical example of the importance of this phenomenon is the critical nature of the alignment of a fibre-optic laryngoscope blade with the handle to ensure the light is effectively transmitted to the end of the fibrescope.

Summary

A little understanding about atomic and subatomic physics is a necessary thing to facilitate understanding of lasers, radioactivity and radiation safety, and the many forms of medical imaging available today; it need not, however, be baffling! To go back to our original case, hopefully you now understand how PET imaging is undertaken to search for distant metastases in these patients. The X-ray CT imaging will give very good anatomical views of the airway and any obstruction for us, ahead of the case, although MRI would give even better soft-tissue imaging. The radiotherapy, meanwhile, we know may cause airway scarring but we now understand that there is no risk to the health of others as a result. The majority of radiotherapy techniques do not rely on introduction of a radioactive source into the patient, rather exposure to a source of radioactivity during therapy. Consequently, there is no ongoing emission of ionizing radiation after therapy.

With particular respect to imaging, we rely on these techniques on a daily basis. Understanding how they work allows an understanding of their strengths and weaknesses. In turn, this allows us to properly request imaging studies to obtain the most useful information with the minimum amount of harmful exposure of our patients.

Questions

MCQs – select true or false for each response

1. Regarding negative exponential processes, such as radioactive decay, which of the following are true?
   (a) The rate of decay depends on the initial amount present
   (b) The half-life expresses the time taken for the amount of substance to halve
   (c) The half-life expresses the time taken for the radioactivity of a substance to halve
   (d) The substance will have entirely decayed after seven half-lives
   (e) The greater the rate of decay, the shorter the half-life
2. Regarding magnetic resonance imaging (MRI), which of the following statements are correct?
   (a) The main magnetic field is around two to three times that of the Earth's magnetic field
   (b) The magnitude of the magnetic field is uniform in the region of the body being imaged
   (c) The electron precession releases radio waves, which are detected to produce the image
   (d) Titanium–niobium alloys are superconductors at temperatures of 4 K
   (e) Gradient magnets are responsible for the characteristic noises in the MRI suite
3. Regarding gamma radiation, which of the following are true?
   (a) Gamma detection is the basis of PET scanning
   (b) Gamma energy has a longer wavelength than ultraviolet energy
   (c) Gamma energy is any energy release associated with nuclear decay
   (d) Unlike X-rays, gamma rays are not ionizing radiation
   (e) SPECT has poorer spatial resolution than PET

SBAs – select the single *best* answer

4. Regarding imaging modality selection for the trauma patient in the first trimester of pregnancy, which one of the following statements is the most accurate?
   (a) CT should be used once ultrasound (FAST) has confirmed free intraperitoneal fluid
   (b) MRI should be used to avoid ionizing radiation exposure
   (c) CT should be used once urine β-HCG has been tested
   (d) Plain films should be employed where possible to facilitate targeted CT imaging with a reduced associated dose
   (e) CT imaging should proceed as usual

Answers

1. TTFFT

   Half-life gives a poor impression of the duration of radiological hazard. Even after many half-lives, a biologically significant quantity of the radionuclide may remain and it may have decayed to substances which are as hazardous as, or more so than, the parent nuclide. Exponential decay is asymptotic – in other words, even at infinity, there will still be a tiny amount of the substance left to decay.

2. FFFTT

   The main field in an MRI scanner is 2–3 T, the magnitude of the Earth's field is measured in micro-tesla. The field has to be different in every region of the scanner – this is necessary for spatial encoding. MRI relies on the behaviour of protons not electrons.

3. TFTFT

   Gamma rays are very much shorter in wavelength and therefore higher in frequency than ultraviolet radiation. Gamma and X-rays are both ionizing radiation.

4. (c)

   Confirmation of pregnancy is useful; a dose-reducing modification can be made to the CT protocol to offer some protection to the fetus. FAST scanning lacks the sensitivity and specificity to reliably triage patients to have CT or not in the setting of major trauma. MRI offers avoidance of ionizing radiation but it is too slow in the hyper-acute setting and offers relatively poor characterization of bony injury. Plain films are relatively slow and insensitive with a high likelihood of needing to reimage the area with CT in the end analysis.

References

1. ICRP. The 2007 Recommendations of the International Commission on Radiological Protection. ICRP Publication 103. *Annals of the ICRP*, 37 (2–4), 2007.

Chapter 16

Electro-biophysiology

Vijay Venkatesh and David Ashton-Cleary

Learning Objectives

- To understand the generation of various electrical signals in the body and the changes they undergo as they are detected on the surface
- To understand how potentials may change as a consequence of disease and how this may be utilized in diagnosis and monitoring of pathology
- To be able to describe various techniques to improve our ability to monitor these potentials, including amplifiers, common mode rejection and filters

Chapter Content

- Biological potentials
- Cardiac potentials and the electrocardiogram
- The electroencephalogram
- The electromyogram
- Amplifiers, common mode rejection and filters

Scenario

A 51-year-old male is admitted via the emergency department after suffering a cardiac arrest and a resulting head injury when he collapsed. Despite arriving in hospital with a stable circulation, he is agitated and very confused. His ECG shows changes consistent with an anterolateral infarction and a CT head does not show any abnormality. He is anaesthetized, undergoes an angioplasty and is admitted to critical care. After failed sedation holds the next day, a CT head is repeated and an EEG is also obtained. The imaging demonstrates cerebral oedema and the EEG shows seizure activity. These are treated medically for a few days and the patient's consciousness improves. However, during this time, he develops ventilator-associated pneumonia, requiring ventilation for a further week. After this, despite improved neurology, there is difficulty in weaning the patient off the ventilator. He is investigated for critical illness weakness and nerve conduction studies. Electromyography confirms critical illness myopathy. With supportive management and appropriate rehabilitation, he eventually recovers.

This is an almost everyday scenario and the understanding of electrical potentials plays a key role in each stage of the case. Think about the ECG on admission: why are there positive and negative waves in the ECG and why does ST elevation suggest infarction? What different types of waves are seen in the EEG and how can they be used in basic interpretation? How can nerve conduction studies and electromyography differentiate between myopathy and polyneuropathy?

Introduction

Biological potentials are perhaps a little mysterious, even daunting, as a topic. Nevertheless, they are vital to anaesthetists and intensivists on a daily basis and this undoubtedly justifies their common appearance in post-graduate exams. Aside from that, a little deeper understanding of the electrophysiology can give you a really helpful insight into ECG interpretation, in particular. This chapter hopes to throw some light on the basic concepts of electro-biophysiology, which are both clinically and academically relevant.

Biological Potentials

Biological potentials are electrical signals generated by the activity within cells. The cell membrane is composed of phospholipids in what is referred to as a bilayer arrangement (Figure 16.1). A phospholipid molecule consists of a hydrophilic head and two hydrophobic tails. The membrane consists of two layers of phospholipids. Because the interior and exterior of cells are mainly comprised of water, the hydrophobic tails align themselves to each other with the hydrophilic heads facing these aqueous

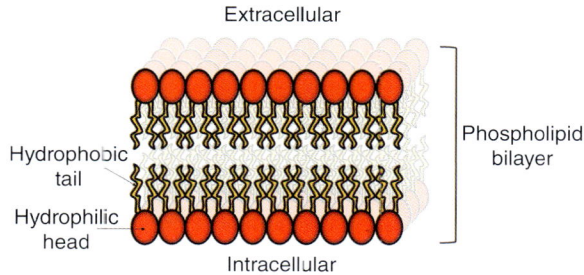

Figure 16.1 Typical phospholipid bilayer of a cell membrane

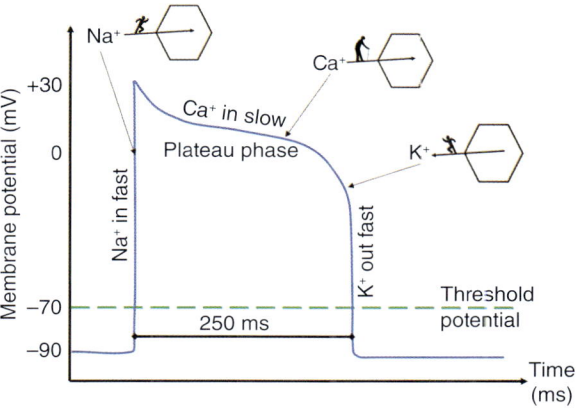

Figure 16.2 Typical cardiac action potential

surroundings. The whole arrangement resembles a sandwich: the hydrophobic tails are the filling between two rows of hydrophilic heads (the bread).

Cell membranes control and facilitate the transfer of ions into and out of the cell by various mechanisms such as pumps, channels, pores and molecular transporters. The differing proportions of anions and cations on either side of the membrane resulting from these mechanisms lead to an electrical potential difference across the membrane of every cell. The interior of the cell is negative in comparison to the exterior. Of course, that can, and does, change; that is the basis for systems which rely on electrical conduction in the body. A cardiac myocyte, for example, has an electrical potential of −90 mV across the membrane at rest. The potential difference changes and totally reverses polarity during initiation of systole. This is depolarization and the interior of the cell becomes less negative and finally positive with respect to the exterior (Figure 16.2). This is brought about through movement of ions (in very brief terms, Na^+ influx followed by K^+ efflux, Ca^{2+} influx then final K^+ efflux to repolarize the cell). These changes are only temporary and, through the action of pumps (which utilize ATP) and ion exchangers, the ionic status quo is regained in preparation for the next cycle. Similar mechanisms are responsible for nerve and neuromuscular signalling.

Of course, the net purpose of all this ionic traffic is to generate a voltage for intercellular communication but there is sufficient conduction through tissues to the skin for us to be able to detect this communication for clinical purposes. The magnitude of the detected voltage, however, is much less compared to the voltage of the actual cell. For example, ECG potentials are of the order of 1–2 mV in comparison to the 140-mV change occurring within the cardiac myocyte itself at the point of depolarization. The tissues are good conductors of electricity but the problem is the high impedance of the final hurdle – the skin. To mitigate this, the electrodes used consist of a silver–silver chloride combination. This maximizes conduction to the sensing lead whilst also preventing the generation of artefactual electrical activity due to interaction between ions in sweat and the electrodes.

Cardiac Potentials and the Electrocardiogram

The electrical activity in the heart is spontaneously generated at the sino-atrial node in the right atrium. This initial depolarization spreads throughout the heart via the atrio-ventricular (AV) node, bundle of His, Purkinje fibres and cardiac muscle. There is a nodal delay at the AV node of around 100 ms, which facilitates sequential contraction of the atria and ventricles in order to optimize the stroke volume.

The electrocardiogram (ECG) is a surface recording of the summation of all electrical activity of the myocardium (Table 16.1). This includes atrial and ventricular contraction and relaxation.

At this point, it's worth pointing out the common misconception about the ECG waves and chamber contraction; one does not coincide with the other. Those who practise echocardiography will be particularly aware of this – if you want to capture an image of end-diastole, you acquire it at the peak of the R wave. The R wave is depolarization of the muscle and it will contract a few milliseconds later. The palpable pulse usually occurs during the T wave. The reason that the R wave is large by comparison

Chapter 16: Electro-biophysiology

Table 16.1 The electrical events within the heart during the cardiac cycle and their ECG counterparts

Atrial depolarization	P wave
AV-nodal conduction	PR interval
Septal depolarization	Q wave
Ventricular depolarization	R and S waves
Atrial repolarization	Wave not seen, submerged within the QRS complex
Ventricular repolarization	T wave

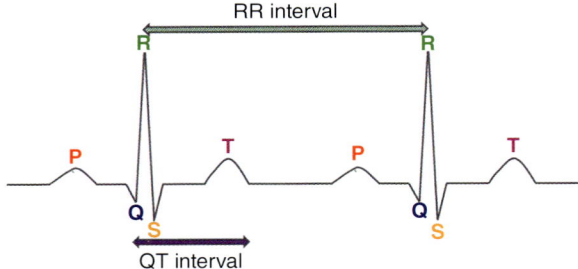

Figure 16.3 Typical component waves of the ECG

to the P wave is not because it represents a larger bulk of muscle contracting but because it is a large bulk of muscle depolarizing. This also explains what you see during a PEA arrest – depolarization may continue in a very orderly fashion but there is no muscular contraction to generate a pulse. The oxygen and energy requirements needed to sustain the conduction system and electrical depolarization are trivial next to the massive requirements of muscular contraction so, in the dying heart, contraction fails before conduction.

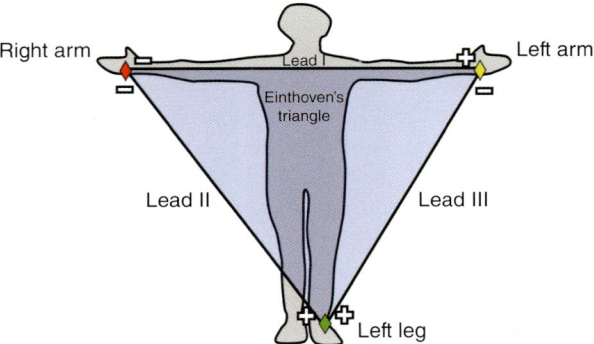

Figure 16.4 Einthoven's triangle

 The nomenclature of the ECG is somewhat arbitrary. It starts with P and runs through the alphabet. Each successive wave is defined as a deflection to the opposite polarity from its predecessor. In other words, the P wave is a positive deflection. A Q wave is, by definition, the first negative deflection to follow a P wave, an R wave is the first positive deflection to follow a Q wave and so on. From this, you can see that the term 'RSR' to describe the pattern of right bundle branch block is not strictly correct but all rules have exceptions!

Typical voltages recorded at the skin are in the range of 1–2 mV with a frequency of 0.5 Hz to 100 Hz. As mentioned, the amplitude of the wave depends on the thickness of the muscle which is depolarizing; this is the basis for the voltage criteria used in the ECG diagnosis of chamber hypertrophy. Figure 16.3 shows a typical ECG with various waves and intervals.

Einthoven's Triangle

William Einthoven (1860–1927) was a Dutch physician and physiologist. He secured the Nobel Prize in medicine in 1924 for his work in devising the ECG.

He postulated that the polarity of electrical signals recorded from the heart depended on the direction of the wave of depolarization relative to the observing lead. Einthoven's triangle is an imaginary inverted equilateral triangle, centred on the chest, with the points defined by standard leads on the arms and leg (right arm, left arm and left foot). In Figure 16.4, which displays the triangle, it can be noted that each of the three leads (I, II and III) has a positive and negative point: the right arm is negative for both I and II; the left foot is positive for both II and III; and the left arm is negative for III and positive for I.

The conventional diagnostic ECG consists of 12 leads in total; three bipolar, three augmented-unipolar and six unipolar-precordial leads. These are generated by combinations of 10 wires (not 12) between the patient and machine (Table 16.2).

ECG Display

Deflection in the ECG depends on the direction of travel of the electrical signal in relation to the electrode position. The deflection is positive or negative depending on whether the wave is travelling towards

Chapter 16: Electro-biophysiology

Table 16.2 The 12-lead ECG. Position of the 10 wires (augmented and precordial leads) and the combinations contributing to the bipolar leads

Bipolar leads		Augmented leads		Precordial leads			
I	Right arm to left arm	aVR	Right arm	V1	Right parasternal, fourth intercostal space	V4	Fifth intercostal space, midoclavicular line
II	Left leg to right arm	aVL	Left arm	V2	Lt parasternal, fourth intercostal space	V5	Fifth intercostal space, anterior axillary line
III	Left leg to left arm	aVF	Left leg	V3	Between V2 and V4	V6	Fifth intercostal space, mid-axillary line

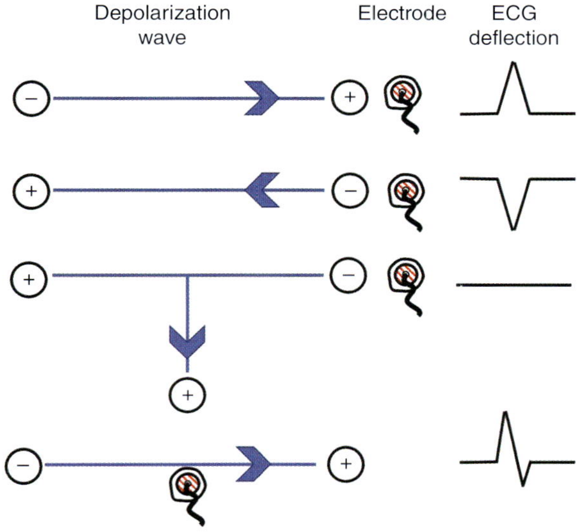

Table 16.3 Monitoring and diagnostic ECG compared

Monitoring	Diagnostic
• Frequency range is 0.5 Hz to 40 Hz • Less susceptible to interference/artefacts • Heavily filtered as bandwidth is narrower	• Frequency range is 0.05 Hz to 150 Hz • Allows accurate ST segments to be recorded • Susceptible to interference from electrical equipment and body movement because of wider frequency range

Figure 16.5 Translation of electrical vectors into ECG waves

or away from the electrode. There is no deflection if the direction of the wave is perpendicular to the direction of the electrode. Also, there can be both positive and negative deflection if the wave travels towards the electrode initially and then continues to move away from the electrode (Figure 16.5).

The ECG is displayed either on an electronic monitor or printout. The standard calibration of the conventional 12-lead ECG recording is 25 mm s^{-1} on the x-axis and 10 mm mV^{-1} on the y-axis.

There are two modes of ECG: monitoring and diagnostic (Table 16.3).

For most purposes, continuous cardiac monitoring utilizes three standard leads, with lead II being superior in detecting arrhythmias. To detect left-ventricular ischaemia, the CM5 configuration (clavicle–manubrium-V5) is used: the right-arm electrode moved to the manubrium, the left-arm electrode at the V5 position and left-leg electrode on the left shoulder/clavicle (the monitor output should be set to read 'Lead I').

Myocardial Ischaemia and Infarction

Following a myocardial infarction, the R wave is classically replaced by a Q wave in the overlying lead. With that piece of myocardium now dead, it cannot generate an R wave (or, indeed, any other components of the ECG). It is also electrically transparent though, so the same lead can now 'look through' the infarct to the depolarization on the opposite wall of the ventricle. Depolarization is always endocardium-to-epicardium, which is why an R wave is an upward deflection: the depolarization wave is travelling towards the electrode. When looking through the infarct, to depolarization on the opposite wall of the chamber, the depolarization wave is effectively moving away from the electrode. In other words, a Q wave is actually an R wave seen from behind and so it is inverted (Figure 16.6).

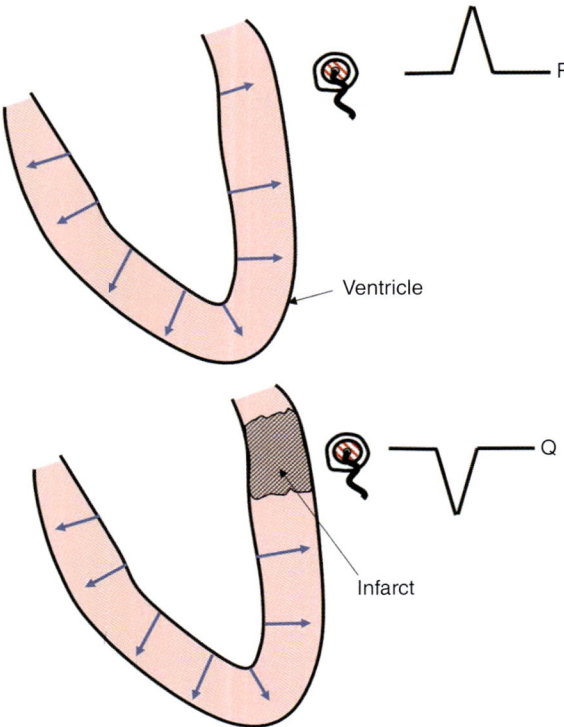

Figure 16.6 Electrophysiology of the pathological Q wave

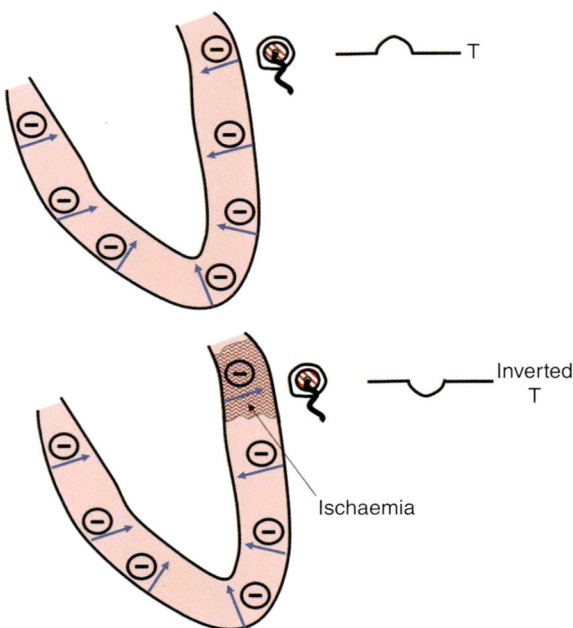

Figure 16.7 The normal T wave and ischaemic T-wave inversion

Now, consider T and ST changes in ischaemia. As described above, the endocardium depolarizes ahead of the epicardium. However, the epicardium action potential is shorter in duration. The net effect is that repolarization starts on the surface of the heart and moves endocardially (the opposite direction to the depolarization wave). Repolarization is a wave of 'increased negativity' so, despite the fact that it is moving away from the electrode, it creates a positive deflection on the ECG: the T wave (Figure 16.7). Ischaemia shortens action potential duration and the endocardium is usually the first place to become ischaemic. That means that in ischaemic conditions, the endocardium will repolarize sooner and so the direction of repolarization is now reversed: endocardium-to-epicardium. This inverts the T wave.

Truly ischaemic endocardium also remains depolarized throughout the cardiac cycle: you can almost think of it as being constantly stuck at the phase II plateau of the action potential, which corresponds to the ST segment. The effect is that, with the rest of the myocardium repolarized at the end of the cardiac cycle, there is an ongoing current between the healthy and ischaemic regions, towards the electrode between PQRST complexes. This appears as ST-segment depression but it's actually the whole baseline of the ECG which is elevated around the ST segment! Only when the rest of the muscle is depolarized will there be no residual current as the whole heart is at +30 mV, either through ischaemia or healthy depolarization.

The situation is different for ST elevation. This results from transmural ischaemia from coronary occlusion. It is important to realize ST elevation is not synonymous with infarction, otherwise, if all the tissue were truly dead, three things would be true. Firstly, we wouldn't rush these patients for coronary intervention because infarcted tissue can't be saved so ST elevation must mean there is still a salvageable state of ischaemia. Secondly, as discussed with Q waves above, an infarct wouldn't generate an otherwise typical ECG as it is dead tissue. Thirdly, if ST segments improve after thrombolysis or angioplasty, that again suggests a reversible problem. This means both ST depression and ST elevation are states of myocardial ischaemia. The only difference is that ST-elevation ischaemia can usually be addressed with coronary intervention. ST depression, on the other hand, reflects endocardial ischaemia and is usually

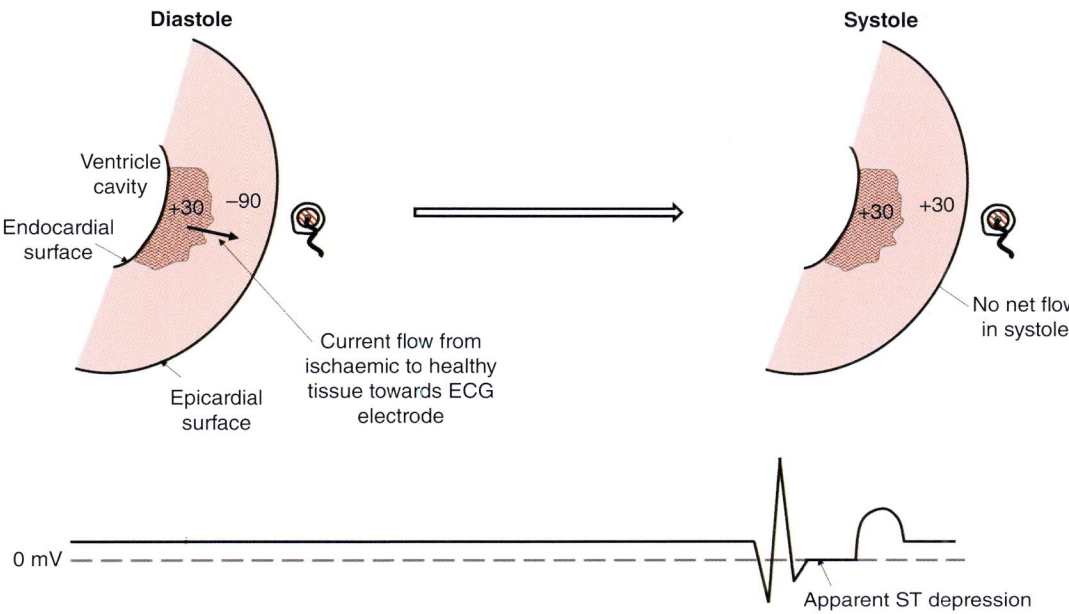

Figure 16.8 The basis of ST changes in endocardial ischaemia (angina)

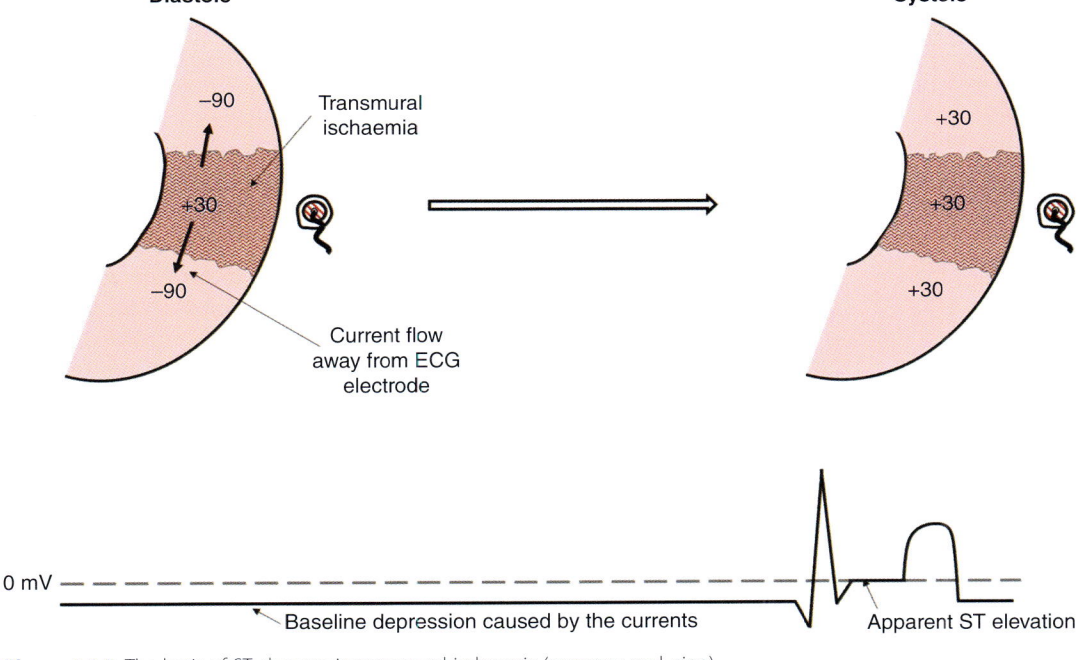

Figure 16.9 The basis of ST changes in transmural ischaemia (coronary occlusion)

demand-related, e.g. exercise-induced angina; it is due to poor flow in myocardial capillaries, which cannot be treated mechanically. As Figure 16.9 demonstrates, a persistent flow of current from the ischaemic myocardium occurs, just as with endocardial ischaemia. The difference is that, because of the shape of the ischaemic region, the overall direction of the current is away from the electrode (see Figure 16.5 again to

Chapter 16: Electro-biophysiology

Table 16.4 EEG wave frequencies and clinical correlates

EEG waves	Frequency (Hz)	Interpretation
δ (delta)	<4	Intracranial lesions, normal in babies
θ (theta)	4–7	Drowsiness
α (alpha)	8–13	Relaxed with eyes closed, coma
β (beta)	14–33	Alert, anxiety

Table 16.5 Graded changes in the EEG associated with deepening plane of anaesthesia

Low doses	↑ amplitude, ↑ frequency (β range)
High doses	↑ amplitude, ↓ frequency
Very high doses	↓ amplitude, ↓ frequency. Burst-suppression or, ultimately, a silent EEG (no activity)

look at current vectors). This results in a continuous negative potential and baseline depression, giving the impression of ST elevation. It is exactly the same electrophysiological mechanism as for endocardial ischaemia (angina) but the currents flow in the opposite direction.

The idea that ST elevation is actually baseline depression, and vice versa, might all seem a little much to accept after years of looking at ischaemic ECGs! Just remember that the ECG only measures currents resulting from differences in potential from one region of the heart to the other. We commonly assume the baseline to represent 0 mV but if you think about it, you will never have seen an ECG or monitor screen which tells you that the baseline is calibrated to an absolute value of 0 mV. Without attaching electrodes to the heart and to earth, the ECG remains a totally relative measurement.

The Electroencephalogram

As with cardiac depolarization, neurological depolarization within the brain can be detected cutaneously. Brain activity is much more complex compared to the somewhat industrial activity of the cardiac conduction system, and the electroencephalogram (EEG) is generated from the summation of post-synaptic potentials across the brain. Principally, those of interest originate from the pyramidal cells of the cerebral cortex in response to discharges from thalamic nuclei.

The electrode placement for this recording is based on the 10–20 international system. It consists of 21 electrodes, placed in a specific pattern based on the reference points of the nasion and the inion. The nasion is the depressed area between the eyes, just above the bridge of the nose; the inion is the lowest point of the skull in the supine patient, in other words the summit of the external occipital protuberance.

> The 10–20 system gains its name from the separation between adjacent electrodes. These are either 10% or 20% of the overall nasion-to-inion or tragus-to-tragus dimensions of the scalp.

EEG waves have a small potential, in the region of 50 μV, and are divided into different frequency bands, which, for the majority of clinically relevant waves, range between 1 and 40 Hz. These can conveniently be remembered with the mnemonic 'DTAB', in order of ascending frequency band: delta (<4 Hz), theta (4–7 Hz), alpha (8–13 Hz), beta (14–33 Hz) (see Table 16.4).

Anaesthetic drugs (both intravenous and inhalational) affect the EEG as described in Table 16.5

Burst-suppression is a particular pattern of the EEG associated with very deep anaesthesia but also pathological states, such as severe brain injury. As the name implies, there are high-amplitude bursts of activity in the δ and θ frequency bands. These typically last up to 10 seconds and are then followed by periods of minimal activity (the suppression phase), which usually last 10 seconds or more.

The EEG is also affected by oxygenation levels, PCO_2, temperature and noxious stimulation. In hypoxia, hypercapnoea and hypothermia, there is an overall decrease in EEG activity with an increase in slow-wave activity, i.e. the EEG tends to consist predominantly of θ and δ waves. During noxious stimulation, α waves are absent and reappear on administration of adequate analgesia.

BIS™ (Bispectral Index) is a method of monitoring depth of anaesthesia. The EEG signal is processed and an algorithm is used to generate a number representing the level of consciousness between 0 (a silent EEG) and 100 (fully awake). The target range of BIS™ values during general anaesthesia is 40–60, which indicates a low probability of awareness with recall. It is extensively studied on healthy volunteers and different patient groups but there is no gold standard for comparison.

Other common forms of processed EEG device include E-Entropy™ and Narcotrend™. E-Entropy™ measures irregularity in brain and facial muscular activity. Data from EEG and FEMG (frontal electromyography) is processed to produce values that indicate depth of anaesthesia. The Narcotrend™ analyzes raw EEGs using spectral analysis, to produce a number of parameters which are then subjected to multivariate statistical methods, providing a visually classified EEG. This classification ranges from stage A (awake) to stage F (very deep hypnosis) with stage E indicating the appropriate depth of anaesthesia for surgery.

Raw and processed EEG data can also be used to predict neurological survival in post-cardiac-arrest scenarios. None of the methods has 100% diagnostic accuracy, however. In this regard, somatosensory evoked potential (SSEP) appears to be the most robust of the electrophysiological tests, with a false positive rate of 0% when checked 1–3 days post-arrest. The main response evaluated is the primary somatosensory cortex potential following electrical stimulation of the median nerve. This is a negative deflection and usually occurs with a latency of 20 ms (which simply means it should take 20 ms for the evoked potential to be generated after the stimulus, provided all the neurological pathways are normal). For this reason, this SSEP is referred to as the N20. Several hundred potentials are usually measured and averaged so as to improve the signal-to-noise ratio and thus exclude artefact. Bilateral loss of this response indicates cortical cell death, provided the rest of the pathway is intact. The remainder of the pathway is tested by checking for an evoked potential at the brachial plexus (N9, otherwise known as Erb's point) and at the cervical spinal cord (N13) following stimulation. This confirms that the absent central response is due to intrinsic neurological damage and not peripheral nerve damage.

The Electromyogram

The electromyogram (EMG) measures electrical activity from muscles. It can be spontaneous or evoked. Potentials range from 50 µV to 30 mV and the range of frequencies from 0 kHz to 4 kHz. The amplitude of the potential is dependent on the number of muscle fibres stimulated. It can be recorded via surface or intramuscular measurement, using surface or needle electrodes, respectively. In simple terms, the key recording is of the motor unit potential (MUP). This is derived by recording the activity of muscle fibres adjacent to the electrode during voluntary contraction. It is also possible to assess how the contraction impulse spreads to other motor units (nerve, motor end plate and muscle fibres) in the muscle; this is referred to as the recruitment pattern.

Nerve conduction studies are performed along with electromyography to accurately localize the part of the pathway affected by pathology. This may prove to be an issue with nerve conduction, the neuromuscular junction or muscle motor units. Stimulation of a motor nerve and measurement of the potential in the contracting muscle gives rise to the compound muscle action potential (CMAP). The latency of this potential includes the conduction interval along the nerve, the signalling interval at the neuromuscular junction and the duration to achieve muscle depolarization. The analogous recording in sensory nerve conduction studies is the sensory nerve action potential (SNAP). This can be recorded in an orthodromic or antidromic manner; orthodromic means in the conventional direction so, for a sensory nerve, the stimulus is applied distally and measured at a more proximal point. Antidromic is the reverse.

Clinically, the EMG is used for monitoring neuromuscular blocking drugs, to diagnose myopathic and neuropathic disorders including types of critical illness weakness (Table 16.6).

Amplifiers, Common Mode Rejection and Filters

Amplification is the augmentation of the amplitude of a wave, in this case the electrical biopotential detected by, for example, the ECG machine. The bandwidth of an amplifier is the range of frequencies over which the amplification is constant. Amplifiers

Table 16.6 Electrophysiological findings in ICU-acquired weakness (Reproduced from: J. Kinsella, R. Appleton. Intensive care unit-acquired weakness. *Continuing Education in Anaesthesia Critical Care & Pain*, 12(2), 2012; 62–66, © Elsevier)

Investigation	Critical illness polyneuropathy (CIP)	Critical illness myopathy (CIM)	Critical illness neuromyopathy (CINM)
Nerve conduction studies	↓CMAP ↓SNAP	↓CMAP Normal SNAP	↓CMAP ↓SNAP
Electromyography	Long duration, high amplitude MUP (re-innervation)	Short duration, low amplitude MUP	Features of either CIP or CIM depending on the dominant pathology
Direct muscle stimulation	Normal CMAP	↓CMAP	Variable depending on relative component of CIP and CIM

can generally be described as either wideband or narrowband. A wideband amplifier increases the amplitude of waves over a large range of frequencies whereas a narrowband device affects only a focused group of frequencies. For our purposes, we need a narrowband device, selectively tuned to increase the amplitude of the frequency of the biological potential of interest. It must be remembered that an amplifier increases the amplitude of all facets of the incoming signal – true signal and any interference, or 'noise'. The characteristics of an amplifier can be quantified in terms of the signal-to-noise ratio, i.e. the amount by which true signal is amplified by comparison to the degree to which electrical noise is amplified. Wideband amplifiers offer convenience and economy – we could open a factory churning out a single wideband amplifier for a range of ECG, EMG and EEG machines. The problem is that they would have a very poor signal-to-noise ratio in all applications. An EEG signal would be swamped by amplified EMG and ECG interference, for example. Narrowband amplifiers offer improved signal-to-noise ratio but at additional cost.

Gain describes the ratio of output voltage to input voltage. Increasing the gain of the amplifier will increase the amount by which the amplitude of the waves is boosted: the volume increases as gain is increased on an audio amplifier, the size of the QRS complex increases as the gain is increased on an ECG amplifier. Don't forget that noise will also increase at high gain: high-frequency clarity on your hi-fi system is lost in crackle at high volume. Similarly, you may lose the P waves in baseline noise of the ECG as you wind up the gain to help see the QRS more clearly.

Amplifiers can also be used to reduce noise, however. A differential amplifier measures the difference between the potential from two different sources. A signal which is common to both inputs can usually be assumed to be noise. The differential amplifier only amplifies the differing component of the signal coming in on the two inputs. This is known as **common mode rejection**. Elimination of interference by the 240-V alternating current mains interference (50 Hz) is a common application. For example, in an ECG machine, 50-Hz noise would be detected by all 10 wires equally and, when connected to a differential amplifier, the machine is able to recognize it as noise and dispense with it.

Filters

Filters remove artefacts and unwanted information from an incoming signal. It is essential to filter biological potentials to secure useful information. Like most noise-attenuation systems, they usually come ahead of the amplification stage. In fact, a series of filters can allow the use of a simple wideband amplifier (rather than a more expensive narrowband amplifier) as the bandwidth of the signal can be narrowed by the filters. There are two types of filters – low-pass and high-pass.

Low-pass filters, as the name suggests, are those which allow low frequencies through but block higher frequencies. These can be used to decrease artefacts from muscle movement (high frequency) and mains electricity. For everyday examples, plasterboard and sunglasses make very effective low-pass filters. Stiff substances reflect high-frequency sound waves. That's why, with loud music playing in the next room, you generally only hear the bass beat (low frequency) through the wall. Sunglasses, meanwhile, allow the lower frequencies of visible light to pass to your eyes whilst screening them from higher-frequency ultraviolet light.

High-pass filters let high frequencies pass but block low frequencies. They are used clinically to remove unwanted signals associated with breathing and other body movements. They are also used in hi-fi speakers to stop the bass signals reaching the tweeters and causing them to explode! A combination of low-pass and high-pass filters is used by most of us every day. The little white telephone splitter plugged into the telephone socket is more accurately known as a 'DSL filter' and uses a low-pass and high-pass filter to separate out broadband and telephone signals which arrive through the same wire from the telephone exchange.

Summary

Every cell in the body exists with a potential difference across the membrane and these are vital in underpinning cellular function and signalling. We have devised methods to measure and display these potentials and how they change with time. This gives rise to the EMG, ECG and EEG. The electrical properties of these different potentials are so different that they represent quite a challenge from an electronics perspective – knowledge of amplifiers and filters is central to understand the limitations of these measuring systems. These signals are all very low in amplitude but this amplitude also differs between the microvolt and the millivolt range between the three modalities. They also differ significantly by frequency range. The result is that it is inevitable that all three have the potential to cause interference with each other. The patient discussed in our opening scenario is a good example of how measurement of all three of these cellular potentials can form a frequent part of clinical practice.

Questions

MCQs – select true or false for each response

1. About EEG measurement and interpretation:
   (a) Theta (θ) waves have a frequency of 14–33 Hz
   (b) The inion is the depressed area between the eyes, just above the bridge of the nose
   (c) At very high anaesthetic doses, EEG waves have decreased amplitude and frequency
   (d) Delta (δ) waves are normal in babies
   (e) A BIS^{TM} value of 100 corresponds to very deep anaesthesia

2. With respect to the EMG and ICU-acquired weakness:
   (a) The EMG has frequencies between 0 kHz and 4 kHz
   (b) The sensory nerve action potential (SNAP) is normal in critical illness myopathy (CIM)
   (c) Direct muscle stimulation in critical illness polyneuropathy (CIP) has normal compound motor action potential (CMAP)
   (d) The amplitude of the EMG depends on the size of muscle being stimulated
   (e) Re-innervation features on the EMG are seen in CIP

3. About cardiac action potentials and the ECG:
   (a) Diagnostic mode is heavily filtered
   (b) Low-pass filters block high frequencies
   (c) The nodal delay of 0.01 s is essential for sequential contraction of the atria and ventricles
   (d) Cardiac cells have an electrical potential of +90 mV inside the cell with respect to the outside
   (e) Ventricular depolarization corresponds to the QT interval

SBAs – select the single *best* answer

4. You are looking after a 56-year-old man undergoing an anterior resection. He has a history of ischaemic heart disease. With respect to ECG monitoring in theatres, the following offers the best option:
   (a) Standard three-lead monitoring
   (b) 12-lead monitoring *in situ* for comprehensive monitoring
   (c) Monitoring through defibrillator pads to offer the option of cardioversion
   (d) The CM5 modification
   (e) 12-lead monitoring with posterior-lead placement

Answers

1. FFTTF
   Beta (β) waves have a frequency of 14–33 Hz whereas that of θ waves is 4–7 Hz. The nasion is the depressed area between the eyes. A BIS^{TM} value of 100 corresponds to a fully awake person.

2. TTTFT

The CMAP is normal in CIP when measured with direct muscle stimulation – it is, however, reduced when measured by nerve conduction studies, so be certain which testing method has been used when interpreting CMAP results. The amplitude of the EMG depends on the number of muscle fibres stimulated and not on the size of the muscle.

3. FTFFF

Monitoring-mode ECG is heavily filtered – diagnostic mode is much less filtered to ensure optimal sensitivity. Nodal delay is 0.1 s (100 ms) although the purpose stated (AV synchronization) is correct. The potential of the interior of the cardiac cell is –90 mV with respect to the extracellular space. Ventricular depolarization corresponds to the R and S waves. The QT interval encapsulates both the depolarization and repolarization phases for the ventricle.

4. (d)

12-lead monitoring is cumbersome in the theatre environment and is often not available as a real-time modality, just as a snapshot printout. Posterior lead placement is useful for detecting posterior ischaemia and infarction but there is nothing in the stem to suggest this is a particular risk for this patient. It is another form of 12-lead monitoring (see earlier) and would also risk pressure injuries for such a long procedure with the patient lying on the cables to the three posterior electrodes. Defibrillator-pad monitoring is probably excessive unless the patient is so prone to malignant arrhythmias that the cardiologists have already elected to insert an ICD which you have then deactivated for the procedure. Standard three-lead monitoring is easy and familiar to work with but CM5 has the advantage of being a relatively straightforward modification, suited for left-ventricular ischaemia detection which would seem most likely given this patient's history (as opposed to arrhythmias to which a standard three-lead is best suited).

References

1. J. Kinsella, R. Appleton. Intensive care unit-acquired weakness. *Continuing Education in Anaesthesia Critical Care & Pain*, 12(2), 2012; 62–66.

Index

absolute risk reduction (ARR), 16
absolute zero, 29–30, 38
acceleration, 32
adiabatic lapse rate, 81
adiabatic temperature rise, 80
air
 pipeline supplies, 84
air compressors, 84
airway pressure release ventilation (APRV), 143
ALARP principle, 231
Allen's Test, 165
alpha radiation, 229
alveolar gas equation, 62–63
amplifiers
 bandwidth, 253–254
 common mode rejection, 254
 differential amplifiers, 254
 gain, 254
 noise reduction, 254
 signal-to-noise ratio, 253–254
 use on biological potentials, 253–254
amplitude of a wave, 209
anaemia with co-existing hypoxia effect on measured SpO_2, 103–104
anaesthesia
 delivering safe mixtures of gases, 113
 delivery at altitude, 126–127
 second gas effect, 67
anaesthetic vapours
 biotransformation, 117
 blood:gas (B/G) partition coefficient, 117–119
 flammable gas mixtures, 148
 global warming potential (GWP), 117
 ideal properties, 119
 key properties of various anaesthetic agents, 117–119
 minimum alveolar concentration (MAC), 117
 oil:gas (O/G) partition coefficient, 117–119
 permitted limits in the theatre environment, 146–147
analysis of variance (ANOVA), 20
anatomical dead-space measurement, 94

anti-neutrinos, 229
Apollo 1 capsule fire and explosion, 149
apparent diffusion coefficients (ADCs), 238
apparent temperature, 46–48
Aristotle, 31
arterial oxygen saturation (SaO_2), 98
arterial waveform analysis, 182
assessment bias, 4
atomic number, 227
atomic structure, 226–228
 nature of matter, 226
Avogadro's constant, 61, 227
Avogadro's law, 61–63

bag squeezer ventilators, 141
bar charts, 5
Barnard, Christiaan, 188
barometers, 72
barotrauma, 124
Bayesian statistics (Bayes' theorem), 14
Beer–Lambert law, 90, 94, 104
Beer's law, 98
bell curve (normal distribution), 6–7
Benedict Roth spirometer, 74
Bernoulli, Joseph, 8
Bernoulli principle, 59–60, 130–131
beta radiation, 229–230
bias, 3–4
 assessment bias, 4
 information bias, 3–4
 observer bias, 4
 publication bias, 4, 21–22
 selection bias, 3
bi-level positive airway pressure (BiPAP) devices, 132
bimetallic strip thermometers, 43
bio-impedance
 cardiac output monitoring, 184
biological potentials, 246–247
biotransformation of anaesthetic vapours, 117
BIS™ (Bispectral Index), 3
blackbody radiation, 43
Bland–Altman plot, 11–12
blinding component of study design, 3

blood
 as a non-Newtonian fluid, 56–57
blood gas analysis
 blood gas machine, 107–108
 Clark (polarographic) electrode, 104
 comparing arterial, venous and capillary samples, 109–110
 derived variables, 107–108
 development of devices, 97
 fuel cell (Hersch or Galvanic cell), 104–105
 oxygen tension (PO_2) electrodes, 104–105
 PCO_2 electrode, 107
 pH electrode, 105–106
 pulse oximetry, 98–104
 Severinghaus electrode, 107
 sources of error, 108–109
  air bubbles, 108
  excess heparin, 108
  hypothermia, 108–109
  patients with haematological malignancy, 108
  protein deposits, 108
  reverse pseudo-hyperkalaemia, 108
 transcutaneous methods, 110
blood:gas (B/G) partition coefficient of anaesthetic vapours, 117–119
blood pressure
 central venous pressure, 160
 components, 160
 definition, 159–160
 diastolic pressure, 160
 isovolumetric contraction, 160
 mean arterial pressure (MAP), 160
 phlebostatic axis, 160
 pulmonary artery pressure, 160
 pulmonary capillary wedge pressure, 160
 systolic pressure SBP, 159–160
 unit of measurement, 159
blood pressure measurement
 DINAMAP (device for indirect non-invasive automatic mean arterial pressure), 160
 Finapres system, 164
 importance in anaesthesia and critical care, 159

Index

blood pressure measurement (cont.)
  invasive arterial blood pressure measurement (IABP)
    additional information from the waveform, 171–172
    Allen's test, 165
    applications, 165
    brachial artery, 165
    components and set-up, 166–167
    contraindications, 165
    damping, 169–170
    femoral artery, 165
    Fourier analysis of arterial pressure waveform, 168–169
    indications, 165
    levelling the transducer, 171
    potential complications, 165
    radial artery, 165
    resonance, 168–169
    sources of error, 167–171
    waveform morphology, 167–168
    zeroing (calibrating the system), 171
  non-invasive, continuous, 164
  non-invasive, intermittent, 160–164
  phlebostatic axis, 163
  radial artery compression, 164
  range of methods, 160–161
  selection of a monitoring technique, 172
  sphygmomanometers, 160–164
Bodok seal, 79
Bohr, Niels, 227
bonding
  covalent bonds, 228
  ionic bonds, 228
  metallic bonding, 228
Bosun's whistle (oxygen failure whistle), 73
Bourdon gauge, 71, 80
Bourdon gauge thermometer, 42–43
box-and-whisker plots, 9–10
Boyle's law, 63–64, 80–82, 124
breathing systems. See ventilators and breathing systems
bremsstrahlung (braking radiation), 229
Brownian motion, 57, 238
Bureau International des Poids et Mesures (BIPM), 26

capacitive hygrometers, 46
capacitors, 30
carboxyhaemoglobin
  effect on measured SpO_2, 104
cardiac assist devices, 204–205
cardiac output monitoring
  arterial waveform analysis, 182
  bio-impedance, 184
  cardiac output monitors, 182
  comparison of different monitors, 174–175
  dilutional methods, 177–178
  Doppler ultrasound devices, 180–182
  Fick principle, 177–178
  lithium dilution methods, 180
  magnetic resonance techniques, 185
  non-invasive finger-cuff technology, 182–183
  pulmonary artery catheter (PAC), 178–180
  selection of an appropriate method, 185
  Stewart–Hamilton equation, 176–177
  transthoracic echocardiography, 183–184
  ultrasound techniques, 184–185
  visual echocardiography, 183–184
  washout curve, 175–176
cardiac pacing
  implantable cardioverter defibrillators (ICDs), 192–193
  implications for anaesthesia, 193
  leadless pacemakers, 192
  pacemaker codes, 192
  permanent cardiac pacing, 190–192
  temporary cardiac pacing, 189–190
  types of cardiac pacemakers, 189
cardiac potentials, 247–249
cardiac support, 187–188
  cardiac assist devices, 204–205
  cardiac pacing, 189–193
  cardiopulmonary bypass (CPB), 198–201
  cell salvage, 188–189
  defibrillators, 194–198
  implantable cardioverter defibrillators (ICDs), 192–193
  intra-aortic balloon pump (IABP), 201–203
  ventricular assist devices (VADs), 204–205
cardiopulmonary bypass (CPB), 198–201
CAT scan, 235
cell membranes
  phospholipid bilayer construction, 246–247
  role in generation of biological potentials, 247
cell salvage, 188–189
  advantages, 189
  disadvantages, 189
  disadvantages of allogenic red-cell transfusion, 188
  indications for, 188–189

centipoise, 54
central venous pressure (CVP), 165
Charles's law, 64
chelation, 239
chi-squared test, 5, 14, 20
chilled mirror hygrometers, 46
chloroform, 117–119
chromatography
  gas concentration measurement, 93–94
circle breathing system, 137
Clark (polarographic) electrode, 104
clinical heat loss, 40
CMAP (compound muscle action potential), 253
Coanda effect, 60–61
Cochrane Q test, 21
coefficient of determination (R^2), 14
Cohen's kappa statistic, 11
colour-change crystal hygrometers, 46
combined gas law, 65
Compton scattering, 235–236
computed tomography (CT), 232–236
conduction, 39–40
confounding, 4
CONSORT (Consolidated Standards of Reporting Trials) statement, 2
contingency tables, 5
continuous positive airway pressure (CPAP) devices, 132
Control of Substances Hazardous to Health (COSHH) regulations (UK), 87
  permitted limits for anaesthetic agents in the theatre environment, 146–147
convection, 39
correlation coefficients, 11
covalent bonds, 228
critical illness myopathy (CIM), 246, 253
critical illness neuromyopathy (CINM), 253–254
critical illness polyneuropathy (CIP), 253–254
critical point, 115
critical temperature, 115
crocodile icefish, 101
crossover study design, 4
Curie, Jacques, 208
Curie, Pierre, 208
Curie temperature, 217
cycles per second (frequency), 18
cyclopropane, 45
  flammability, 148

Dalton, James, 226
  law of partial pressures, 62–63
Darwin, Charles, 207

Index

data representation, 5–8
  bar charts, 5
  contingency tables, 5
  exponential distribution, 7–8
  graphical representations, 5
  histograms, 5
  normal distribution, 6–7
  skewed distributions, 6–7
dead-space measurement, 94
decibel (dB), 209
Declaration of Helsinki, 4
decompression chambers, 125
decompression sickness, 66, 125
  risk at high altitude, 125–126
defibrillators, 30, 194–198
  cardioversion, 194
  components, 194–198
  defibrillation procedure, 194
  electrodes, 198
  functions of a defibrillator, 194
  implantable cardioverter
    defibrillators (ICDs), 192–193
  types of, 194
  waveforms, 198
desflurane, 117–119
dew point, 45
diastolic blood pressure (DBP), 160
diffusion, 58
DINAMAP (device for indirect non-
    invasive automatic mean
    arterial pressure), 163
direct injection vaporizers, 122
divers
  decompression sickness, 66
  See also hyperbaric systems; scuba
    diving.
dog whistle, 207
Doppler, Christian, 180, 219
Doppler effect, 219–220
Doppler shift, 221
Doppler ultrasound, 219–222
  cardiac output monitoring, 180–182
  colour Doppler, 222
  continuous-wave Doppler (CWD),
    221–224
  development of, 208
  oesophageal Doppler monitor
    (ODM), 221–222
  pulse-wave Doppler (PWD),
    221
double-blinded studies, 3
draw-over vaporizers, 122
DWI (diffusion-weighted imaging),
    238
dynamos, 36

E-Entropy™, 253
Earth
  magnetic field, 34–35

echocardiography, 247
echolocation, 207
Edison, Thomas, 29
Einthoven's triangle, 248–249
electric motors, 35–36
electric shock
  risk in the operating theatre, 48
electrical equipment
  ignition sources, 148–149
electrical safety, 150–155
  effects of different currents on the
    human body, 150–151
  IEC standards for medical electrical
    equipment, 152–154
  macroshock, 150–152
    capacitive coupling, 152
    determinants of clinical effect,
      150–151
    equipotential bonding, 154–155
    leakage currents, 151–152,
      154–155
    resistive coupling, 151–152
  microshock, 152
  physics of, 150
  protection against shock, 152–154
electrical volume meter, 75–76
electricity
  alternating current (AC), 29–30
  ampere (SI unit), 28
  capacitance, 30
  definition of electric current, 28
  direct current (DC), 29–30
  electromotive force (EMF), 30–31
  galvanometers, 28
  historical observations, 28
  impedance, 30
  inductance, 30–31
  parallel circuits, 29
  potential difference (voltage), 28
  reactance, 30
  resistance, 28
  series circuits, 29
  simple circuits, 28–29
  symbols of common electrical
    components, 29
  transformers, 31
electro-biophysiology, 246
  amplifiers, 253–254
  biological potentials, 246–247
  cardiac potentials, 247–249
  electrocardiogram (ECG), 247–249
  electroencephalogram (EEG),
    252–253
  electromyogram (EMG), 253–254
  filters, 254–255
  myocardial ischaemia and infarction,
    249–252
  uses and limitations of measuring
    systems, 255

electrocardiogram (ECG), 247–249
  display, 248–249
  Einthoven's triangle, 248–249
  myocardial ischaemia and infarction,
    249–252
electroencephalogram (EEG),
    252–253
  BIS™ (Bispectral Index), 253
  E-Entropy™, 253
  effects of anaesthetic drugs, 252
  Narcotrend™, 253
  somatosensory evoked potential
    (SSEP), 253
  wave frequencies and clinical
    correlates, 252
electroluminescence, 240
electromagnetic energy, 32
electromagnetic waves
  properties of, 208–209
electromagnetism, 35–36
  construction of electromagnets,
    35
  dynamos, 36
  electric motors, 35–36
  transducers, 36
electromagnets, 34
electromyogram (EMG), 253
electrons
  energy levels, 227–228
  valence shells, 227–228
electrostatic discharge risk
  humidity and, 155
energy, 31–32
  definition, 31–32
  electromagnetic energy, 32
  forms of, 32
  kinetic energy, 32
  laws of thermodynamics, 38–39
  phase change and, 115–117
  potential energy, 32
  power and, 32
  sound energy, 32
  thermal energy, 32, 39
  work and, 31–32
enflurane, 117–119
enthalpy
  phase change and, 117
Entonox
  latent heat of evaporation, 116
  pseudo-critical temperature,
    116–117
  storage and use, 82
  two-stage Entonox valve, 72–73
entropy, 38
  phase change and, 117
equipotential bonding, 154–155
Erb's point, 253
ether (diethyl ether), 117–119
ether inhaler, 122

Index

ethics committee
  consideration of clinical study design, 4
Euler, Leonhard, 8
Euler's constant, 8
Euler's number, 8–14
evidence-based medicine
  appraisal process, 22
explosions. See fires and explosions
exponential distribution, 7–8
extra-corporeal CO_2 removal ($ECCO_2R$), 143–144
extra-corporeal life support (ECLS), 199
extra-corporeal membrane oxygenation (ECMO), 143–144, 199

Faraday, Michael, 35
  law of electromagnetic induction, 34
FDG (^{18}F-fluorodeoxyglucose), 236
fibre-optic thermometers, 44–45
fibre optics, 242–244
Fick principle, 177–178
Fick's law, 66–67
filters (for signals), 254–255
Finapres system, 164
finger-cuff technology, 182–183
fires and explosions, 148–150
  attempts to extinguish fire, 150
  components required for fire, 148
  evacuation of fire-affected areas, 150
  explosion risk in the operating theatre, 48
  explosions of flammable gas mixtures, 148
  factors implicated in higher risks, 149
  flammable gas mixtures, 148
  flammable substances in the theatre environment, 149
  fuel sources, 149
  hazards in the operating theatre, 148
  ignition sources, 148–149
  laser safety issues, 148–149
  management of fires, 149–150
  minimizing the risk of fire, 149
  oxidizers, 149
  recognizing fire, 149–150
  safety of electrical equipment, 148–149
Fisher's exact test, 20
FLAIR (fluid attenuation inversion recovery) imaging, 238
Fleiss's kappa statistic, 11
flowmeters. See gas flow measurement
FlowTrac/Vigileo™, 182
fluid mechanics, 53, 58
  Bernoulli principle, 59–60
  Coanda effect, 60–61
  Pascal's principle, 58–59
  Venturi effect, 60
fluids
  blood as a non-Newtonian fluid, 56–57
  Brownian motion, 57
  definition of a fluid, 53–54, 114
  diffusion, 58
  dynamic viscosity, 56
  Hagen–Poiseuille equation, 54–55
  kinematic velocity, 56
  laminar flow, 54–55
  movement and mixing, 57–58
  Newtonian fluids, 54–56
  non-Newtonian fluids, 56–57
  osmosis, 58–59
  Poiseuille's law, 54–55
  properties of fluids, 53–54
  Reynolds number, 56
  turbulent flow, 55–56
  viscosity, 54
fluorescence, 239–240
force, 32
Forest plot, 21
Fourier analysis of arterial pressure waveform, 168–169
fragility index, 18
frequency
  definition, 209
Fresnel equations, 211
fuel cell (Hersch or Galvanic cell), 104–105
funnel plot, 21–22

gadolinium contrast agents, 238–239
Galilean thermometer, 45
galvanometers, 28
gamma radiation, 229–230
  nuclear medicine, 236
gamma scintigraphy, 236
gas concentration measurement
  chromatography, 93–94
  infrared gas analyzer, 88–89
  mass spectrometry, 90–91
  nitrogen meter, 94
  paramagnetic oxygen analyzer, 87–89
  piezoelectric absorption, 92–93
  Raman gas analyzers, 90–91
  refractometry, 92
  role in anaesthesia, 87
  summary of methods and uses, 94–95
  ultraviolet absorption, 93–94
gas flow measurement
  flowmeters, 76–77
  hot-wire anemometer, 79
  mechanical strain gauge flowmeter, 78–79
  peak-flowmeters, 77
  pitot-tube pneumotachograph, 77–78
  pneumotachograph, 77–78
  variable-orifice flowmeters, 76–77
gas laws
  Avogadro's law, 61–63
  Boyle's law, 63–64
  Charles's law, 64
  combined gas law, 65
  Dalton's law of partial pressures, 62–63
  Fick's law, 66–67
  Gay-Lussac's law, 64
  Graham's law, 66
  Henry's law of solubility, 66
  ideal gas concept, 61
  ideal gas laws, 61
  universal gas law, 61, 65–66
gas pressure
  definition of pressure, 70
  manipulation of high-pressure gases, 72–73
  oxygen failure whistle, 72–73
  pressure-reducing valves, 72
  units of measure, 70
gas pressure measurement, 71–72
  absolute or total pressure, 71
  barometers, 72
  Bourdon gauge, 71
  gauge pressure, 71
  manometers, 71–72
gas supply, 79
  cylinders, 79–82
    avoiding adiabatic temperature rise, 79–80
    identifying the gas within the cylinder, 79
    safety features, 79–82
    volume of gas within a cylinder, 80–82
  pipeline gas supplies, 82–84
    air, 84
    nitrous oxide, 82–83
    oxygen (vacuum-insulated evaporator, VIE), 82–84
    oxygen concentrator, 84
gas volume measurement, 74
  Benedict Roth spirometer, 74
  electrical volume meter, 75–76
  Vitalograph®, 74
  Wright respirometer, 74–75
gases
  saturated vapour pressure (SVP), 66
Gauss, Carl Friedrich, 26
Gay-Lussac's law, 64, 80, 83
global warming potential (GWP) of anaesthetic vapours, 117
good clinical practice (GCP) standards, 4
Graham's law, 66
graphical representations of data, 5
gravimetric hygrometers, 46
gray (Gy), 231

Index

haemoglobinopathies
    effect on measured SpO_2, 103
Hagen–Poiseuille equation, 54–55, 210
hair hygrometers, 46–47
Hales, Stephen, 165
halothane, 93, 117–119
hazard, 17
hazard ratio (HR), 17
heat
    definition, 39
    relationship to temperature and humidity, 46–48
    thermal energy, 39
heat and moisture exchangers (HMEs), 48–49
heat capacity, 41
heat transfer
    clinical heat loss, 40
    conduction, 39–40
    conduction coefficients, 40
    convection, 39
    insulators, 40
    latent heat of fusion, 41
    latent heat of vaporization, 40–41
    mechanisms, 39
    radiation, 39–40
Heliox, 125
Henry's law, 66, 93, 104–105, 125, 201
Hertz (Hz), 209
high altitude
    delivering anaesthesia at altitude, 126–127
    drop in atmospheric pressure with increasing altitude, 125
    risk of decompression sickness, 125–126
    risk of flying after diving, 126
high-flow nasal oxygen (HFNO) devices, 132
high-frequency oscillating ventilator (HFOV), 142–143
high-intensity focused ultrasound (HIFU), 223
histograms, 5
hot-wire anemometer, 79
Hounsfield scale, 235
humidification in clinical practice
    avoiding static electricity build-up, 48
    benefits for theatre patients and staff, 48
    reducing explosion risk, 48
    reducing the risk of electric shock, 48
humidification methods, 48–50
    active and passive methods, 48
    heat and moisture exchangers (HMEs), 48–49
    nebulizers, 49–50
    water-bath humidifiers, 49
humidity
    absolute humidity, 45
    apparent temperature and, 46–48

definition, 45
dew point, 45
electrostatic discharge risk and, 155
relationship to temperature and heat, 46–48
relative humidity, 45
safety issues in clinical practice, 45
specific humidity, 45
ways to express, 45
humidity measurement, 45–46
    capacitive hygrometers, 46
    chilled mirror hygrometers, 46
    colour-change crystal hygrometers, 46
    gravimetric hygrometers, 46
    hair hygrometers, 46–47
    psychrometers, 46
    Regnault's hygrometer, 46–47
    resistive hygrometers, 46
    wet and dry bulb hygrometers, 46
Humphrey ADE system, 136
hydrostatic pressure equation, 72
hygrometers, 45–46
hyperbaric oxygen therapy, 125
hyperbaric systems
    barotrauma, 124
    dangers of, 124–125
    decompression chambers, 125
    decompression sickness, 66, 125
    hyperbaric oxygen therapy, 125
    narcosis, 124
    oxygen toxicity, 124–125
    uses for, 124
hypergolic substances, 148
hypothesis testing, 18–19
hypothesis tests, 19–20

I^2 statistic, 21
implantable cardioverter defibrillators (ICDs), 192–193
    implications for anaesthesia, 193
indocyanine green
    effect on measured SpO_2, 103
inductors, 30–31
inertia, 33
information bias, 3–4
infrared gas analyzer, 88–89
infrared radiation, 39–40
infrared thermometers, 43
insulators, 40
intention-to-treat analysis, 4
intermittent positive pressure ventilation (IPPV), 138–139
International System (SI) of units, 25–28
interquartile range (IQR), 9–11
intra-aortic balloon pump (IABP), 201–203
inverse piezo effect, 92
ionic bonds, 228

ionizing radiation, 40
    See also radiation
Ionizing Radiation (Medical Exposure) Regulations (IRMER) UK, 231
ions, 227
isoflurane, 117–119
isotopes, 227

jet entrainment, 60

Kaplan–Meier chart, 17
kinetic energy, 32
Kolmogorov–Smirnov test, 7
Kouwenhoven, William Bennett, 194
kurtosis, 7

Lambert's law, 98, 104
Laplace's law, 160
lasers, 239–244
    common laser systems and their applications, 240
    lasing process, 240–241
    lasing threshold, 241–242
    optical discs, 242
    optical fibres, 242–244
    population inversion, 241–242
    properties of laser light, 240
    safety issues, 148–149
    stimulated emission, 240–241
latent heat, 41
latent heat of evaporation, 116
latent heat of fusion, 41, 115–116
latent heat of vaporization, 40–41
Le Chatelier's principle, 115
LEDs (light-emitting diodes), 240
LiDCO™, 182
light
    properties of, 208–209
    spontaneous emission, 239
Likert scale, 3
linear regression, 13
liquid crystal thermometers, 43
lithium dilution
    monitoring cardiac output, 180
lithotripsy, 223
logistic regression, 14
log-linear regression, 14

magnetic-resonance-guided focused ultrasound (MRgFUS), 223
magnetic resonance imaging (MRI), 236–239
    components of the MRI scanner, 236–238
    contrast agents, 238–239
    principles, 236–238
    types of imaging sequences, 238
magnetism, 33–34
    definition, 34
    definition of a magnet, 34
    diamagnetism, 34

Index

magnetism (cont.)
  Earth's magnetic field, 34–35
  electromagnetism, 35–36
  electromagnets, 34
  inventions using, 34
  magnetic fields, 34–35
  magnetic flux density, 34
  paramagnetism, 34
  strength of a magnetic field, 34
Manley MP3 ventilator, 140–141
Mann–Whitney U test, 20
Mann–Whitney–Wilcoxon (MWW) test, 20
manometers, 71–72
Mantel–Haenszel procedure, 21
Mapleson classification of breathing systems, 133–136
mass, 33
mass number, 227
mass spectrometry
  gas concentration measurement, 90–91
mean (measure of central tendency), 8–9
mean arterial pressure (MAP), 160
measurement
  SI (Système Internationale) units, 25–28
mechanical strain gauge flowmeter, 78–79
mechanical ventilation, 137–141
  'bag squeezer' ventilators, 141
  classification by cycling, 138–140
  classification by mode of operation, 140–141
  intermittent blower ventilators, 141
  intermittent positive pressure ventilation (IPPV), 138–139
  'mechanical thumb' ventilators, 140
  minute-volume dividers, 140–141
  negative versus positive pressure ventilation, 138
  positive end-expiratory pressure (PEEP), 138–139
  positive pressure ventilators, 138–141
  pressure-control ventilation (PCV), 140
  volume-control ventilation (VCV), 139–140
mechanics
  acceleration, 32
  force, 32
  inertia, 33
  mass, 33
  momentum, 33
  Newton's laws of motion, 32–33
  pressure, 32–33
  velocity, 33
  weight, 33

median (measure of central tendency), 8–9
meta-analysis, 21
metallic bonding, 228
methaemoglobinaemia
  effect on measured SpO_2, 102–103
methylene blue
  effect on measured SpO_2, 103
MIBI scanning, 236
minimum alveolar concentration (MAC) of anaesthetic vapours, 117
mode (measure of central tendency), 8–9
molar heat capacity, 41
mole, 227
  Avogadro's constant, 61
momentum, 33
motor unit potential (MUP), 253
multivariate regression, 13–14
myocardial ischaemia and infarction
  ECG findings, 249–252

Napier's number, 8
narcosis related to hyperbaric systems, 124
Narcotrend™, 253
nebulizers, 49–50
  ultrasonic nebulizers, 223
negative predictive value (NPV), 12–13
neutrinos, 229
neutrons, 226–227
Newton, Isaac, 31
  laws of motion, 32–33, 200
Newtonian fluids, 54–56
nitrogen meter, 94
nitrous oxide
  as a fuel and an oxygen source, 149
  key properties, 117–119
  latent heat of evaporation, 116
  pipeline supply, 82–83
  volume of gas in a cylinder, 80–81
non-invasive finger-cuff technology, 182–183
non-Newtonian fluids, 56–57
normal distribution, 6–7
nuclear medicine, 236
nucleons, 226–227
nuclides, 227
null hypothesis, 18
number needed to harm (NNH), 16
number needed to treat (NNT), 16
Nyquist limit, 222

observer bias, 4
Occupational Health and Safety Act (OHSA) (USA)
  permitted limits for anaesthetic agents in the theatre environment, 146–147

odds, 16–17
odds ratio (OR), 16–17
oesophageal Doppler monitor (ODM), 221–222
Ohm's law, 30, 150
oil:gas (O/G) partition coefficient of anaesthetic vapours, 117–119
open or open-label studies, 3
optical discs, 242
optical fibres, 242–244
osmosis, 58–59
oxidizers
  fire and explosion risk, 149
oxygen
  oxygen concentrator, 84
  paramagnetic oxygen analyzer, 87–89
  vacuum-insulated evaporator (VIE), 82–84
  volume of gas in a cylinder, 80
oxygen failure whistle, 72–73
oxygen toxicity
  related to hyperbaric systems, 124–125

p-value, 11, 19
pacemakers. See cardiac pacing
paramagnetic oxygen analyzer, 87–89
parameters of populations, 10
Pascal's principle, 58–59
PCO_2 electrode, 107
peak-flowmeters, 77
Pearson's correlation coefficient, 11
Penaz principle, 164
Pendelluft ventilation, 143
periodic table of elements, 227
PET (positron emission tomography), 236
pH electrode, 105–106
phase of a cycle, 209
phases of matter
  condensation, 115
  critical point, 115
  critical temperature, 115
  definition of vapour, 115
  deposition, 115
  energy and phase change, 115–117
  enthalpy, 117
  entropy and phase change, 117
  evaporation, 115
  fluids, 114
  gas phase, 113
  latent heat of evaporation, 116
  latent heat of fusion, 116
  liquid phase, 113
  melting, 115
  phase changes, 114–115
  phase diagram, 114–115
  plasma, 113
  principal phases, 113–114

Index

pseudo-critical temperature of gas mixtures, 116–117
saturated vapour pressure, 115
solid phase, 113
temperature and phase change, 115–117
triple point, 115
vapour pressure, 115
phlebostatic axis, 160, 163
phosphor thermometry, 45
phosphorescence, 240
photoelectric effect, 235–236
photons, 230
photoplethysmograph, 164
PiCCO^{TM}, 182
PICO model, 1–2
piezoelectric absorption
gas concentration measurement, 92–93
piezoelectric effect, 92–93, 208, 216–217
pitot-tube pneumotachograph, 77–78
Plank's constant, 228, 239
platinum resistance thermometers, 43–44
plenum vaporizers, 119–121
pneumotachograph, 77–78
PO_2 electrodes, 104–105
Poiseuille's law, 54–55
Poisson distribution, 14
Poisson regression, 14
portable ventilators, 141–142
positive end-expiratory pressure (PEEP), 138–139
positive predictive value (PPV), 12–13
potential energy, 32
powders
properties of, 54
power, 32
Poynting effect, 82
pressure, 32
definition, 70
units of measure, 70
pressure (mechanics), 33
pressure-control ventilation (PCV), 140–144
pressure-reducing valves, 72
probability, 14–15
conditional probability, 14
frequentist statistical approach, 14–15
objectivism, 14–15
posterior probability, 14
prior probability, 14
quantifying, 15
subjectivism, 14
protons, 226–227
pseudo-critical temperature
mixtures of gases, 116–117
psychrometers, 46
publication bias, 4, 21–22
pulmonary artery catheter (PAC), 178–180

pulmonary artery pressure, 165
pulse-echo principle, 218
pulse oximetry, 98–101
causes of incorrect SpO_2 readings, 100, 102–104
development of devices, 97
SaO_2 (arterial oxygen saturation), 98
SpO_2 (pulse-oximetry oxygen saturation), 98
pulse-oximetry limitations, 102–104
anaemia with co-existing hypoxia, 103–104
carboxyhaemoglobin, 104
fingernail polish, 103
haemoglobinopathies, 103
intravenous pigmented dyes, 103
methaemoglobinaemia, 102–103
movement artefact, 103
poor perfusion, 103
sulph-haemoglobinaemia, 103
venous pulsations, 103
Pythagoras, 207

quantum mechanics, 226–227

radiation (ionizing), 40
radiation (thermal), 39–40
radiation and decay, 228–229
alpha radiation, 229
beta radiation, 229–230
gamma radiation, 229–230
half-life, 229–230
X-ray radiation, 229–230
radiation safety, 230–232
Raman effect, 90–91
Raman gas analyzers, 90–91
randomization, 3
avoiding selection bias, 3
range, 9–11
Rayleigh refractometer, 92
Rayleigh scattering, 90, 92, 212–213, 222
reflection, laws of, 211
refractive index, 92, 242–243
refractometry
gas concentration measurement, 92
Regnault's hygrometer, 46–47
regression, 13–14
resistive hygrometers, 46
reverse piezoelectric effect, 216
Reynolds number, 56
rheology, 57
risk, 15–17
absolute risk (AR), 15
risk ratio (relative risk), 15–16
Ritchie oxygen failure whistle, 72–73

safety
electrical safety, 150–155
fires and explosions, 148–150

humidity and electrostatic discharge prevention, 155
issues relating to humidity, 45
lasers, 148–149
scavenging systems, 146–147
sampling, 3
saturated vapour pressure (SVP), 66, 115
scatterplots, 11
scavenging systems, 146–147
adjuncts to scavenging, 147
collecting system, 147
components, 147
disposal system, 147
exterior port, 147
permitted limits for anaesthetic agents in the theatre environment, 146–147
receiving system, 147
transfer system, 147
Schimmelbusch mask, 122
Schrader connectors, 84
Schrader sockets, 82
scuba diving
equipment, 105
rebreathing systems, 137
risk of flying after diving, 126
See also hyperbaric systems.
Sechrist Bird VIP ventilator, 140
second gas effect, 67
Seebeck effect, 44
selection bias, 3
Severinghaus electrode, 107
sevoflurane, 117–119
SI (Système Internationale) units, 25–28
ampere (electric current), 26
base units, 25–27
candela (luminescence), 26
derived units, 27–28
kelvin (temperature), 26
kilogram, 25–34
metre, 25–26
mole (amount of substance), 26
reporting style conventions, 27–28
second (time), 26
sievert (Sv), 231
Simpson's rule, 184
skewed distributions, 6–7
smoke detectors, 229
SNAP (sensory nerve action potential) 253
Snell's law, 214
somatosensory evoked potential (SSEP), 253
SONAR, 208, 223
sound energy, 32
sound intensity level (SIL), 209
sound pressure level (SPL), 210

263

Index

Spearman's rank correlation coefficient, 11
specific heat capacity (SHC), 41
specific latent heat, 41
SPECT (single-photon emission computed tomography), 236
spectroscopy, 228
sphygmomanometers, 160–164
   aneroid sphygmomanometers, 162
   auscultatory method, 161
   digital sphygmomanometers, 163
   DINAMAP (device for indirect non-invasive automatic mean arterial pressure), 163
   elements required for BP measurement, 160–161
   factors affecting accuracy of measurement, 163–164
   less commonly used methods, 161
   mercury sphygmomanometers, 161–162
   oscillometric method, 161
   phlebostatic axis, 163
   Von Recklinghausen oscillotonometer, 162–163
SpO_2 (pulse-oximetry oxygen saturation), 98
standard deviation (SD), 7, 9–11
standard error, 10
standard error of the mean (SEM), 10
standards
   IEC standards for medical electrical equipment, 152–154
static discharge
   lightning bolts, 48
   risk in the operating theatre, 48
statistics
   absolute variation, 9
   agreement, 11–12
   analysis of variance (ANOVA), 20
   association, 11
   average, 8–9
   box-and-whisker plots, 9–10
   categorical data, 5
   chi-squared test, 19–20
   confidence intervals, 17–18
   continuous variables, 5
   correlation, 11
   correlation coefficients, 11
   data representation, 5–8
   data types, 4–5
   deductive statistics, 14–20
   descriptive statistics, 4–8
   dichotomous data, 5
   discrete variables, 5
   distinction from population parameters, 10
   exponential distribution, 7–8

Fisher's exact test, 20
Forest plot, 21
fragility index, 18
funnel plot, 21–22
goodness-of-fit measures, 14
hazard, 17
hazard ratio (HR), 17
hypothesis testing, 18–19
hypothesis tests, 19–20
importance in medicine, 1
interquartile range (IQR), 9–11
interval variables, 5–14
Mann–Whitney U test, 20
mean, 8–9
measures of central tendency, 8–9
measures of spread, 9–11
median, 8–9
metric data, 5
mode, 8–9
negative predictive value (NPV), 12–13
nominal data, 5
normal distribution, 6–7
null hypothesis, 18
odds, 16–17
odds ratio (OR), 16–17
ordinal data, 5
p-value, 11, 19
positive predictive value (PPV), 12–13
power calculation, 18–19
probability, 14–15
qualitative data, 5
quantitative data, 5
range, 9–11
ranked data, 5
ratio variables, 5–14
regression, 13–14
risk, 15–17
risk ratio (relative risk), 15–16
scatter plots, 11
sensitivity, 12–13
skewed distributions, 6–7
specificity, 12–13
standard deviation (SD), 9–11
standard error, 10
standard error of the mean (SEM), 10
summary statistics, 8–14
t-test, 19
type 1 error, 18
type 2 error, 18
types of variables, 4–5
variance, 9
Wilcoxon signed rank sum test, 20
statistics in clinical practice
   evidence-based medicine, 22
   meta-analysis, 21

   publication bias, 21–22
   systematic review, 21
Stewart–Hamilton equation, 176–177
STIR (short T1 inversion recovery) imaging, 238
study design
   allocation of participants to study groups, 3
   avoiding selection bias, 3
   bias, 3–4
   blinding, 3
   case–control studies, 2
   causes of incorrect recording of measurements, 3–4
   clinical standards, 4
   cohort studies, 2
   confounding, 4
   consideration by an ethics committee, 4
   crossover, 4
   cross-sectional studies, 2
   defining the research question, 1–2
   double-blinded studies, 3
   experimental studies, 2
   intention-to-treat analysis, 4
   key questions, 1
   observational studies, 2
   open or open-label studies, 3
   outcome measures (endpoints), 2
   PICO model, 1–2
   publication bias, 4
   randomization, 3
   sampling, 3
   uncertainty around outcome measures, 2
sulph-haemoglobinaemia, 103
Swan–Ganz catheter, 178
systematic review, 21
systolic blood pressure (SBP), 159–160

t-test, 19
technetium-sestamibi-99m, 236
temperature
   absolute zero, 41
   apparent temperature, 46–48
   continuous variables, 5–14
   definition, 41
   laws of thermodynamics, 38–39
   phase change and, 115–117
   relationship to heat and humidity, 46–48
   thermometric properties, 42
   triple point of water, 41–42
   units of measurement, 41
temperature measurement, 42–45
tesla (T), 34
theatre environment
   electrical safety, 150–155
   fires and explosions, 148–150

Index

humidity and electrostatic discharge prevention, 155
scavenging systems, 146–147
thermal energy, 32, 39
thermistors, 44
thermochromism, 43
thermocouples, 44
thermodynamics
  first law, 31–32
  laws of, 38–39
  second law, 117
thermometers, 42–45
  alcohol thermometers, 42
  bimetallic-strip thermometers, 43
  Bourdon gauge thermometer, 42–43
  electrical devices, 42
  fibre-optic thermometers, 44–45
  Galilean thermometer, 45
  infrared thermometers, 43
  liquid crystal thermometers, 43
  liquid thermometers, 42
  mercury thermometers, 42
  non-electric thermometers, 42
  phosphor thermometry, 45
  platinum resistance thermometers, 43–44
  thermistors, 44
  thermocouples, 44
  tympanic-membrane thermometers, 43
thermometric properties, 42
thermometry, 42
Torricellian vacuum, 72
total internal reflection (optical fibres), 242–243
transducers, 36
transformers, 31
trans-oesophageal echocardiography (TOE), 183
transthoracic echocardiography, 183–184
transthoracic electrical bio-impedance (TEB), 184
triple point, 115
triple point of water, 41–42
tympanic-membrane thermometers, 43
type 1 error, 18
type 2 error, 18

ultrasonic nebulizers, 223
ultrasonic scalpels, 223
ultrasound
  3D and 4D ultrasound, 222
  A-mode (amplitude mode), 217
  acoustic impedance for human tissues, 210
  applications outside of clinical imaging, 223
  artefacts, 218–219
  attenuation coefficients of human tissues, 210–211
  B-mode (brightness mode), 217–218
  basic image generation, 217–219
  Doppler imaging, 219–222
  fundamentals, 208–213
  high-intensity focused ultrasound (HIFU), 223
  history of development, 207–208
  image processing, 219
  M-mode (motion mode), 218
  piezoelectric effect, 216–217
  probe construction and behaviour, 213–216
  propagation velocities for human tissues, 210
  properties of ultrasound waves, 208–210
  pulse-echo principle, 218
  reflection of energy, 211–213
  reverse piezoelectric effect, 216
  timed gain compensation (TGC), 211
ultraviolet absorption
  gas concentration measurement, 93–94
universal gas law, 61, 65–66

vacuum-insulated evaporator (VIE) oxygen supply, 82–84
vacuum-insulated oxygen evaporator action of the superheater, 116
vaporizers, 119
  direct-injection vaporizers, 122
  draw-over vaporizers, 122
  entropy and phase change, 115
  ether inhaler, 122
  hazards associated with, 123–124
  operation with the circle breathing system, 137
  plenum vaporizers, 119–121
  safety features, 122–123
  saturated vapour pressure, 115
  Schimmelbusch mask, 122
  systems of historical interest, 122
  vapour-injection vaporizers, 121–122
vapour
  definition, 115
  See also anaesthetic vapours.
vapour-injection vaporizers, 122
vapour pressure, 115
variable-orifice flowmeters, 76–77
velocity, 33
ventilators and breathing systems, 130
  airway pressure release ventilation (APRV), 143
  alternative modes of ventilation, 142–144
  Bernoulli principle, 130–131
  bi-level positive airway pressure (BiPAP) devices, 132
  circle breathing system, 137
  classification systems, 132
  components of breathing systems, 132
  continuous positive airway pressure (CPAP) devices, 131–132
  extracorporeal CO_2 removal (ECCO$_2$R), 143–144
  extra-corporeal membrane oxygenation (ECMO), 143–144
  high-flow nasal oxygen (HFNO) devices, 132
  high-frequency oscillating ventilator (HFOV), 142–143
  Humphrey ADE system, 136
  ideal characteristics, 132–133
  Mapleson A system, 133–134
  Mapleson B system, 134–135
  Mapleson C system, 135
  Mapleson classification, 133–136
  Mapleson D, E and F systems, 135–136
  mechanical ventilation, 137–141
  non-invasive ventilation (NIV), 131–132
  open, semi-open, semi-closed and closed systems, 133
  portable ventilators, 141–142
  Venturi effect, 130–131
ventiPAC™ ventilator, 141–142
ventricular assist devices (VADs), 204–205
Venturi effect, 60, 130–131
Venturi masks, 131
Venturi oxygen masks, 60
viscosity
  dynamic viscosity, 56
  kinematic velocity, 56
visual echocardiography, 183–184
Vitalograph®, 74
volume-clamp method, 164, 182
volume-control ventilation (VCV), 139–140
Von Recklinghausen oscillotonometer, 162–163
voxels, 233

washout curve, 175–176
water
　triple point, 41–42
water-bath humidifiers, 49
Water's bag, 135
wavelength, 209
waves
　properties of, 208–210
weber (Wb), 34
weight (mechanics), 33
wet and dry bulb hygrometers, 46
Wheatstone bridge, 166–167
Wilcoxon rank sum test, 20
Wilcoxon signed rank sum test, 20
Wood's metal, 82

work
　definition, 31–32
　energy and, 31–32
World Health Organization (WHO)
　Surgical Safety Checklist, 149
Wright respirometer, 74–75

X-ray radiation, 229–230